Studying for a Foundation Degree in Health

Edited by Mary Northrop,
Jayne Crow and Sarah Kraszewski

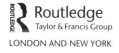

Routledge
Taylor & Francis Group

LONDON AND NEW YORK

First published 2016
by Routledge
2 Park Square, Milton Park, Abingdon, Oxon OX14 4RN

and by Routledge
711 Third Avenue, New York, NY 10017

Routledge is an imprint of the Taylor & Francis Group, an informa business

© 2016 M. Northrop, J. Crow and S. Kraszewski

British Library Cataloguing-in-Publication Data
A catalogue record for this book is available from the British Library

Library of Congress Cataloging in Publication Data
Studying for a foundation degree in health / edited by
Mary Northrop, Jayne Crow, and Sarah Kraszewski.
        p. ; cm.
    Includes bibliographical references and index.
    I. Northrop, Mary, editor. II. Crow, Jayne, editor.
    III. Kraszewski, Sarah, editor.
    [DNLM: 1. Health Personnel—education—Great Britain.
    2. Clinical Competence—Great Britain. 3. Education, Professional—
    Great Britain. W 18]
    R735
    610.71—dc23   2015004359

ISBN: 978-0-415-73411-0 (hbk)
ISBN: 978-0-273-78620-7 (pbk)
ISBN: 978-1-315-68463-5 (ebk)

Typeset in Times
by Keystroke, Station Road, Codsall, Wolverhampton

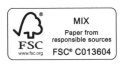

MIX
Paper from
responsible sources
FSC® C013604
www.fsc.org

Printed and bound by CPI Group (UK) Ltd, Croydon, CR0 4YY

Studying for a Foundation Degree in Health

Studying for a Foundation Degree in Health is designed to provide clear, relevant knowledge and to support appropriate skills development amongst students enrolled on foundation degree and equivalent level courses, in health and social care. Combining academic study skills, work-based learning skills and practice-focused content in one volume, this is the first textbook to focus specifically on the Band 4 role of associate and assistant practitioner within the health sector.

Features include:

* 13 chapters that cover the core topics students will be expected to demonstrate proficiency on by the end of their degree, including health promotion, healthcare delivery, safeguarding, quality in healthcare and research and evidence-based practice;
* learning outcomes and activities, enabling students to actively engage with their course content;
* content written by authors from a broad range of health disciplines, including nursing, radiography, physiotherapy, dentistry and public health, accurately depicting the dynamic field of healthcare in the UK today.

Written by authors with a wealth of experience in running foundation degrees in health, the book aims to provide students with lifelong learning skills that will benefit them while on their course, during future study and in the workforce.

Mary Northrop is a Senior Lecturer in the Faculty of Health, Social Care and Education at Anglia Ruskin University, UK.

Jayne Crow, having been a Senior Lecturer at Anglia Ruskin University for many years, is now a freelance workshop facilitator and lecturer in Health and Social Care.

Sarah Kraszewski is Head of Department Midwifery, Child and Community Nursing at Anglia Ruskin University, UK.

Contents

List of figures and tables   xi
List of contributors   xv
Preface   xvii
Acknowledgements   xix
List of abbreviations   xxi

1   Preparing for study   **1**
JANE SHELLEY AND IAIN JOHN KEENAN

Introduction 1
Reading skills 1
Reading effectively 3
Vocabulary 6
Assessments 7
Using the library effectively 9
Finding information – literature searching 16
Evaluating information 30
New technology and social media 31
Note taking 32
Writing skills for academia 34
Referencing 38
Glossary compilation 47
Chapter summary 47
Glossary 48
Further resources 49
Further reading 49
References 49

2   Work-based learning   **51**
CLAIRE THURGATE

Introduction 51
Lifelong learning 51
Work-based learning: what is it? 52
Making sense of work-based learning 54

Personal development plans 56
The role of your mentor/supervisor 60
Demonstrating your work-based learning 61
Reflection 63
Chapter summary 67
Further resources 68
Further reading 68
References 68

3 Communication   **69**

MARY NORTHROP AND DAVID HINGLEY

Introduction 69
Definitions of communication 70
Methods of communication 71
Modes of communication 72
Principles of communication 79
Communicating with clients 83
VERA – a framework for compassionate communication 84
Applying communication skills 88
Models of communication 89
Reflecting on communication 89
Chapter summary 91
Further resources 92
Further reading 92
References 92

4 Working in teams   **93**

JAYNE CROW AND IAIN JOHN KEENAN

Introduction 93
Understanding relationships within teams 94
Reflection and developing empathy with colleagues 96
Communication within teams 97
Strategies for improving communication in teams 98
Non-defensive communication 98
Offering constructive criticism 99
Avoiding blame culture 100
Influencing other people's behaviour in teams 100
Role modelling 101
Whistleblowing 101
Tribalism related to teams 101
Collaboration 103
Leadership in teams 104
Leadership and management 104
Recognising burnout in our colleagues 106
Chapter summary 107
Further resources 108

Further reading 108
References 108

5 Valuing people: Fostering dignity and respect   **109**
VICKI ELLIOTT AND JAYNE CROW

Introduction 110
Values, attitudes and culture 110
Dignity 115
Ethics 117
Ethical theories 118
Ethical principles 119
Ethical theories and principles applied to decision-making 120
Diversity and equality 120
Discrimination 122
Chapter summary 124
Further resources 124
Further reading 124
References 124

6 Healthcare delivery   **126**
MARY NORTHROP

Introduction 126
Demographics 126
Epidemiology 127
Social policy 128
Healthcare policy 133
Healthcare delivery 135
Chapter summary 140
Further resources 141
References 141

7 Quality in healthcare   **144**
SARAH KRASZEWSKI

Introduction 144
What is quality assurance? 145
Quality assurance programmes 145
Further thoughts about quality 148
Quality assurance agencies: the CQC 150
Understanding clinical governance 150
Patient safety 154
Health and safety 160
Chapter summary 161
Further resources 161
References 162

8   Legal aspects of healthcare delivery   **164**

PATRICIA MACNAMARA

Introduction 164
Utilitarianism 164
Duty-based ethical thought 166
The Four Principles approach 168
Human rights 169
Key Articles of the Human Rights Act 170
The NHS Constitution (2013) 172
The Mental Capacity Act 2005 173
The Mental Health Act 1983 178
Parental responsibility 179
Confidentiality 180
Chapter summary 181
Further reading 182
References 182
Table of statutes 183
Table of cases 183

9   Research and evidence-based practice   **184**

SHIRLEY JONES

Introduction 184
Developing knowledge using research 186
Understanding the research process 187
How to read a research article 188
Step 1 – identify the title of the research article 189
Step 2 – read the abstract 189
Step 3 – read the introduction 189
Step 4 – identify the research questions 190
Step 5 – understanding the methodology 191
Step 6 - identifying the participants in the study – the sample 198
Step 7 – what method is used to gather information – data collection tools 202
Step 8 – confirming the validity and reliability of data collection tools 207
Step 9 – consider the protection of participants in the study – research ethics 208
Step 10 - reading and understanding the results 208
Step 11 – focus on the discussion and conclusion 212
Step 12 – finally, the references 213
Conclusions 213
Chapter summary 214
Further resources 214
Further reading 214
References 215

10 Improving public health   **216**

DR ANDY STEVENS AND SARAH KRASZEWSKI

Introduction 216
History 217
Definition 217
Theoretical approaches 219
Assessing determinants of health 223
Immunisation 229
Legislation 230
Chapter summary 232
Further resources 232
References 232

11 Health promotion   **235**

DR FIONA MCMASTER

Introduction 235
Thinking about healthy living 235
Behaviour choice and health promotion 237
What is health promotion? 239
Approaches to health promotion 239
Theories and models can help 240
Controversies of health promotion 249
How to promote health with patients 249
Priority areas for health promotion 253
Chapter summary 254
Further resources 255
Further reading 255
References 255

12 Safeguarding individuals and families   **257**

DR CHRIS THURSTON

Introduction 257
Abuse statistics 258
Reasons for abuse 259
Risk factors 259
Process of protecting vulnerable individuals 262
Types of abuse 264
Inter-professional working 270
Chapter summary 278
Further resources 278
Further reading 278
References 278

13   Teaching and assessing   **280**
DR ANNE-MARIE REID

Introduction 280
Approaches to teaching and learning 281
Assessing others 296
Chapter summary 303
Further resources 303
Further reading 304
References 304

Index   305

List of figures and tables

Figures

1.1	Example of a QR code	10
1.2	Key tips for using your university library	11
1.3	Mind map for booking a holiday	18
1.4	Mind map for the essay topic 'Communication Issues in the Healthcare Environment'	19
1.5	Example reading list	23
1.6	Example of a journal reference from a database	27
1.7	Use of Boolean AND	27
1.8	Use of Boolean OR	28
1.9	Use of Boolean NOT	28
1.10	Tips for doing a good search	32
1.11	Example of book chapter for secondary referencing	42
2.1	The cyclical process involved in PDP (Quality Assurance Agency (QAA) 2009)	56
2.2	SWOT analysis	57
2.3	Sources of evidence for your portfolio	59
2.4	Portfolio content	62
2.5	Cycle of reflective practice	64
2.6	Structured reflective process, adapted from Jasper (2003)	64
2.7	Gibb's reflective cycle, adapted from Gibb (1988)	65
3.1	Face-to-face communication	73
3.2	Non-verbal communication	75
3.3	Email communication, adapted from Talktalk (n.d.). Do's and don'ts and good practice, adapted from Emailogic workshop on How to get better results from your email (Emailogic n.d.)	78
3.4	Communication barriers	80
3.5	Speech and language problems	83
3.6	VERA acronym	85
3.7	Understanding emotions – some of the many words that can be associated with anger	86
3.8	Model of communication	90
4.1	Some possible power relationships within teams	95
4.2	Communication behaviours within teams	97

5.1   Your attitude affects the service user's experience   109
5.2   Our family and upbringing are the foundations for our values   111
5.3   We develop our own value system through education and experience   112
5.4   Values inform our decision-making   113
6.1   Decision process for developing a social policy   131
6.2   Healthcare delivery in England   137
6.3   Roles within healthcare delivery   138
6.4   Patient and public involvement in healthcare   140
7.1   Quality assurance programme levels, adapted from WHO (2006)   145
7.2   Quality dimensions, adapted from WHO (2006)   146
7.3   Quality measurement domains, adapted from Leatherman and Sutherland
      (2003)   146
7.4   Quality objectives   148
7.5   The audit cycle   152
7.6   Clinical audit stages   153
7.7   Medication errors   158
9.1   Components of evidence-based practice   185
9.2   Common phrases to describe research   187
9.3   The research cycle, adapted from Ellis (2013)   188
9.4   Experimental study design   193
9.5   Selecting a sample   199
9.6   Representative sample   200
9.7   Example of a bar chart indicating patient satisfaction with care provided in
      a maternity hospital   210
10.1 Dahlgren and Whitehead's Rainbow Model of Health, adapted from Dahlgren
      and Whitehead (1991)   220
10.2 Model of accumulated risk of cancer, adapted from Uauy and Solomons
      (2005)   221
10.3 Two bivariate graphs, adapted from an annual HSCIC (2012) report   224
11.1 Example responses from Anglia Ruskin Public Health students   236
11.2 Do you always make the healthiest choice?   237
11.3 Reasons for inactivity   238
11.4 Dahlgren and Whitehead's Rainbow Model of Health, adapted from Dahlgren
      and Whitehead (1991)   241
11.5 Social Cognitive Theory, adapted from Bandura (1973)   242
11.6 The Health Belief Model, adapted from Hochbaum (1958)   242
11.7 Stages of change   245
11.8 Self-Determination Theory, adapted from Deci and Ryan (1985)   248
11.9 Tannahill's Model of Health Promotion, adapted from Downie et al. (1990)   249
12.1 Specific risk factors for abuse, adapted from Rogers (2003) and Walker and
      Thurston (2006)   260
12.2 Signs of physical abuse   265
12.3 Signs that psychological abuse is taking place, adapted from Walker and
      Thurston (2006) and Local Government Association (LGA) (2015)   266
12.4 Signs that sexual abuse may be taking place, adapted from Walker and
      Thurston (2006) and LGA (2015)   267
12.5 Signs that neglect and acts of omissions may be occurring   268

12.6	Signs that discrimination may be taking place, adapted from LGA (2015)	269
12.7	Signs that financial abuse may be occurring, adapted from LGA (2015)	269
13.1	The Kolb cycle, adapted from Kolb (1984)	283
13.2	Peyton's four-stage model for teaching practical skills, adapted from Walker and Peyton (1998)	288
13.3	Stakeholders in professional and vocational education	297
13.4	Miller's Pyramid, adapted from Miller (1990)	299
13.5	What we assess, adapted from Miller (1990)	300

Tables

1.1	Information sources chart	12
1.2	Scope of a literature search	21
1.3	Examples of some key health and social care databases	26
1.4	Refining your search	29
1.5	Example of recording your search results	30
1.6	Points to consider when writing assignments	35
1.7	Types of essays and writing	35
1.8	Bibliography or reference list – what is the difference?	39
1.9	What information do I need to record for my references?	43
2.1	Example of a learning agreement	55
2.2	A completed PDP using SMART principles	58
3.1	Planning communication	88
4.1	Positive and negative aspects of being in a 'tribe'	103
6.1	Reports and policies and what they hope to achieve	134
9.1	Summary of qualitative research approaches	195
9.2	Main differences between quantitative and qualitative research	197
9.3	Advantages and disadvantages of questionnaires	203
9.4	Advantages and disadvantages of interviews	204
9.5	Example of a highly structured observation schedule	205
9.6	Advantages and disadvantages of participant and non-participant observation	206
9.7	Criteria for trustworthiness	207
9.8	Example of a frequency distribution table	210
11.1	Ewles and Simnett's Five Categories for health promotion approaches (1999)	240
12.1	Advantages and disadvantages of inter-professional working, adapted from Walker and Thurston (2006)	272
12.2	The potential safeguarding plan summary for the Jones family	277
13.1	Positive and negative descriptions of learning	281
13.2	Steps in planning teaching: Elaine and Louise's case study	287
13.3	Steps in planning teaching: John and Edith's case study	292
13.4	Steps in planning teaching: Rahima's case study	295
13.5	Formative and summative assessment	298
13.6	Giving feedback, adapted from Norcini and Burch (2013)	303

Contributors

Jayne Crow, having been a Senior Lecturer at Anglia Ruskin University for many years, is now a freelance workshop facilitator and lecturer in Health and Social Care.

Vicki Elliott, now retired, was formerly a Senior Lecturer in the Department of Allied and Public Health in the Faculty of Medical Science at Anglia Ruskin University.

David Hingley is a Senior Lecturer in the Department of Adult and Mental Health Nursing at Anglia Ruskin University.

Shirley Jones is a Senior Lecturer in the Faculty of Medical Science at Anglia Ruskin University.

Iain John Keenan is a Senior Lecturer in the School of Health and Human Sciences at the University of Essex.

Sarah Kraszewski is Head of Department Midwifery, Child and Community Nursing at Anglia Ruskin University.

Patricia Macnamara is a Senior Lecturer in the Faculty of Health, Social Care and Education at Anglia Ruskin University.

Fiona McMaster is a Senior Lecturer and Course Leader MSc Public Health at Anglia Ruskin University.

Mary Northrop is a Senior Lecturer in the Faculty of Health, Social Care and Education at Anglia Ruskin University.

Anne-Marie Reid is a Senior Lecturer and Head of Curriculum Development in Leeds Institute for Medical Education at the University of Leeds.

Jane Shelley is a Subject Librarian: Health and Social Care at Anglia Ruskin University.

Andy Stevens is a Fellow of the Royal Society of Public Health and was Principal Lecturer in Public Health at Anglia Ruskin University (now retired).

Claire Thurgate is Director of the Centre for Work-Based Learning and Continuing Development at Canterbury Christ Church University.

Chris Thurston is Head of Department Adult and Mental Health Nursing at Anglia Ruskin University.

Preface

One of the many changes in health and social care over recent years has been the enhancement of skill mix and with this has come new, and most welcome, educational opportunities for the workforce. One such opportunity has come in the form of Foundation Degrees (FD) to support the role of assistant or associate practitioners across many specialities in health and social care. The editors and chapter authors are all health professionals experienced in facilitating learning for the health and social care workforce, so when we set out to produce this book we began by asking our own Health and Social Care FD students what they would like to see in a textbook. What would help them get the most out of their studies and help them to succeed? The scope, direction and format of this textbook was born out of their feedback to us and under their direction we have included case studies, examples, activities and tips which will help you engage actively with the text and promote learning. We also hope it will encourage you to step back and reflect frequently; to take that long hard look at practice and consider how things can be improved and to go on to strive for excellence in your work.

The authors offer a wealth of experience in the different topic areas and chapters cover core issues such as public health, health promotion, quality in healthcare, team-working, teaching and assessing, policy perspectives and communication skills. Each chapter can be read either as standalone or in conjunction with others, and we have signposted where possible to ease navigation. A text of this nature cannot cover all topics in depth but aims to provide a useful introduction and to direct you to other useful resources where you can extend the depth and breadth of your knowledge. You will note some overlap between chapters in places and it is hoped that this 'building block' effect will be helpful in making the links between important concepts and integrating the material in a way that reflects practice in the real world. For example, the role of ethics, whilst it is raised in the Valuing People chapter, is considered again from a legal stance and in relation to teamwork and research in other chapters

A recurrent theme in the feedback from our students, many of whom had not studied for a long time when they started on the course, has been the importance of 'sorting out' how to go about their studies. So to provide a helpful structure we have begun each chapter with a set of learning outcomes and ended them with a chapter summary of key points. This enables the reader to focus upon what they can achieve from reading each chapter and to assist in selecting what to read when. You will notice that there are two larger chapters – Preparing for Study, and Research and Evidence-Based Practice. This is because our students have identified to us that these are the topic areas that need particular emphasis at their level of study. We wish you every success with your studies.

Mary Northrop, Jayne Crow and Sarah Kraszewski

Acknowledgements

For help with producing this text, we would like to thank Dave Kraszewski for his time, patience, IT skills and critical eye throughout.

We would also like to thank all our chapter authors for their valuable contributions. Chapter 7 contains public sector information published by the Health and Safety Executive and licensed under the Open Government Licence.

List of abbreviations

A & E	Accident and Emergency
CAPI	Computer Assisted Personal Interviewing
CCG	Clinical Commissioning Group
CHM	Commission on Human Medicines
CPS	Crown Prosecution Service
CQC	Care Quality Commission
CV	Curriculum Vitae
DfCSF	Department for Children, School and Families.
DH	Department of Health
EBP	Evidence-based Practice
EMO	Emotional
FD	Foundation Degree
FII	Fabricated or Induced Illness
FTT	Failure to Thrive
FPH	Faculty of Public Health
GMC	General Medical Council
GP	General Practitioner
IT	Information Technology
IVF	In Vitro Fertilization
HAI	Hospital Acquired Infection
HCPC	Health and Care Professions Council
HPV	Human Papilloma Virus
HRA	Human Rights Act
HSCIC	Health and Social Care Information Centre
HSE	Health and Safety Executive
LINKs	Local Involvement Networks
LLL	Lifelong Learning
LOLER	Lifting Operations and Lifting Equipment Regulations
MHRA	Medicines and Healthcare Products Regulatory Agency
MS	Multiple Sclerosis
NHS	National Health Service
NICE	National Institute for Clinical Excellence (1999)
NICE	National Institute for Health and Clinical Excellence (2005)
NICE	National Institute for Health and Care Excellence (2013)
NMC	Nursing and Midwifery Council

NPSA	National Patient Safety Agency
NRLS	The National Reporting and Learning System
NSPCC	National Society for the Prevention of Cruelty to Children
NVQ	National Vocational Qualification
ONS	Office for National Statistics
OSCE	Observed Clinical Examination
PALS	Patient Advice and Liaison Services
PDP	Personal Development Plan
PPIfs	Patient and Public Involvement in Health forums
PSI	Patient Safety Incident
QAA	Quality Assurance Agency for Higher Education
QOF	Quality and Outcomes Framework
RCT	Randomised Controlled Trial
RIDDOR	Reporting of Injuries Diseases and Dangerous Occurrences Regulations
RoSPA	Royal Society for the Prevention of Accidents
SCIE	Social Care Institute for Excellence
SOCAT	Social Capital Assessment Tool
SMART	Specific, Measurable, Achievable, Realistic and Time-bound
SWOT	Strengths, Weaknesses, Opportunities and Threats
UK	United Kingdom
VLE	Virtual Learning Environment
VTE	Venous Thromboembolism
WBL	Work-based Learning
WHO	World Health Organisation

Chapter 1

Preparing for study

Jane Shelley and Iain John Keenan

LEARNING OUTCOMES

By the end of this chapter you will be able to:

1 Understand the importance of effective reading and the skills involved.
2 Understand the importance of literature searching and the skills involved.
3 Understand the importance of writing academically and the skills involved.

Introduction

To be successful in your studies you must be competent in three main academic areas; reading, writing and literature searching. These skills will underpin all your academic studies and will be important to you achieving your goals. This chapter provides key prompts and guidance to help you understand these skills and aid you in developing them.

Reading skills

When you study for a course you will undoubtedly be required to read, read and read some more. The need to read a great deal of material in what is usually a restricted amount of time is a major challenge for students and one that requires you to learn new skills and brush up on the use of old ones. In this age of information there will not be time for you to read everything published on a subject even if you wanted to. You would be quickly overwhelmed. So what follows are some ideas on how to manage your reading on your course.

Reading is a neglected skill. If asked, we would probably all say we are competent readers but reading isn't just the ability to understand and interpret individual words it is also about comprehending the meaning of the words and putting them into context.

When reading we have to use many skilful thought processes to successfully understand the meaning of what we are reading and put it into the right context. This is why reading is a skill, and why, like any skill we wish to master, we must ensure that we practice it frequently.

ACTIVITY – THE VARIETY OF THINGS YOU READ

Reading material comes in a variety of different styles and the style is often related to the purpose of the material. In the left-hand column below make a list of all the different things you read. Then in the right-hand column identify the reason (purpose) for reading that particular material. The first one has been done for you.

Style of material	Purpose
Newspaper	To keep up to date with current national and international issues

From your list you can see that reading is a purposeful activity. We read for very specific purposes – sometimes to inform, sometimes for instructions and sometimes for our own entertainment. Everday reading material comes to us in a variety of ways. How about when we are at work though? Now look at the table below. It lists the variety of work-based reading you may come across. Fill in the right-hand column with the purpose for reading that material. The first one has been done for you.

Style of material	Purpose
Uniform/dress policy	To confirm to the correct standard
Service users notes	
Measurement chart	
Health and safety guidelines	
Referral letter	

When you read at work it tends to be far more specific than everyday reading. Reading at work tends not to be optional but essential.

When you study for a course you will be expected to undertake a lot of reading. You will mainly be reading **journal** articles or books but within each of these you will find similar styles.

ACTIVITY

Here is a list of academic-based reading. See if you can work out the purpose of each style of material. Enter in the right-hand column the purpose for reading that particular material. The first one has been done for you.

Source of material	Purpose
Practice guidance article in a journal	To understand the step-by-step procedure for undertaking a task
Research paper	
Anatomy and physiology book	
Study guide book	
Opinion piece in a journal (an article that is not a research report or literature review but contains a discussion of the authors opinion on a subject)	
Course module guide	

You can see that there is a wide range of reading for academic studies and that the purpose of that reading varies greatly as will the style and the way the information is presented. To be successful you must master all these varieties and be comfortable in navigating your way through them.

STUDENT TIP

Keep reading throughout your course. Not just the academic books but newspapers, magazines, novels and anything you find interesting; it really helps improve your reading speed and vocabulary.

Reading effectively

To help you navigate the vast amount of reading material available to you, you will have to develop some specific key reading strategies. Two such strategies are skim reading and scanning:

- **Skim reading** is what you do when you are searching quickly to get an overview of the reading material so you can decide whether its suits your purpose. This may involve reading any summary provided and looking at titles and headings, but you will also cast your eyes over the body of the text to take note of subheadings.
- **Scanning** is when you have a specific purpose in mind or a specific topic in mind and you are searching through the text to find keywords or phrases. You are most likely to do this on a content or index page but will also do it in the text itself by casting your eyes over the text more carefully.

Both of these strategies are used at the beginning of any attempt to engage in reading so as to ensure you utilise your time efficiently and do not read unnecessary material.

ACTIVITY

Now try these skimming and scanning activities.

Let's look at a contents page. A contents page is usually located at the front of a book and gives you a broad overview of subject headings and chapters that can be found in the book.

Contents

Introduction	ii
List of tables	viii
Notes on contributors	xi
Glossary	xiii
Chapter 1 – What is health and social care?	1
Chapter 2 – Child and adolescent health and care	3
Chapter 3 – Community services for children and adolescents	21
Chapter 4 – Adult health and care	40
Chapter 5 – Community services for adults	80
Chapter 6 – Professional nursing services	122
Chapter 7 – Carers	143

Look at the contents page and try to answer the following questions:

1   In which chapter are you most likely to find information on adults with diabetes?
2   In which chapter might you find a definition of social care?
3   In which chapter are you most likely to find information on family planning?

Now let's look at an index taken from a book. An index is found at the back of a book and is an alphabetical list of names, places and subjects mentioned in the book. The index provides the page number where each item is mentioned. Have a look at the index and then answer the questions below.

A
Abuse 70,
 Alcohol 71, 72
 Drug 73
 Sexual 70, 89
Accident and Emergency 12, 20, 32
Adoption and fostering 32–44
Adult protection 90, 91
Alcohol *(see abuse)*
Alzheimer's 55
Asthma 20, 44, 82, 97
Attendance allowance 130, 131
Autism 18, 20–22

B
Babies 2, 4, 6, 67
Back pain 43
Benefits 2, 23, 91
Bereavement 62, 63
Blind people 94
Breast cancer 57
Breastfeeding 17

C
Cancer 11, 42
Care 1, 4, 66, 143–145
Care and carers 10, 88, 143, 145
Care homes 3, 11, 45, 102, 125, 143
Carer's self-assessment 146–148
Chemists 144
Child protection 7, 21, 23
Children's services 2, 24
Chronic pain 52
Community nursing 122
Condom service 24

D
Death 60, 91, 94, 150
Dementia 62
Depression 37, 92, 101, 152–153
Diabetes 77
District nursing 123–127
Domestic violence 90, 91, 94
Drugs *(see abuse)*
Dying 90, 37, 149

1 On which page can you find information on chronic pain?
2 On which pages can you find information on adoption and fostering ?
3 On which page can you find information on drug abuse?

Once you have found the relevant page you will need to find the actual material that is of use to you.

 Now read the following passage and locate where the information about drug abuse is contained.

> Abuse is the term given to the inappropriate use or treatment of a person, object, substance or situation. Abuse has many forms such as verbal, emotional, sexual, physical, drug and alcohol to name but a few. Abusers typically misuse, mistreat, degrade or show no concern or regard for the integrity, safety, purpose, function or value of the person, object, situation or substance that they are involved with. Their behaviour seeks to manipulate and control what they are abusing to 'fall in line' with their own objectives, morals or purpose. When we talk about drug abuse we are referring to a destructive pattern of using a substance for the purpose of seeking a 'high' (sense of euphoria). Drugs that are abused are typically ones that have a legitimate medical purpose but have been altered, tampered with or modified and are administered incorrectly or by hazardous or harmful means. Alternatively, when we talk about verbal abuse we are referring to the act of speaking to someone in an intimidating or aggressive way or by using our words to manipulate or misguide a person into changing their behaviour, beliefs or attitudes

so that they benefit the abuser. From these two examples we can see that abuse as a defining term comes in different guises and can be applied to a multitude of lived experiences.

Did you find the section on drug abuse easily?

LEARNING POINT

Can you see how an index links to specific words, not always chapters or page headings? If you use the contents page and index correctly and practice your skimming and scanning techniques you can obtain the relevant information quickly and efficiently. You'll then be able to be selective in locating the information on the page and therefore will not waste time reading through unrelated information.

WEB LINK

BBC Skillswise (2014) provides some excellent resources to help improve your reading. Available at: www.bbc.co.uk/skillswise/topic-group/reading.

Vocabulary

Once you understand the style of what you are reading and its purpose you will notice that the vocabulary differs greatly.

Let's see if you can identify the different styles of material. Below are four sections; one is taken from a novel, one from a policy document, one from a research paper and one from an opinion piece in a journal.

ACTIVITY

Can you identify which piece is taken from a NOVEL, a POLICY DOCUMENT, RESEARCH PAPER and an OPINION PIECE?

1   'The study is descriptive in nature and requires research data relating to the experiences of participants rather than their behaviours. This is therefore qualitative data and an individual interview method will be used to gather and interpret it. An unstructured interview technique will be used.'
2   'Cautiously he approached his victim, stepping softly as he crept nearer, slowing his breathing as he reached within an arms length of her shoulder.'

3 'Whilst it is obvious to the experienced professional that standards have waned in the past ten years it would seem that the authorities have not taken notice. Whilst the professionals have continued to advocate a fundamental change in the structure of education and staff development the authorities seem to still be insisting on financial investment in capital initiatives.'

4 'Staff must maintain a high level of personal hygiene presenting a clean, neat and tidy appearance at work. Hair must be off the shoulder and tied back when appropriate. Hands and nails must be clean and nail varnish is strictly forbidden.'

REFLECTION POINT

Make a list of the key differences between these styles of material.

Can you identify how the language and vocabulary differs in each style?

Did you correctly identify which was which?

The first is taken from a research paper, the second a novel, the third an opinion piece and the fourth is from a policy document.

As a student you will need to be able to see the differences in the material you read so that you can select the right reading material for the right purpose. For example, if you were writing an essay you may need to read factual material such as a policy document or a research paper rather than an opinion piece.

Understanding varying styles and vocabulary will also help you with your writing style. Students need to adopt an appropriate style of writing and to do this they need to recognise what that looks like.

STUDENT TIP

The most important part of being able to write a good essay is reading. You cannot begin to write an essay until you have done all the necessary background reading.

Assessments

Most students when they start a course of study understandably focus on the assessment that they will need to undertake. Within every course there exists a range of assessments to test your knowledge and understanding of the subject. These assessments range from the traditional essay or assignment to presentations and, more commonly these days, practical classroom assessments. To help you understand the range and purpose of the assessments on the course, your tutors will provide you with various resources that are essential reading for you. These documents will help you to understand and navigate your way around the assessments and the course. . .

. . . so make sure you find them and make good use of them.

Below are listed a few key resources that you will need to familiarise yourself with:

Course guide – this guide provides you with a complete overview of the course, the modules/ units, the learning outcomes and a broad outline of the assessments within the course. You should be provided with this guide at the very beginning of your programme and should refer to it throughout.

Student handbook – this is usually provided at the start of the course and provides you with key information about your responsibilities as a student and key organisational policies and procedures that you, as a student, will be expected to abide by. It will include information on how to hand in assessments and the policy on plagiarism, attendance, student support information and also information on the appeals process should you wish to appeal any assessment grade you have received.

Assessment guidelines and marking grids/criteria – these are generally provided for each course and should provide you with a clear, detailed explanation of what is expected of you for the assessment and how the assessment is going to be marked. Students frequently overlook the marking grid/criteria but it is an invaluable resource, providing you with a clear outline of what the examiner is looking for.

Different types of assessment

As mentioned previously, there are a number of different assessment methods used within any course. Listed below are the common assessment methods that you will come across:

Assignment/essays – assignments are the traditional form of assessment and you can expect to be asked to write many of these during your studies. The number of words you are asked to write will vary considerably. Perhaps from 1,000 to 6,000 words. This can sound scary to students writing a first essay but in fact once you get going you will find that it is often the case that you feel you need a larger word allowance for an assignment, not a smaller one. The three main styles you will be expected to produce will be a theoretical piece, a reflective account or a case study (see section below).

Examinations – usually carried out in exam conditions similar to those you may have been used to at school. Exams can be multiple-choice, short-answer or essay-type questions.

Presentations – with presentations you tend to choose a specific topic from broad guidelines that are given to you by the course leader. You will then usually be required to talk about the subject in front of the examiners and maybe your fellow students.

Portfolio – portfolios represent a collection of various learning materials that have been completed by the student along with some explanatory notes, reflective accounts or commentaries. Portfolios can either be structured (clear guidelines as to what is to be included) or they can be informal (no set guidelines) and they tend to be used in subjects with very broad themes, such as health promotion, or for evidence of personal development.

Skills book – on most vocational courses there is an element of practical assessment. This is usually carried out with the use of a skills book that clearly outlines the practical skills that you need to achieve and the level to which they need to be obtained. Some elements of the skills book can be completed by students but the assessment elements of the particular skills must be completed by the person identified as the mentor in practice, assessor or supervisor. Make sure you check who has to sign which parts of your skills book.

Learning logs – learning logs are like diaries of learning, where the student records the type, duration and outcome of the variety of learning activities they have undertaken.

Observed Structured Clinical Examinations (OSCEs) – OSCEs are practical assessments of skills involving service users, a set scenario and equipment. They are generally carried out in skills laboratories and there is a clear timeframe and brief set out for you at the start. These assessments allow you to show off your practical skills. This can be considered a 'role play' situation and for that reason a lot of students find them uncomfortable but if you treat them like real-life practical situations then you will succeed in showcasing your practical ability.

Whatever the assessment it is important to check the learning outcomes in the course guide. In order to pass it is necessary to utilise all the appropriate learning material which you will be guided to by the course leader. To successfully retrieve the learning material you will need to learn how to use the library effectively.

Using the library effectively

This section will introduce you to using your university library and library website effectively during your course. Whatever you are studying you will need to find information to help you complete your assessed work. The library and library website are good places to start.

Your library website

Libraries are no longer just physical buildings with rows of books and other materials on shelves; they are also online 'digital libraries'. Library websites provide an increasing amount and range of full text resources online for you to use for free – electronic books (e-books), electronic journals (e-journals), quality websites and a wide variety of digital resources to support your course. Online resources are usually available 24/7 – all the time, day and night, all year round and anywhere you have access to the Internet.

Your library website will also be the place to renew and reserve books and obtain help in finding and using information so it is a good idea to become familiar with your library website early in your course.

Logins and passwords

While a student at your institution you will be given usernames and passwords. You will need these to log in to and access services available to you as a student, such as course resources via **Virtual Learning Environments (VLEs)**, library resources and email.

STUDENT TIP – PASSWORDS

Your institution may have a number of usernames and passwords for various services, e.g. library, IT, email, VLE, or may use just one for everything.

Keep all necessary usernames and passwords in a safe place.

Borrowing books and avoiding fines

As soon as possible obtain your library card and find out how to borrow books and how many books you can borrow. Make a note of how to renew your books, how to contact the library and what fines, if any, are charged. Always remember you may not be able to renew – another student may have reserved the books which you have borrowed!

STUDENT TIP

I got a £50 fine for overdue books. Now I always make sure I put a reminder on my mobile phone a few days before they are due...

Undertake the following activity for your own university library.

ACTIVITY – LIBRARY TREASURE HUNT

- Make a note of the opening times of the library/libraries and IT facilities.
- Note down the website address (also known as a **Uniform Resource Locator or URL**) of your university library.

You might find it useful to bookmark (favourite) the website or if you have a suitable mobile device you might be able to make use of your QR reader and QR codes for the library (QR codes or Quick Response codes are like barcodes allowing you to access websites via smartphones and devices with QR code readers). Here's an example of what they look like:

Figure 1.1 Example of a QR code.

- How many books can you borrow from the library?
- How long can you borrow items for?
- Can you renew books? If yes, how do you do this?
- Take a look at your library website and note down some useful links or guides for future use.
- Practise logging into your library account or the online library.
- Does the library provide an online enquiry/chat/contact us link? Note down the details.
- Bookmark or favourite some useful help pages or guides from the website.

You will see from this activity that your university library provides lots of help, much of it in the form of self-help and online guidance. Make use of this and any training sessions and online tutorials to help you get the best support for your course.

STUDENT TIP

Keep your ID/library card safe and always carry it when you visit the library.

Figure 1.2 contains some key tips for using your university library.

Information sources

Information is available from a variety of sources – from the people we chat to in the corridor or an email we receive, to reading a scholarly textbook or research paper. It is often said that we now live in the age of information overload, but remember that information can

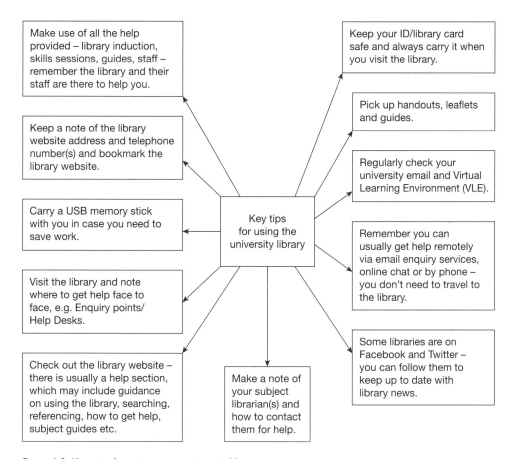

Figure 1.2 Key tips for using your university library.

vary greatly in type and quality. A search on a search engine such as Google for the topic 'communication' finds many thousands of hits of varying usefulness and accuracy. Not all of the results would be helpful in writing an academic essay on communication in the health and social care environment. Information can come from many sources. Table 1.1 is not an exhaustive list but just some examples of types of information.

Quality of Internet resources

Internet sources can vary widely in quality, reliability and accuracy and can range from personal biased opinion lacking any accuracy or truth, to **peer-reviewed** scholarly research

Table 1.1 Information sources chart

Source of material	Format	Purpose/why use	How to find
Dictionaries, **thesauruses**, directories, yearbooks and encyclopaedias	Print Electronic/online	Useful for spellings, meanings, facts and quick overview of subject.	Library catalogues and library search/discovery tools. These will provide you with the location number (shelf number) where the item is shelved, or provide you with a link to the online version where available. Some freely available online via the Internet.
Books Edited books and chapters of books	Print Electronic/online (e-books) Audio	Books can vary in depth and coverage. Generally books are good for providing an introduction and overview of a topic or subject. They can vary from broad topic coverage to a niche focus on a specific area. Most books go through a rigorous editorial process by publishers before they are made available. This helps to ensure academic credibility and authority. Use contents pages and indexes to track down detailed information.	Library catalogues and library search/discovery tools. Search by author and/or title for specific books or by subject/topic for a variety of books. Catalogues will provide the location number (shelf number) where the book is shelved or provide you with a link to the online e-book. Most university libraries now provide access to full text e-books online. Additionally publishers' websites sometimes provide free chapters and Google books may provide excerpts from books To search for chapters within books search for the book title and editor. When you locate the book the chapter will be inside the book (check the content pages).

Source of material	Format	Purpose/why use	How to find
Journals	Print and/ or electronic (e-journals/ online journals) Also known as **magazines, periodicals, serials** Published in successive individual volumes and parts on a regular basis, e.g. weekly, bi-weekly, monthly, quarterly etc., or irregular basis, e.g. April 2012 or volume 10 part/issue 5 Journal articles: Journals are made up of a variety of articles or papers of variable length written by different people	Useful for providing more up-to-date information on topics. Can provide a variety of information including: news, commentaries, opinions, primary or original research studies and in-depth research papers and reviews including literature reviews and systematic reviews. Some journals are peer reviewed, e.g. *Social Science and Medicine*. This is where experts in the subject area have critiqued and reviewed the material to ensure it is acceptable for publication. They are a good source of current research in many health topics and can help you to keep up to date.	Library catalogues and library search/discovery tools. Search by the title of the journal, e.g. "Community Care" "Health and Social Care in the Community" "New Scientist" "British Medical Journal". To find journal articles use your library website search/ discovery tools and databases and indexes. Examples of databases for health and social care include ASSIA (Applied Social Science Index and Abstracts). You can search databases for articles on a variety of topics.
Newspapers	Print Electronic	Can be useful for current events. Watch for bias and lack of in-depth coverage or sensationalism.	Library catalogues and library search/discovery tools. Your library may also have specific newspaper databases and resources. Some newspapers are also available freely online, e.g. *The Guardian*.
Reports (government/ professional bodies/charities/ official enquiries etc.)	Print Electronic	E.g. Department of Health, Royal College of Nursing, Joseph Rowntree Foundation, Diabetes UK all provide a wealth of information. Summaries are often available for you to read.	The Internet is usually the best place to search for government reports and documents or charity websites. Use a search engine. Library subject guides or your course guides may include specific quality websites and links for you to use.

Table 1.1 continued

Source of material	Format	Purpose/why use	How to find
Policy/guidelines/ protocols	Print Electronic	Examples of organisations producing guidelines and policies: National Institute for Health and Care Excellence (NICE) – includes links to policies, guidelines and care pathways. Skills for Health or Skills for Care. Social Care Institute for Excellence (SCIE).	The library catalogue search/ discovery tool or Internet search engines are usually the best place to search for policies, guidelines and protocols. Library subject guides or your course guides may include specific titles for you to use. Your employer's intranet or website (internal network) is useful for locating internal, local and work related policies/guidelines/protocols.
Charity/service user websites	Electronic	Useful for up to date and increasingly full text material/ visual/sound etc. (watch for bias), e.g. MIND, Age UK, British Heart Foundation, Cancer Research UK. Note that such information is often at a level for and for the perspective of the public/ patient/client/lay person.	Internet search engines. Your library website, library subject guides or your course guides may include specific charities or organisations for you to use.
Legislation	Print Electronic	Acts of Parliament, e.g. Mental Capacity Act 2005 can be useful in providing the current law. Note there are usually books, journal articles and codes of practice that will help you to understand and put into practice current legislation.	Library catalogues and library search/discovery tools. Online via the government's legislation website (all acts since 1988 and many from earlier) at: www.legislation.gov.uk/.
Websites	Electronic	Websites of a great variety including official sites like government departments and official organisations like the World Health Organization to personal Web pages including blogs and wikis. Websites can be useful sources of information but remember anyone can create – so watch for quality and accuracy. Blogs are a type of online diary providing regularly updated articles written by someone or an organisation	Use an Internet search engine to locate these. Your library website is the best place to start finding websites to ensure quality sources and full text access where available. Library subject guides or your course guides may include specific quality websites and examples for you to use.

Source of material	Format	Purpose/why use	How to find
		with either an interest or expertise. Examples include conference and organisational blogs, e.g. Department of Health, Kings Fund. A wiki is a type of website with collaboratively written content.	

papers and journal articles. Locating and using information based on correct and reliable evidence is crucial. Therefore you must always evaluate what you find before using it. Remember, anyone can create and make public a website, so use such sources with care and always evaluate what you read, especially anything found on the Internet (see Chapter 9: Research and evidence-based practice for further information on this subject).

ACTIVITY – WHY CAN'T I RELY ON GOOGLE FOR ALL MY INFORMATION?

Most of us use an Internet search engine such as Google and sometimes it can be helpful in locating useful information quickly. However, for your course and essays you cannot rely on it!

Try out a search for either 'communication and health' or 'communication and social care' in:

(a) Google
(b) Your library search box (catalogue or discovery tool)

Compare the results and spend a few minutes reflecting on the differences. Note and compare:

•   The number of hits/results
•   Type of results

From the previous activity you should have noted that your library search tool and library website resources provide you with a wide variety of resources which are of a good quality and available in full text for you to either borrow or read online. Your Google search may have found more results but often you are unable to identify the author and quality of what you have found and it is therefore less useful to you for academic work. Additionally you may not be able to access the full text.

STUDENT TIP

Always use your university library as your starting point for finding and accessing material for your course and assignments. If in doubt about using any material you find for an assessment or essays always check with your tutors. For example, many institutions would suggest you do not use sources like your PowerPoint lecture slides or Wikipedia in your essays.

Finding information – literature searching

Searching for information for your coursework is known as literature searching or information retrieval and is the process of searching effectively for information and literature on your topic. This could involve searching for a variety of resources: books, journal articles, key documents and websites. A good starting point is to look at any reading list you have been given for your course either in the form of a reading list or module guide or examples from your lecturers. This will usually include lists of books, journals or journal articles and websites and other materials for you to look at. Links to key readings and materials may be made available for you on your VLE. Although you can start with your reading list you will usually need more information. So how do you start to find more information on your topic?

Searching

ACTIVITY – REFLECTION

Think of the last time you had to search for information? What was your topic?

- How successful were you?
- Where did you search?
- What word/words did you search for?
- How much information did you find?
- Were any of the results useful?
- Reflect on your search and the results you got.
- How successful were you and why?
- What went wrong and why?

Come back to this activity after reading the rest of this chapter and say what you might now do to improve your search.

Good searching is a mix of many things. Think of putting together a DIY flat-packed piece of furniture or cooking a recipe. For a good result you need to use the right ingredients or the correct instructions in the correct way. Miss something out or do something in the wrong order and the results may not be as good as you want. The key to a successful search is using the right words in the right place. To do a good search whether it is personal or academic related uses a similar methodology.

Key elements for a search

Plan your search

Planning your search is very important and saves you time in the long run. **Do try to avoid the temptation to jump straight into your search on the computer.**

Start with your topic/subject/essay question or title – what is it about? Ask yourself what you already know about and around your topic. You may think that you have no experience of looking for information but if you think about this for a moment you will realise that you do this in your everyday life all the time. For example you use these skills when you book a holiday or go shopping.

Think about going on your next holiday – most people do not just book up. You think and plan beforehand. For example you consider when you want to go, location, costs, type of holiday, accommodation and activities available. So if you have been set the following essay title: '**Discuss the issues around communication in the healthcare environment**', you will need to think around this topic, e.g. are you going to cover all aspects of communication in all healthcare settings? Are you going to include communication with families and/ or colleagues?

Mind map

One way of helping yourself in the initial stage is 'mind mapping'. Try to resist the temptation to jump onto the computer and search Google. Start with spending some time thinking about what you want to find out about. Some kind of mind map or spider diagram may be useful or write down lists under key headings if you find that easier. Paper and pen is fine for this purpose although you might want to save it on your computer using a word processor or make use of mind mapping software. There are many packages available, some of which are free and some of which are not or are only available via your institution.

A mind map for 'Booking and going on holiday' might look something like Figure 1.3.

Now let us apply this same method to writing an essay on the communication topic mentioned above. You might mind map it in a similar way but the information required would be different.

You can see in Figure 1.4 that for this essay there are three main elements or concepts: 'issues', 'communication' and 'healthcare environment'. Can you think of anything else you might want to cover? Note that for an essay you will probably have to be selective in which areas of this mind map you focus on, e.g. communication with adults in an acute ward.

Identify alternative words or phrases for the key concepts

The key concepts for your essay can often be expressed in different ways. It is easy to get tunnel vision and only use the first word that you think about. Always spend a few minutes creating a list of keywords to use in your search and thinking of alternative words you could use.

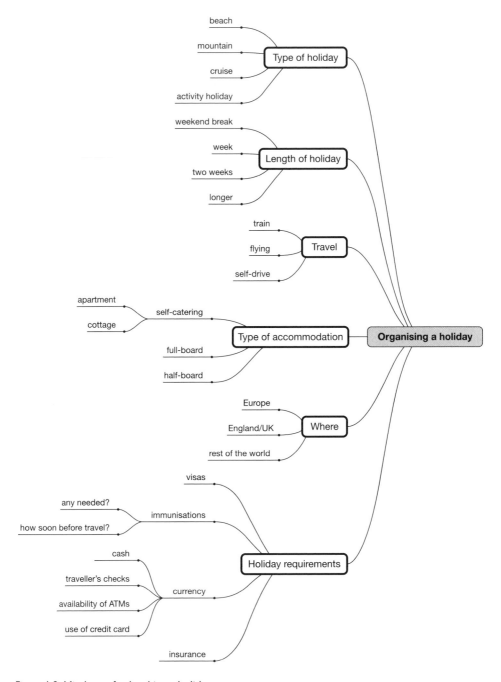

Figure 1.3 Mind map for booking a holiday.

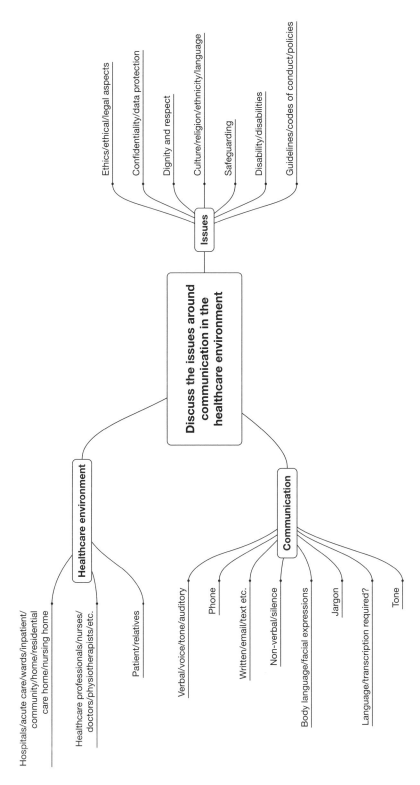

Figure 1.4 Mind map for the essay topic 'Communication Issues in the Healthcare Environment'.

Points to think about when creating your list of keywords:

- synonyms (words which have the same meaning), e.g. vacation/holiday, teenager/adolescent, old people/elderly/elder/older
- variant/alternative spellings, e.g. healthcare/health care, paediatric/pediatric
- singular and plurals, e.g. patient/patients
- acronyms and abbreviations/full words, e.g. NHS/National Health Service, MS/Multiple Sclerosis
- broader/narrower terms, e.g. hospital/ward, looked after children/fostering
- phrases, e.g. 'informal carers'
- scientific/medical vs. common/lay term
- words used in particular countries, e.g. accident and emergency department/A & E/ emergency room.

STUDENT TIP

Use a dictionary and a thesaurus to help with terms and meanings. As you start your search new words may emerge. Add these to your list to use in your search.

You will see from Table 1.2 that the scope of your search and possible synonyms and alternative words can be variable and quite large. Can you think of any others?

STUDENT TIP

If in doubt about aspects of the scope of your search such as currency of material and limiting to the UK focus – always check your assignment guidelines or ask your tutor.

Where to search?

You will need to use and search for appropriate sources. See Table 1.1: Information sources chart for full details of information sources and how and where to find them.

Searching for books

Even though so much is available online, books are a good starting point. Holiday guides to the country you are thinking of visiting or a textbook on communication in health would be good starting points for our example searches.

For your academic work always remember to start with your reading list or module guide or books suggested by your lecturers. Your reading list will show details of the material you need to read and you need to understand what the different sources are and how to locate them.

Table 1.2 Scope of a literature search

Stage of the search	Issues around communication in the healthcare environment
Mind map the topic	See above
Key concept(s)	'issues', 'communication', 'healthcare'
Keywords (alternative words) and synonyms for each of your concepts (alternative search words)	**Issues:** Ethics/ethical/legal/confidentiality Dignity and respect Culture/religion/ethnicity/language Safeguarding Disability/disabilities Guidelines/codes of conduct/policies **Communication:** Communication/communicate/interpersonal relations/ interpersonal relation/interpersonal relationships/ interpersonal skills/non-verbal/non verbal/nonverbal/body language Verbal/voice/tone/auditory Phone/written/email/text etc. Silence/body language/facial expressions/tone Jargon Language/translation required? **Healthcare environment:** Nurse/nurses/nursing/health professionals/care workers/ doctor/doctors /physiotherapists etc. Health care/healthcare/hospitals/acute care/wards/ inpatient/community/home/residential care home/nursing home Healthcare professionals/nurses/doctors/physiotherapists/ patients/relatives/family
Scope of search:	
How current?	How far back in time do you need information from, e.g. last 5/10/25 years?
Type of publication/source of information/level	E.g. professional, patient/public focused, research, official/ government policy?
Language	English language material only or are you able to get translations?
Geographical area	Do you want UK-relevant material only? European? Exclude US? Sometimes you may wish to undertake a comparison of a number of countries.

Table 1.2 continued

Scope of search:	Issues around communication in the healthcare environment
Focus	Age: adults only? Children only? Older people? All/ any age...
	Gender: male or female or both...
	Specific subjects: smoking, health promotion, healthcare approaches, clinical aspects etc.

Interpreting your reading lists

Figure 1.5 shows an example of a reading list. Take a look at the entry details for a book and a chapter from a book. You should also be able to see on your reading list that books will usually include the following details:

- Author(s)
- Publication date
- Title
- Edition
- Publisher information (place/publisher name).

You will need to use the library website search facility or library catalogues to search for books and edited books. Most libraries, including your academic library, provide an online search or discovery tool or catalogue where you can search for books and find out where books are located.

You can search in many different ways such as by author/title/keyword (you could take the keywords from your mind map). For the examples in Figure 1.5 you could type the keywords into the search box in the following ways:

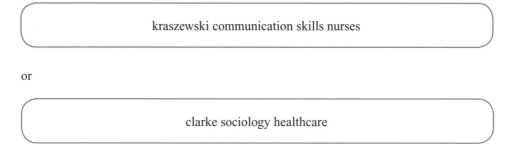

kraszewski communication skills nurses

or

clarke sociology healthcare

The results screen should tell you if the library has the book, if it is available to borrow (on the shelves) and where it is located (shelf number).

Note down the location number (shelf number where you will find the book on the shelves).

Make use of your library's reservation system for books on loan.

Make use of your library's Inter-Library Loan service for items not available.

Example of Book List

Book:

Author   Title   Edition

Clarke, A. 2010. *The Sociology of Healthcare,* **2nd edn. Harlow: Pearson.**

    Date of publication   Place of publication and publisher

Chapter From A Book:

Author   Date of publication   Title of chapter   Book editors

Crow, J. 2010. 'Communication: The Essence of Care', in Kraszewski S. and McEwan A., eds., *Communication Skills for Adult Nurses.* **Maidenhead: Open University Press, Chapter 3.**

      Title of book   Place of publication and publisher   Chapter number

Journal Article:

Authors   Date of publication   Article title

Reed, J. and Stanley, D. 2013. 'Improving Communication Between Hospitals and Care Homes: The Development of a Daily Living Plan for Older People', *Health & Social Care in the Community* **11(4), 356–63.**

Volume/part (issue)   Page numbers   Journal title

Internet Resource:

Author   Date of publication   Title of document

Department of Health. 2010. Essence of Care 2010: Benchmarks for Communication. [online]. Available at:
http://www.dh.gov.uk/prod_consum_dh/groups/dh_digitalassets?@dh/@en/@ps/documents/diitalass et/dh_119973.pdf [Accessed 22 April 2013]

          Accessed date (for website)   Web address (URL)

Figure 1.5 Example reading list.

E-books

An e-book is an online version of a book allowing you to read online (over the Internet, on a mobile device or e-book reader). Currently not all book titles are available to buy in electronic format and not all e-books are downloadable to e-book readers. Your university library will provide you access to e-books for your studies, normally via the library website. Technology is rapidly changing and will vary from library to library and from supplier to supplier. Always check out your own library to see what is possible.

ACTIVITY

Find the catalogue or search tool for your university library and search for some books on your reading list.

What book did you search for?

Are there copies available to borrow?

At what shelf number in your library is the book shelved at?

Go to the shelves and try to find the book.

How to locate journal articles

If your lecturer has suggested a journal article to read, probably the easiest way of reading it is to find the journal via the journal title, e.g. *Age and Ageing, Community Care*. Remember your university library will provide you with access to a wide range of both print and electronic journals.

Take a look at the journal article entry in the reading list in Figure 1.5. The easiest way to locate the journal article is to find the journal *Health & Social Care in the Community* on the shelves or online via the library website, then go to 2013 and find volume 11 and then issue/ part 4, then locate page 356.

Finding Internet resources from your reading list

Look at the Internet resource listed on the reading list in Figure 1.5. The easiest way to locate this document is either:

(a) Use a search engine like Google to search for the document using search words like:

---

department of health essence care communication

(b) Type in or copy and paste the website address (URL) into your address bar on your Internet browser.

How do I find journal articles?

The easiest way to find articles, such as for your essay on communication in healthcare, is to use **databases**.

What is a database?

Databases are a type of index accessed via computers. They give you access to thousands of journal articles on health and social care topics and, where available, will provide the full text of the article to save, print and read. These databases allow you to search for articles using your keywords from your mind map and search plan. The database will include details of the journal articles found for your topic and give you information about the authors, date published, article titles, name of the journal it is located in, and volume and part (issue/month) and page details. They may also provide an abstract or summary of the content.

Key health and social care databases

Your university will provide you with access to a variety of databases. Some you need to access via your library website with your library username and password, others are freely available via the Internet. Table 1.3 provides a list of some examples of health and social care databases. Note that your library may not provide access to all of these databases.

ACTIVITY

Take a look at your own university library website and make a list of the key health databases you are able to use.

Searching databases

We are now going to search the Pubmed database for information for our essay on issues around communication in the healthcare environment.

ACTIVITY

Go to your Internet browser and access Pubmed by searching for pubmed – http://www. ncbi.nlm.nih.gov/pubmed

Try searching for some journal articles for our essay on issues in communication in healthcare.

What keywords did you type into the search?

Note some results:

How might you refine your search or search words?

Table 1.3 Examples of some key health and social care databases

Name of database	Subject coverage	Access
ASSIA (Applied Social Sciences Index and Abstracts)	Applied social sciences	Via library website
British Nursing Index	Nursing, health, mental health, midwifery (UK focus)	Via library website
CINAHL	Nursing and allied health	Via library website
EMBASE	Medicine and pharmacology	Via library website
Maternity and Infant Care	Midwifery and neonates	Via library website
Medline	Medicine	Via library website
PsycArticles	Psychiatry	Via library website
PsycInfo	Psychology and psychological aspects of medicine, psychiatry, nursing, pharmacology, physiology, anthropology	Via library website
Science Direct	Science, medicine, health	Via library website
Web of Science	Science	Via library website
Cochrane Library	Evidence-based healthcare	www.thecochranelibrary.com/
Google Scholar	General	http://scholar.google.co.uk/
Pubmed	Medicine/biomedical	www.ncbi.nlm.nih.gov/pubmed/
Europe PubMed Central	Medicine	http://europepmc.org/
Social Care Online (from SCIE Social Care Institute for Excellence)	Social care	www.scie-socialcareonline.org.uk/

You should hopefully have found that typing words like communication and health care or communication and healthcare into the search box found you a list of details for a variety of journal articles.

How to interpret your search results from a database

Figure 1.6 shows a fictitious example for the detailed information (**citation** or **reference**) for a journal article found in a list of search results from a database like Pubmed. Within a database you would click on the title link from the results screen to find out more information about the article, including whether it is available for you to view on the shelves or online as an e-journal. To locate the example below we are looking for the journal *Journal of Health and Social Care* for 2014. You will need to check your library catalogue or library search tool to see if they have access to the journal for the particular issue you require – 2014, volume 25, issue or part 6.

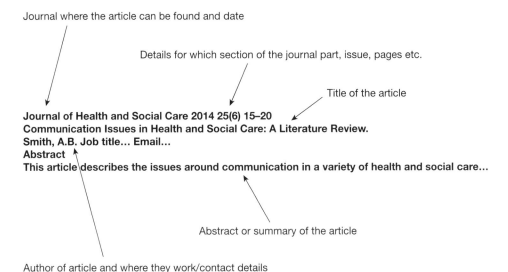

Journal where the article can be found and date

Details for which section of the journal part, issue, pages etc.

Title of the article

Journal of Health and Social Care 2014 25(6) 15–20
Communication Issues in Health and Social Care: A Literature Review.
Smith, A.B. Job title... Email...
Abstract
This article describes the issues around communication in a variety of health and social care...

Abstract or summary of the article

Author of article and where they work/contact details

Figure 1.6 Example of a journal reference from a database.

Search strategies and tips

There are a number of search strategies you can use to improve your search.

Combining words

Combining words (also known as **Boolean** operators) can be helpful to link your key search words or phrases. There are three main ways to combine words:

1 **AND**

   AND focuses your search on results which only include all the search terms you have used. A search for 'communication AND healthcare' will bring back results which contain both words. See Figure 1.7 for an example.

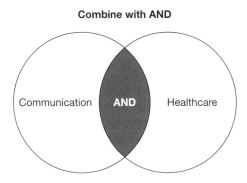

Figure 1.7 Use of Boolean AND.

2 OR

OR broadens your search and brings back results containing any of the search terms. A search for 'communication' OR 'interpersonal skills' will bring back results which contain either term. See Figure 1.8 for an example.

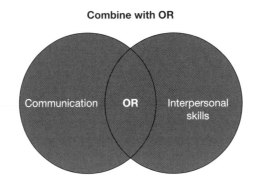

Figure 1.8 Use of Boolean OR.

3 NOT

NOT excludes all the results containing the specified search term. A search for 'communication' NOT 'children' will exclude any results containing the word children.

Note – use NOT with caution as you may lose relevant results! See Figure 1.9 for an example.

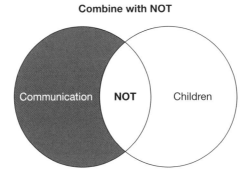

Figure 1.9 Use of Boolean NOT.

ACTIVITY

Access Pubmed – www.ncbi.nlm.nih.gov/pubmed/

Continue your search on the topic of communication in healthcare, this time trying out some of the techniques such as combining your search words with AND

What do you notice?

You should notice that by combining your search words with combining terms like AND helps to focus your search results on your topic.

Advanced searching

There are a number of additional searching techniques which you might want to try out for a more effective search. Many search screens in the databases will allow you to undertake either a basic or an advanced search:

- The advanced search screen can help to improve the structure and effectiveness of your search.
- There are also a number of techniques you can apply to your search. See the search tips and help links within the database for full details of how they work with the database you are using.

STUDENT TIP

Always consult the on-screen help within the database or guides produced by your library for tips on searching the individual databases effectively.

Refining your search

Depending on your search results, be prepared to change your search. Searching is rarely a nice straight motorway journey, rather a country route along roads with bends and junctions. If you find too many records, too few records or results that are not relevant you will need to refine your search. You could try out some of the refining tips shown in Table 1.4.

Are your results relevant?

You may need to filter out certain results that are not relevant to answer your essay. For example you may find an article on telephone answering systems in nursing homes which may not

Table 1.4 Refining your search

Do I have too few results?	Do I have too many records?
Check your typing and spelling! It is easy to mistype and miss-spell words.	Try changing your search words to be more specific, e.g. acute care rather than care.
Combine your search words with OR.	Combine your search words with AND.
Change your keywords and try out other words or synonyms, e.g. teenager rather than adolescent.	Check and change the scope of your search, e.g. adults/children
Broaden your search words, e.g. hospital rather than wards.	Change the range of years, e.g. narrow to the last 5 years.

Table 1.5 Example of recording your search results

Date	Where searched, e.g. name of database/ search engine etc.	Search words or keyword(s) used	Scope/remit used, e.g. UK only, last 5 years	Items found	No. of useful items	Full references	Notes (optional)
1/4/13	CINAHL	Communication/ healthcare/nurses/ patients	UK	60	30	Write in the full reference details	Article x particularly useful for...
7/4/13	ASSIA	Communication/ healthcare/nurses/ patients	UK	50	10	Write in the full reference details	Article x particularly useful for...

be useful if you are looking at communication between healthcare professionals and patients in an acute care setting. Additionally you may wish to ignore articles not relevant to the UK.

Recording your search

Recording your search is important. You need to keep track of your literature search as you may search over a number of days and for some assignments you may be asked to include information on how and where you found the literature you used in your assignment. How you record this is up to you as there is no perfect way – just do not rely on memory! You might find a table or spreadsheet helpful to record your search and results. See Table 1.5 for an example of a table format.

Evaluating information

Evaluating the information sources you find is vital. You can use the five 'Ws' framework to help to do this by asking questions about the sources you find: where, who, what, when, why.

Where has the information come from?

- Is it from an academic publisher?
- Did you find it via an academic database or library catalogue or Google?
- Is it from a peer-reviewed journal?
- Is it from an official source, e.g. government, Royal College, conference?

Who wrote or published the information?

- Do you know who wrote the source and whether they are an expert in the subject area?
- Can you find out where they work?
- Has the author published other works?
- Are they an expert in the field?

What is the content and coverage?

- Is the content and coverage suitable to your level?
- Is it relevant to your area of practice and study?
- Can you check for the accuracy and quality of the information?
- What is the purpose of the source and what audience is it targeted at?
- How does it compare with other sources?
- How good are the references – are they up to date, accurate, good quality etc.?

When was it written?

- When was it written, published, updated?
- Is it current?
- Is it too old to be relevant today?

Why was it written?

- Why was the information written/published? Make sure it is not trying to sell you something.
- Are there any obvious biases? E.g. organisational viewpoint, political, commercial interest, religious etc.

As you can see, the process of searching and evaluating the literature needs to be careful and painstaking but it is a very worthwhile use of your study time. Figure 1.10 provides you with some useful tips on undertaking an effective search.

New technology and social media

Technology, IT and information production and exchange is constantly changing at an increasingly fast pace. This includes the emergence of Web 2.0, a group of technologies which allows for increased collaboration and sharing by making use of social media. These tools are more flexible, participatory and interactive than traditional Web resources and can help you keep up to date and in communication with other people.

There are a wide range of tools, from RSS feeds, email alerts and blogs, social bookmarking and tagging, to Facebook and Twitter. Some students may be used to using things like Facebook and Twitter to keep up with family and friends but often organisations like the World Health Organization and universities and libraries have Facebook pages and Twitter feeds to help you to keep up to date.

STUDENT TIP

Check out your local library for help and watch out for relevant symbols showing links to tools like Facebook and Twitter. Do think about your 'digital footprint' though and remember the appropriate use of such tools for both personal and family spheres and your academic and professional life – these tools can be very public!

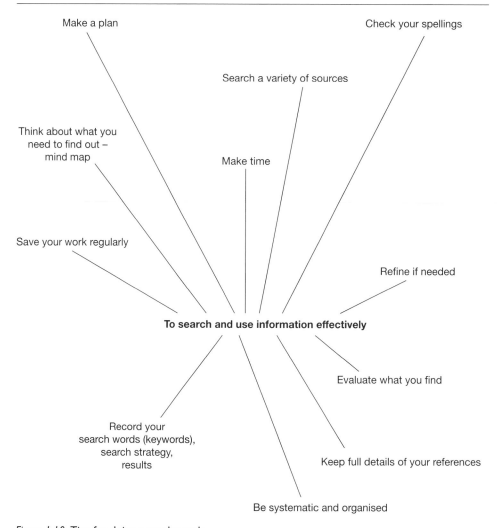

Make a plan

Check your spellings

Search a variety of sources

Think about what you
need to find out –
mind map

Make time

Save your work regularly

Refine if needed

To search and use information effectively

Evaluate what you find

Record your
search words (keywords),
search strategy,
results

Keep full details of your references

Be systematic and organised

Figure 1.10 Tips for doing a good search.

You should now have an understanding of the importance of reading, how to use the library and search for information effectively and how to make your reading and searching purposeful. However, with the best will in the world remembering information and retaining it is a difficult task and you will need help.

Note taking

It is a good habit to take notes when reading for academic study so that you have something to refer back to and also to jog your memory (it is also an essential component when it comes to writing an essay or assignment). As you can imagine this is another skill in itself and takes practice.

When reading a piece of writing you should follow these easy steps:

Step 1 – Read enough that you get a clear understanding of the material. Depending on what you are reading this could be a sentence, a paragraph or a page.

Step 2 – Put the material to one side and try to put the main points together in your head in your own words. Think of the meaning, message and motive of the material.

Step 3 – Now attempt to write down on paper in your own words (paraphrase) the idea or ideas of the piece you have just read. Also add in any additional points of your own that will help you to understand.

Step 4 – Make a note of the key identifying features of the material so you can easily return to the exact page and point at a later date if needed (see section on Referencing, p. 38).

Avoid trying to copy the material word for word as although it may help you remember what was said this method does not help you to understand the meaning. In fact copying out chunks of text can be done without really engaging the brain at all! It is a PASSIVE activity and you can waste a lot of valuable study time doing it and feeling virtuous but not learning anything at all. The key to effective note taking is to keep the brain ACTIVE and paraphrasing regularly when you are reading is a good way to do this.

Here is an example of a passage from a book and below it is the type of note you might take. On reading this you might put it into your words and make the following notes:

> An important part of social interaction is affirmation. We affirm and recognise the other person in and through our interactions and thereby give him or her, a sense of security and importance.
>
> (Taken from Thompson, N., 2009. *People Skills*. 3rd edn. Basingstoke: Palgrave Macmillan. Page 5)

Affirmation – a type of social interaction where we recognise (affirm) someone through interacting with them. This gives that person a sense of security and makes them feel good.

Read in the Thompson, N 2009 book People Skills 3rd edition Basingstoke, Palgrave Macmillan page 5.

Taking notes in this way guides you to seek the meaning in what you are reading and provides you with valuable information you will be able to use when writing an essay or assignment.

LEARNING POINT

Make sure that you record all the information related to the reading material you require so that you can easily locate it and reference it appropriately in your assignment.

Writing skills for academia

Writing an essay for academic courses can be an anxious and frightening experience for a lot of students especially those who have not done any academic study since school. Having said that, academic writing is a skill and as such has certain rules and guidelines that need to be followed. Once you have mastered the rules and guidelines it will become second nature.

When you are writing your assignments you need to consider the following points shown in Table 1.6.

STUDENT TIP

Once you start to construct your essay make sure that you keep track of all the reference material you have used so that it can be easily located. You may need to go back and forth between your reading material and notes as you start to put your essay together.

The structure of your writing (reflective, case study, theoretical)

When asked to write an academic essay you will be instructed as to the style (or structure) it is to be written and presented in. Generally, essays are either reflective accounts, case studies or theoretical pieces. Knowing and understanding the rules that apply to these different types of styles is vitally important if you are to do well. Table 1.7 explains some of the rules

Supporting your written work with facts

Trying to understand the difference between what is fact and what is opinion is difficult but it is an essential skill when writing, as you need to make sure that you base your academic work on facts rather than opinions.

ACTIVITY

In the list of statements below, identify which are FACTS and which are OPINIONS:

- Curry is the best dish in the world.
- London is the capital of England.
- Manchester City is a great football team.
- Manchester City won the FA Cup in 2011.
- Mount Everest is the highest mountain in the world.
- Dogs are better pets than cats.
- It is colder in winter than in summer in Britain.
- War is always wrong.
- In England only 17% of men and 13% of women aged 65–74 are physically active.
- According to the Amateur Swimming Association 2012 report, 51% of children aged 7–11 surveyed cannot swim 25 m of a pool unaided.
- Despite its faults the NHS is a well-run and efficient service.
- Almost two-thirds of hospital acute beds are used by people over 65.

Table 1.6 Points to consider when writing assignments

	Comments
Audience	Be clear who your audience is and the level at which your essay should be pitched. Understand what knowledge can be assumed and what needs to be made explicitly clear. Clarify with your tutor if you are unsure.
Objectives	Make sure you understand what the assessment objectives are. You will find these in the assessment guidance provided by the tutor. Also look at the marking criteria so you know exactly what you will need to demonstrate to gain marks. This will help you maintain your focus and concentrate on the key aspects.
Structure	The assessment guidance will instruct you on how to structure your essay and what style it should be in (see section below). Make sure you understand the rules of writing for the structure required of you.

Table 1.7 Types of essays and writing

Style	Focus	Perspective
Reflective account	Personal experience in practice around a specific incident, skill or activity	Improving personal practice through looking back at the actions and decisions you took then evaluating and analysing them using evidence
Case study	Identifying a specific individual from your own area of practice that can be used as a reference point to explore a wider topic	Widening your knowledge and understanding of a specific condition or topic by examining the topic from the perspective of an individual experiencing the condition
Theoretical piece	Exploring a topic in a broad sense	Gathering and examining all available information and evidence related to a specific topic

When writing academically it is preferable to discuss factual information and support any ideas or views you have with factual information.

Tense

The importance of writing in the correct tense cannot be overstated. Get it wrong and in most cases the meaning of your essay could be misinterpreted. The reason it is so important is down to the evidence and supporting information you have to include in your essays. When you write an essay the marker will expect that you have engaged with the current 'body of evidence' that exists, in book or article form, around that subject or issue and that you bring some of that evidence into your essays to support any key points that you make. If you introduce or discuss other people's viewpoints using the **past tense**, such as:

   '**Jones (2012) believed. . .** ' or '**Jones (2012) suggested. . .** '

their viewpoint seems dated and their viewpoint may have since changed. Whereas if you introduce or discuss other people's viewpoints using the **present tense**, such as:

> **'Jones (2012) believes. . . '** or **'Jones (2012) suggests. . . '**

it is clear that their viewpoint is current and up to date. However, this rule can change if you are writing a reflective account about yourself and describing a past event. In this situation using the past tense is acceptable.

Future tense is generally only used in the introductory sections of essays when you wish to tell the reader what you hope to achieve in the essay; for example;

> 'This essay will demonstrate. . . '

Paraphrasing

We have already mentioned the importance of note taking. Taking notes forms the basis for constructing your essay as you turn those notes into meaningful information. One of the most important skills to master in essay writing is paraphrasing. Paraphrasing is when you put someone else's ideas into your own words. This is in contrast to directly quoting; when you write exactly, word for word, what someone has written in a book or journal. When paraphrasing you still need to identify where you obtained the information (reference/citation). Changing only one or two words from a sentence you have read in a book is not paraphrasing. You must rephrase the idea entirely whilst still conveying its essence and meaning. The benefit of paraphrasing over directly quoting is that it clearly demonstrates to the reader that you have understood what you have read and this is key to achieving a good mark.

Direct quotes

As mentioned, a direct quote is when you write exactly word for word what someone has written in a book or journal and provide the reference/citation. You should use direct quotes sparingly and only use them for information that cannot be conveyed (paraphrased) in any other meaningful way. Using lots and lots of direct quotes in your essay will lose you marks as it only demonstrates that you can copy out of a book or journal.

Critical thinking

Writing essays is more than just conveying the ideas of published authors or conveying factual information. You will be expected within your essays to show a degree of critical thinking (maybe referred to as critical analysis). The need for you to demonstrate critical thinking will increase as you progress through your course and as you go on to higher levels of study. Critical thinking is the process you undertake when you gather, process, apply, analyse and skilfully weave together key concepts, ideas and theories and put them together into a logical structure that clearly conveys understanding of the issues to the reader. It is the skill of linking together the ideas and concepts that you have read and finding connections and comparisons that may not always be obvious. To achieve higher marks in your essays you will be expected to demonstrate critical thinking in your writing.

STUDENT TIP

I thought writing an essay was about pouring my opinions out into a piece of writing. I now realise that good academic writing is about pulling evidence together from different sources and showing that I have read widely and can understand how information links together.

As an example, have a look at these two paragraphs and think about which one is written critically and which remains at a descriptive level:

- Burton and Dimbleby (1988) suggest that from the moment we are born we start communicating with others. Darley (2002) suggests that communication is a simple term when a message of any form is passed from one person to another. Harris (1990) believes that communication can be conveyed with emotions, behaviours, through words, gestures or simply by listening. Barker (2006) suggests that the reason for communication is to create a relationship with the other person.
- Burton and Dimbleby (1988) believe that from the moment we are born we start communicating with others. This belief is supported by Darley's (2002) view that communication is a simple term when a message of any form is passed from one person to another. Harris (1990) summarises this succinctly by explaining that communication can be conveyed with emotions, behaviours, through words, gestures or simply by listening. Harris's view provides a wider understanding of communication and links closely with Barker's (2006) opinion that the reason for communication is to create a relationship with the other person.

The writer has paraphrased in both paragraphs but you can see that in the second paragraph the writer has weaved information and linked it together, with some evaluative and comparative comment of their own, thus demonstrating to the reader a clearer understanding of the material and subject.

LEARNING POINT

Beware the spellchecker!

Although an invaluable tool to help you correct spelling mistakes there are some things you need to be wary of.

Make sure your spellchecker is set to UK English and not USA English as there are numerous variations in spellings between the USA English and UK English; especially with verbs where we use 's' the Americans tend to use 'z', i.e. 'organize' (USA) and 'organise' (UK).

Homophones (words that sound the same but are spelt differently). These words will not be picked up by a spellchecker as you will have spelt them correctly. Be careful of the following:

'there' or 'their'
'bear' or 'bare'
'dye' or 'die'
'hole' or 'whole'
'write' or 'right'
And be wary of words such as 'quite' and 'quiet'.

Use the grammar checker!

Most word processor software has a grammar checker. Usually if an error in grammar is picked up it is underlined. If you click on the sentence that is underlined you should be provided with an explanation. Take time to read the explanation as this will help you improve your grammar. However, be careful because sometimes it makes mistakes so you can ignore the advice!

Making use of feedback

After any assessment you will receive feedback along with your mark. Students have a tendency to ignore the written feedback and focus just on the mark. Get into the habit of reading the comments the marker has made about your work and take on board the constructive criticism. This is the best way of improving your work. If you are unsure about any aspect of the feedback make an appointment to see the marker so they can clarify their comments with you and elaborate.

Referencing

What is referencing?

Referencing is writing and including in the text the details of every source you use in completing your assignments. The details of every book, article, website, DVD or information source you mention or *refer* to (this is sometimes also known as **citing**) in your assignment usually need to be included in two places.

- within the text of your assignment (an in-text reference or citation)
- in a detailed list, usually at the end of your assignment (your reference or citation list).

Remember: all sources you refer to or cite within your piece of work must be included in your reference list.

Bibliography or reference list – what is the difference?

Depending on where you are studying and the demands of your course assignments you may have to produce reference lists and/or bibliographies for your pieces of work. So what is the difference? Table 1.8 will help explain.

Table 1.8 Bibliography or reference list – what is the difference?

	What is the difference?	Notes
Reference list	A **reference list** is a complete list of all the items (books, journal articles, newspaper articles, Web pages, government documents, sources etc.) **that you refer to and use in the text of your assignment**	All assignments MUST have a reference list. You must always include a list of the resources that you have referred to in the text of your assignment A reference list means everything you REFER to in your assignment
Bibliography	A **bibliography** is a list of items (books, journal articles, Web pages, documents etc.) that you read during the preparation of your assignment **but did not actually use and refer to in the text of your assignment**	Not all assignments will need a bibliography – check with your course tutor/guide

Sometimes you may be asked to produce a reference list and a bibliography list and occasionally you may be asked to produce one list which includes your references (items you actually refer to and use in your assignment) and other items you also read during producing an assignment. The most important thing to get used to is keeping and producing a list of all the items you refer to in your assignment, as these items become your reference list.

STUDENT TIP

Always refer to your own institutional guidelines, course guide or tutor for guidance on whether you need to produce a reference list, bibliography, combined list, or both for your assignments.

Style of referencing

There are many types or styles of referencing. **Make sure you use the style set by your university or course.** Common styles used in UK universities include:

- Harvard system (sometimes known as the author/date system)
- Vancouver system (also known as the numerical system).

The guidance here will be on good referencing principles but will provide some examples using the Harvard system. If you would like examples of the use of the Vancouver numerical system there are examples in free health and medical journals via Biomed Central – www.biomedcentral.com/ and Free Medical Journals – www.freemedicaljournals.com/.

ACTIVITY

Find out what style of referencing you have to use.

Locate the guide your library or institution provides to help with referencing and keep details to use in the future.

Why do I need to reference?

You might be asking yourself, why the need to reference? Well you need to reference in order to:

1. **Identify the sources you have used in your assignment:**
   To show your marker the range of resources you have read and used in your work. And to help other people to locate the sources you have used.
2. **Avoid plagiarism**
   Plagiarism is stealing ideas or information and is seen as cheating!
      It occurs when you present the ideas and work of someone else as your own, either deliberately or by mistake. This includes material that you may use in an assignment and then fail to acknowledge the source of information and reference correctly. This could include copying or putting into your own words any of the following:

   - text and words
   - images, pictures, graphs, tables
   - data
   - sound recordings and performances.

Remember – how would you feel if someone else used something you had published without acknowledging you as the author and tried to pass it off as their own? You would be rather annoyed.

Key tips for avoiding plagiarism

- Keeping track of what you read is crucial to helping you avoid plagiarism.
- Always note down the author(s) of any information, including quotes that you want to use in your work. For quotes, note down the page you found the quote on. Additionally record where it came from (e.g. book, journal article and website details).
- Always keep full details of all your sources as you search, read and write your assignment.
- Good management of your sources of information throughout your time studying is good practice.
- Most universities provide guides to referencing and offer sessions on referencing – keep an eye out for them.

STUDENT TIP

You will not remember everything you read.

ALWAYS keep a note of the full details. Don't add to your stress levels by having to find the full details of your references as you are finishing off your assignment just before you hand it in!

In-text referencing

In-text referencing is what you do within the writing of your assignment (essay, presentation etc.). Whatever system you use you will need to record where you use a reference and then at another part of your assignment provide the full reference – the full details of the information source you used. This could be the author details or a number to identify the information source.

Primary and secondary referencing (second-hand references)

Sometimes when you read a book, article or other source of information the authors will make reference to literature they have read in writing their own work. If you wish to use these sources, ideally it is good practice to track down the sources referred to in what you read and go back to the original. To do this take a look at the reference list at the end of the work, search for them in your university or other library, via the Internet (if it is an online source) or obtain them via your library's Inter-Library Loan service. If you are not able to do this then you can use the references but you need to do this in a particular way as these are secondary references or second-hand references. You need to acknowledge and refer to the original source of the information and then the publication source which you actually read.

Take a look at the section of text in Figure 1.11 by Crow in Chapter 3 of the book edited by Kraszewski and McEwan.

Crow, J., 2010. 'Communication: The Essence of Care', in Kraszewski, S. and McEwan, A., eds, *Communication Skills for Adult Nurses*. Maidenhead: Open University Press, Ch.3.

In this example Crow uses other authors' material in writing the book chapter. On p. 44 of this book we can see that Crow makes reference to two sources in writing their own book chapter – Elaswarapu 2007 and Walsh and Kowanko 2002. If you wish to refer to information from these sections without tracking down and reading the Elaswarapu 2007 and Walsh and Kowanko 2002 works then you need to acknowledge the authors, Elaswarapu 2007 and Walsh and Kowanko 2002, and the book chapter by Crow you are reading in the book edited by Kraszewski and McEwan 2010. Using a Harvard style of referencing in your work you need to put the following information within the text:

Elaswarapu 2007 cited in Crow 2010
Walsh and Kowanko 2002 cited in Crow 2010.

Taken from page 44 of a book:

[Crow, J. 2010. 'Communication: The Essence of Care', in Kraszewski, S. and McEwan, A., eds, *Communication Skills for Adult Nurses*. Maindenhead: Open University Press, Ch. 3.]© Open University Press. Reproduced with the kind permission of Open University Press. All rights reserved.

44 Communication Skills for Adult Nurses

Threats to good communication

There is evidence that patients and staff agree about the elements of care that communicate dignity and respect in healthcare. However, although both groups agree that it is important, it seems that staff may give it a lower priority (Elaswarapu 2007) It has been suggested that lack of interpersonal communication skills on the part of health professionals can be a problem (Walsh and Kowanko 2002). It also seems that there are times when even staff who possess these communication skills find they are likely to be compromised. The danger times are when interactions become routine and staff cease to see patients as individuals and more as a task in a long line of other tasks. Communication skills can also fail when staff are stressed or working under time pressures. There are so many competing demands on staff attention and targets to meet, that it is easy for them to lose sight of the way in which they are communicating. At these times it must be remembered that good communication skills conveying dignity and respect to patients and carers are not 'optional extras', but a fundamental and essential part of any healthcare professional's role.

Figure 1.11 Example of book chapter for secondary referencing.

In your reference list at the end of your essay you then just put in the details of the book you actually read, i.e. Chapter 3 written by Crow found in the book edited by Kraszewski and McEwan on communication. So in your reference list you include the chapter and book details, e.g.:

> Crow, J. 2010. 'Communication: The Essence of Care', in Kraszewski, S. and McEwan, A., eds, *Communication Skills for Adult Nurses*. Maidenhead: Open University Press, Ch.3.

It is important to remember that sometimes key information can be lost as it passes through a **secondary source** (second-hand source) so to be clear about the information it is always best practice to obtain it from the original (**primary**) source where possible.

What you need to record for your references

STUDENT TIP

My assignment is due in tomorrow and I've still got my reference list to do. . . I wish I'd kept a record of all my books and articles at the time, now I've forgotten what I used – help!

Unlike this student you want to make sure the details of all the books, articles, government reports and other materials you used in your assignment are ready to create a reference list for you to be able to hand in your assignment on time.

So the question is – just what do you need to include in each reference? Have a go at this activity to start thinking about what you need to include:

ACTIVITY – WHAT DO I INCLUDE IN A REFERENCE?

1   Think about a book you are reading either for your course or a hobby – what type of information do you think you might need to record for this book?
2   Think about a magazine or journal article – what type of information do you think you might need to record to reference the article?
3   Think about something you have looked at on the Internet – what type of information do you think you might need to record to reference the website?

What you come up with on your list may include some of the elements listed in Table 1.9 in the next section. You might not have thought of them all but the more you reference the easier it will get.

How do I record information for my references?

Whatever reference style your institution or course uses there are key pieces of information that you need to make a note of so that you can produce a reference list for your assignments. Table 1.9 shows what information about each resource you need to keep.

Table 1.9 What information do I need to record for my references?

Type of resource	Author(s)	Date	Title	Edition	Other information
Book	Surnames and initials of all authors	Date of publication/ edition (year), e.g. 2013. NOTE: Do not use the date of printing/ reprints	Full book title including subtitle	Include the edition, e.g. 2nd, 3rd etc. If the first edition, do not include	Name of the publisher and place of publication, e.g. London: Routledge Note: Place is usually a town or city not a county, state or country
Edited book	Editors of the book	Date of publication/ edition (year), e.g. 2013. NOTE: Do not use the date of printing/ reprints	Full book title including subtitle	Include the edition, e.g. 2nd, 3rd etc. If the first edition, do not include	Name of the publisher and place of publication, e.g. London: Routledge Note: Place is usually a town or city not a county, state or country

Table 1.9 continued

Type of resource	Author(s)	Date	Title	Edition	Other information
Chapters of books	Author(s) of the chapter used AND the editor(s) of the book the chapter is found in	Date of publication/ edition (year), e.g. 2013 NOTE: Do not use the date of printing/ reprints	Title of the chapter used AND the full title of the book the chapter is in	Include the edition, e.g. 2nd, 3rd etc. If the first edition, do not include	Name of the publisher and place of publication, e.g. London: Routledge Note: Place is usually a town or city not a county, state or country Note the chapter number and/or pages for the chapter, e.g. Ch. 3 pages 90–140
Journal articles	Author(s) of the article	Date of the article (year), e.g. 2013	Title of the journal article AND the title of the journal	Not required	Note the volume, part (or issue) or month and the pages where the journal article is located, e.g. volume 10 part/issue 5 pages 15–20
Newspaper articles	Author(s) of the article	Date of the article (year), e.g. 2013	Title of the article AND the title of the newspaper	Not required	Note the day and the pages where the article is located, e.g. 31 May 2013, volume 10 part/ issue 5 pages 15–20
Web resource	Author(s) of the Web page or online document	Date of the Web page or online document (year), e.g. 2013	Title of the Web page or online document	Edition if not the first edition	Note the fact that it is online/pdf etc. Note full Web address (URL) for the Web page or online document, e.g. http://www...etc... Note the date you accessed or viewed the page/online document, e.g. 1 June 2014

From Table 1.9 you will see that you have to keep quite a few pieces of information. Most sources you reference will usually have an author or authors, publication date and title. Get into good practice of always keeping the full details of every resource you look at, read or make notes from.

Note about authors

The author(s) of a source you use could be a person, e.g. John Brown, or an organisation, e.g. Department of Health, Joseph Rowntree Foundation.

How many authors do I include? This will depend on the referencing system you are using and your local university guidelines. Some referencing systems allow you to use the word 'et al.', meaning 'and others' for additional authors. This means that if the book, article or document you are referencing includes many authors (sometimes you may see up to ten or more) you are able to note the first author and then et al., e.g. Brown, J. et al. rather than all of them.

Note about editions

It is important you tell your assignment marker what edition of a book or resource you used. You may only need to note and provide edition information if the book or resource is not the first edition as often the first edition is not noted, it being assumed that the book is the first or only edition unless otherwise stated. If you are using the second or subsequent editions make sure you record this and add it to your reference list entry, e.g.:

Bloggs, A. 2012. *Communication in Health*, 2nd edn. London: Bloggs Press.

Note about place of publication

The place of publication is usually a town or city, e.g. London, rather than a country, county or state.

Note about Web resources

For websites, Internet resources, electronic version of books (e-books), journals (e-journals) and newspapers you *may* also need to add the following additional detail:

• Medium, e.g. online, e-book, e-journal, PDF etc.
• Website address or URL for the resource.
• Date you accessed the resource.

If in doubt, always be guided by the referencing style guide for your course or institution.

ACTIVITY – REFERENCING

Using the referencing guidance provided by your course tutors or your university, practise referencing some sources:

Part 1

Book
Find a book on your library catalogue/search.
How would you cite this book within the text of your essay?

Journal article
Find and reference a journal article from your own library and reference an article from within it:
  How would you cite this journal article within the text of your essay?

Website
Find the following document on the Internet:

Commissioning Board Chief Nursing Officer and DH Chief Nursing Advisor 2012 Compassion in Practice.
    www.england.nhs.uk/wp-content/uploads/2012/12/compassion-in-practice.pdf

How would you cite this online document within the text of your essay?

Part 2

Now create a reference list for these sources (from Part 1) using the guidelines recommended by your course tutors or your university.
  Mark your own practice by checking against the guidelines you have been given:

* Have you included all the information?
* Have you followed the guidelines exactly as to the punctuation and use of italics?
* Have you listed the items in the correct order as prescribed by the guidelines?

Manage your references

You may feel overwhelmed with information sources. You need to work out a way of managing the references you find and storing them ready to use in your work and creating reference lists. **Make a system that works for you.** This could be creating your own lists saved on paper or computer using a Word or Excel spreadsheet or increasingly many universities provide you with free access to referencing management (citation) tools such as RefWorks or Endnote, Microsoft Office referencing application, Mendeley, CiteUlike or Zotero to name just a few. The advantages of these tools are that they not only allow you to keep track of your reference sources they also create your reference lists as well in the style required. **Work out what works best for you.** This may take time but remember that referencing the recording and use of your references takes time whatever method you use, but the more you do it the easier it should become and it will save you time in the end!

Recording your references

Whatever method you use it is important that you correctly record all the details for each of your references. You may find a table format useful to keep your references and to remind you how to reference. See Table 1.9: What information do I need to record for my references? (on p. 43) to remind you what information to record. It is also an example of a table you could use to record your own references.

Key tips for referencing

- Keep records of all the information sources you use.
- Keep all the information you need for each resource, e.g. authors, date, full title, publisher, URL etc.
- Be consistent in your in-text referencing and your reference list.
- Check your reference list – would you be able to find all the resources you list?
- References to websites or Internet documents include more than just the website address/URL and need to provide information on author, date, title etc.
- Check that all the references you mention in your essay match up and are included in your reference list and vice versa.
- Remember if you use a quote you need to include the page numbers in the text.
- Always proofread – undertake a final check before you submit your work.
- **Always reference using the style and guidelines required by your course or university.**

Glossary compilation

As you progress through your studies you are bound to come across terms and phrases that are unfamiliar to you and a good way to familiarise yourself with these terms is to compile your own glossary. This is a list, usually in alphabetical order, of terms written alongside their meaning or definition. Writing this in your own words will help you remember and learn. Below you will find an example of a glossary that we have compiled for this chapter. We suggest you do the same for each chapter as you read this book.

Chapter summary

- Effective reading is the key to effective learning. You may use different reading strategies to suit different purposes and reading should constitute the majority of your preparation for most assignments.
- Writing styles vary according to the purpose of the author.
- Assessments take many forms so make sure you understand the required format and content required and make full use of the guidance available to you.
- Using the library competently is key to effective study. You need to practise to become comfortable and competent in searching, accessing and evaluating the range of resources provided.
- Searching the literature effectively requires good planning, a systematic approach and careful record keeping. It will save you time in the long run.
- Referencing is a key skill within academic writing and demonstrates that you have accessed, read and understood a range of evidence and utilised it within your writing to support your viewpoints.
- Referencing your work correctly involves following a set of prescribed rules which are readily available. Failing to do so may be interpreted as plagiarism.

Glossary

Bibliography–A list of resources you might have read while undertaking an assignment but which you may not actually have used and cited or referred to in the final version. A bibliography can also mean a list of resources on a topic suggesting further reading.

Boolean–Boolean operators also known as Boolean logic created by George Boole. They can improve searches and help to combine search words using the linking words AND, OR and NOT, e.g. health AND ethics.

Citation (reference)–Mention or make reference to (cite) a source used in a piece of work, e.g. Department of Health (2014). These citations (references) are then listed in a Reference list at the end of the work.

Database–An electronic store of information which is searchable. Library databases provide access to sources of information such as journal articles. Databases include details of the articles (author, title, journal, volume, issue, pages etc.), often including abstracts (summary of the content). Additionally some databases will include access to the full text for free.

Journal (or magazine, periodical, serial)–A publication which is usually published in regular issues, weekly, monthly, quarterly etc. and often published in volumes and issues or parts. Increasingly available online as e-journals.

Magazine see **Journal**

OPAC (Online Public Access Catalogue)–An electronic searchable list of all the resources that can be found in a library. Increasingly OPACs include access to electronic resources including e-books and e-journals. It may also just be called 'library catalogue', library search tool etc.

Peer review–Refers to articles published in journals which have gone through a review and approval process by subject peers or experts. This improves quality and reliability. Such journals are known as peer-reviewed journals.

Periodical–see **Journal**

Plagiarism–The offence of using or quoting someone else's work as your own. This can be done deliberately or by mistake by failing to include the references for the sources used in your work.

Primary source–A source written directly by people such as researchers or experts which are in their original form. Examples include newspaper articles, artwork, music, poems, letters, research reports, certain journal articles and some books (those containing original research or ideas). The definition of a primary source and examples of primary sources varies between different subject disciplines.

Reference (alternatively known as citation) see **Citation**

Reference list–List of all the references or citations used within your piece of work, usually at the end. A reference list provides full details for the sources used within the piece of work in the referencing style for the institution or organisation where you are studying.

Secondary source–Secondary sources are those which describe, discuss, analyse, comment on, adapt and interpret information from primary sources and can include encyclopaedias, books and journal articles such as literature reviews.

Serial see **Journal**

Thesaurus–There are two meanings for thesaurus. First, it is a list of words and their synonyms or related words, e.g. teenagers/adolescents. Second, it is a list of preferred subject headings, usually controlled, which are used in publications like databases and other information sources.

Uniform Resource Locator (URL)–The unique address for a website or Web page, e.g. your university, library, Department of Health, usually beginning http://. . . or www. . .

Virtual Learning Environment (VLE)–An online learning resource for your course and modules hosted by your academic institution. It may include links to materials such as your module guides, lecture notes, course reading, learning and assessment activities, discussion boards etc.

Further resources

Useful material/follow up for using libraries and finding information

Your own institution may have online tutorials to help you learn more about study skills and also library, searching and referencing skills. Take a look at it.

Safari–An expedition through the information world (the Open University's guide to searching for and using information). See www.open.ac.uk/safari/index.php [Accessed 1 December 2014].

Virtual Training Suite–Developing Internet Research Skills (variety of online tutorials to learn the skills of Internet Searching). See www.vtstutorials.co.uk/ [Accessed 1 December 2014].

Internet Detective–A self-paced interactive online tutorial for you to learn more about evaluating websites. See www.vts.intute.ac.uk/detective/ [Accessed 1 December 2014].

Further reading

Allen, K., ed. 2005. *Study Skills: A Student Survival Guide.* Chichester: John Wiley.

Aveyard, H. 2014. *Doing a Literature Review in Health and Social Care: A Practical Guide.* 3rd edn. Maidenhead: McGraw Hill Education.

Cottrell, S. 2013. *The Study Skills Handbook*, 4th edn. Basingstoke: Palgrave Macmillan.

Godfrey, J. 2013. *How to Use Your Reading in Your Essays*, 2nd edn. Basingstoke: Palgrave Macmillan.

Maslin-Prothero, S. 2010. *Bailliere's Study Skills for Nurses and Midwives*, 4th edn. Edinburgh: Bailliere Tindall.

References

Barker, A. 2006. *Improve Your Communication Skills*, 2nd edn. London: Kogan Page.

BBC Skillswise. 2014. *Skillswise English & Maths for Adults* [online]. Available at: www.bbc.co.uk/skillswise/topic-group/reading [Accessed 1 December 2014].

Biomed Central. Available at: www.biomedcentral.com/ [Accessed 1 December 2014].

Burton, G. and Dimbleby, R. 1988. *Between Ourselves: An Introduction to Interpersonal Communication.* London: Edward Arnold.

CitUlike. Available at: www.citeulike.org/ [Accessed 1 December 2014].

Clarke, A. 2010. *The Sociology of Healthcare*, 2nd edn. Harlow: Pearson.

Commissioning Board Chief Nursing Officer and DH Chief Nursing Advisor. 2012. *Compassion in Practice: Nursing, Midwifery and Care Staff Our Vision and Strategy* [PDF]. London: Department of Health/NHS Commissioning Board. Available at: www.england.nhs.uk/wp-content/uploads/2012/12/compassion-in-practice.pdf [Accessed 1 December 2014].

Crow, J. 2010. 'Communication: The Essence of Care', in Kraszewski, S. and McEwan, A., eds, *Communication Skills for Adult Nurses*. Maidenhead: Open University Press, Ch. 3.

Darley, M. 2002. *Managing Communication in Health Care: Six Steps to Effective Management Series*. Edinburgh: Bailliere Tindall.

Department of Health. 2010. *Essence of Care 2010: Benchmarks for Communication* [online]. Available at: www.gov.uk/government/uploads/system/uploads/attachment_data/file/216695/dh_119973.pdf [Accessed 1 December 2014].

Endnote. Available at: http://endnote.com/ [Accessed 1 December 2014].

Facebook. Available at: www.facebook.com/ [Accessed 1 December 2014].

Free Medical Journals. Available at: www.freemedicaljournals.com/ [Accessed 1 December 2014].

Google. Available at: www.google.co.uk/ [Accessed 1 December 2014].

Harris, S. 1990. *Human Communication*, 2nd edn. Oxford: Blackwell.

Legislation.gov.uk. Available at: www.legislation.gov.uk/ [Accessed 1 December 2014].

Mendeley Referencing Manager. Available at: www.mendeley.com/ [Accessed 1 December 2014].

National Library of Medicine, Pubmed database. Available at: www.ncbi.nlm.nih.gov/pubmed [Accessed 1 December 2014].

Reed, J. and Stanley, D. 2013. 'Improving Communication between Hospitals and Care Homes: The Development of a Daily Living Plan for Older People', *Health & Social Care in the Community* 11(4): 356–63.

RefWorks. Available at: www.refworks.com/ [Accessed 1 December 2014].

Thompson, N. 2009. *People Skills*, 3rd edn. Basingstoke: Palgrave Macmillan.

Twitter. Available at: https://twitter.com [Accessed 1 December 2014].

Wikipedia. Available at: www.wikipedia.org/ [Accessed 1 December 2014].

Zotero. Available at: www.zotero.org/ [Accessed 1 December 2014].

Chapter 2

Work-based learning

Claire Thurgate

LEARNING OUTCOMES

By the end of this chapter you will be able to:

1   Discuss how work-based learning contributes to your lifelong learning.
2   Define what work-based learning means to you.
3   Identify work-based learning opportunities within your workplace.
4   Discuss how you may demonstrate work-based learning.

Introduction

The aim of this chapter is to give you an overview of the principles of work-based learning (WBL) and how this contributes to your lifelong learning (LLL). This chapter will:

- Consider the concept of LLL.
- Discuss a range of definitions and aspects of WBL.
- Make sense of learning in the workplace through the use of learning agreements and personal development plans (PDPs).
- Discuss the role of mentors/supervisors in supporting your WBL.
- Use portfolios and reflection to demonstrate WBL.

Lifelong learning

The concept of LLL is based on the premise that learning occurs all the time and is not just the result of undertaking a programme of learning. Therefore learning in, from and through the workplace or WBL is a fundamental component of LLL. Engaging in LLL will ensure that you remain employable, that the knowledge and skills which you require to undertake your role safely and effectively are current and that you keep abreast of changes both within the workplace and nationally. LLL, therefore, requires different skills from those required to undertake more traditional forms of learning and includes the following:

- You identify the learning which you need to achieve and negotiate this with your workplace so that you are able to identify clear learning goals. This could be in the form of a PDP.

- You are in control of what learning should take place but you may want to discuss with a colleague in the workplace to ensure that you have considered all aspects required to achieve your learning needs.
- You will engage in reflection, reflective practice, problem-solving and action learning to ensure that there is depth to your learning. This gives your learning meaning and ensures that your learning becomes embedded within your practice.
- You are an active recipient in the learning process.

This approach to learning may appear unfamiliar but as you engage in WBL you will see that the skills required to engage effectively are similar to those skills required for LLL, namely motivation and the ability to be a self-directed learner. This is important and will ensure you develop the knowledge, skills, behaviours and attitudes required to develop and enhance your career.

Work-based learning: what is it?

This section will consider the concept of WBL and some of the many definitions which are used to describe this approach to learning. In 2008 the Department for Children, Schools and Families (DfCSF) defined WBL as:

> planned activity that uses the context of work to develop knowledge, skills and understanding useful in work, including learning through work, learning about work and work practices and learning the skill for work.
>
> (DfCSF 2008: 8)

While this definition identifies the role of learning in the workplace it appears to be related more to a work placement or the experience of work for a short duration. This, it could be argued, is a similar model to pre-registration nursing programmes in the United Kingdom (UK) where student nurses experience placements as part of their learning to link theory with practice and practice with theory. Or Foundation Degrees (FDs) where placements are incorporated as part of the programme of learning rather than being in employment which is the norm in a large proportion of health and social care FDs. Eraut (2004), on the other hand, included non-informal learning in his definition of WBL:

> learning for work, learning at work and learning through work.

Eraut's concept of non-formal learning is not fully understood but it is an important component of WBL which will help you engage in experiential learning as you give meaning to experiences at work and develop the skills necessary to become a lifelong learner. Rhodes and Shiel (2007) believe that WBL 'focuses on learning in and from the workplace' and through the use of reflection and critical reflection you will be able to extend your 'capability and individual effectiveness'. Raelin's (2008) definition of WBL is similar to Rhodes and Shiel's (2007), as he believed that WBL arises from the world of work, merges theory with practice, knowledge with experience and is centred around conscious reflection on actual work experiences.

Based on the definitions above it appears that learning and reflection from experience and/or practice within the world of work, which may be paid or non-paid, is fundamental to the success of WBL. WBL, therefore, may be part of your everyday work as either alone or with colleagues you try and make sense of experiences which have arisen at work. This may be achieved through informal discussions with peers or personal reflection/thoughts or through more formal supervision sessions with a colleague who will help you make sense and give meaning to the situation. However, as you engage in a programme of learning and development which incorporates WBL you will receive academic recognition for this learning. Hence the purpose of this chapter is to support your understanding of WBL, help you identify WBL opportunities and to make sense of your WBL through the use of a portfolio. Therefore, your programme of learning and development will require you to integrate theory and practice and demonstrate a change of attitudes and behaviours within your workplace.

ACTIVITY

Having read the above definitions regarding WBL, what does WBL mean to you?

Have your thoughts changed as a result of reading these definitions?

Are you aware of how WBL is addressed in your programme of study?

You may find that during your programme of learning and development you experience these two differing approaches to WBL as well as other forms of WBL. In the beginning your learning may be prescribed in that you are given tasks to complete in the workplace, specific reading and reflections. As you progress through your programme you may be asked to identify skills which you would like to develop that are appropriate to your role in the workplace or additional learning opportunities i.e. attending a multidisciplinary planning meeting or working with a specialist within a particular field. By the end of your programme you may have the opportunity to identify the learning for a module. This could include identifying the learning outcomes (what you will achieve), how these will be achieved and in some cases the assessment that you will produce. This will allow you flexibility in fusing theory and practice and meeting your own learning needs. It will also give you the freedom to link your learning specifically to your individual development, but you will need to be motivated and self-directed to make the most of this form of learning.

ACTIVITY

Think about how you learn in the workplace.

What has helped you achieve this learning?

What has hindered your learning?

The aim of the next section is to help you make sense of WBL through the use of learning agreements and PDPs and the role of mentors/supervisors.

Making sense of work-based learning

Learning agreements

During your programme of learning and development you may be required to complete a learning agreement (or learning contract) in partnership with your tutor and workplace mentor/supervisor or manager. The aim of this is to allow clear learning goals to be set which link specifically to your job description, competency and skill development or the application of new knowledge within your workplace. Using a learning agreement will allow you to identify specific areas of learning linked to either programme or module learning outcomes and in the spirit of WBL it requires you to be motivated and take an active role in your learning. In return it means that the learning is personalised to your learning and development needs, that you develop the ability to learn by yourself and that you link new knowledge to your workplace (Munroe *et al*. 2008). Alongside your mentor/supervisor and with support from your tutor you will need to identify what you want/need to learn, what resources will be required to support your learning, what activities you will need to undertake to achieve your learning, how you will be assessed and how you will demonstrate your learning and development.

ACTIVITY

Think about what you would like to learn.

How will you achieve this learning and how will you demonstrate your learning?

This structured approach to a learning agreement is demonstrated in Table 2.1.

You will note that the learning agreement has a number of identified sections:

- Your name and programme – this is the unique identifier to ensure the correct outcomes are used.
- Module and date – this ensures that the learning outcomes match the outcomes for the module.
- Learning outcomes – this may reflect the module learning outcomes to ensure that they are appropriate and meet your specific learning needs.
- Resources – these include people and available resources, i.e. specialists, workplace protocols/policies, library.
- Learning activities – these may include visiting other departments/teams, working with specialists, undertaking specific activities.
- Assessment – this may be a mix of academic activities and competencies.
- Evidence required – this may be completed competencies, care plans, record of discussions/reflections.

This is an example of what a learning agreement may look like but please note there may be other ways of presenting your learning agreement. What is important is that it identifies a learning outcome, how you will achieve the learning and the mode of assessment you will use and the evidence required to demonstrate that you have achieved your learning outcome. For your learning agreement to be successful you will need to lead your learning, to liaise at the outset with your mentor/supervisor and tutor and then throughout the module you will need to ensure you have frequent meetings with your mentor/supervisor to gain feedback on your learning and ensure that your learning agreement is completed in the agreed timescale.

Table 2.1 Example of a learning agreement

Name: S. Walters	**Programme**: FD Health and Social Care
Module: Infection Prevention	**Date**: October–December
Learning outcomes	Module learning outcome: examine the role of the healthcare worker in the prevention and control of infection.
	My learning outcome: explore my role in the prevention and control of infection in a community setting.
Resources	Workplace protocols, infection control nurse, mentor, library, intranet – local policies.
Learning activities	Care plans, observed practice especially hand-washing technique, infection precautions and safe disposal of sharps and waste products.
Assessment	Demonstrate competency in hand washing, portfolio completion, case study demonstrating infection control precautions, integration and application of new knowledge in practice.
Evidence required	Portfolio: completed hand-washing competency, completed disposal of sharps competency, competence statements, observed practice for infection control precautions, case study, example care plans, reflections.

Mid-module review date:

Mid-module review:

Final comments:

Learner's signature:	Date:
Mentor/supervisor signature:	Date:
Tutor signature:	Date:

ACTIVITY

Using Table 2.1 as a template, create your own learning agreement.

Personal development plans

If you work in the health and social care sector you may already have a PDP. Like a learning agreement it is personal to you but, unlike a learning agreement, a PDP may not be linked to a module. Instead it is a means for you to demonstrate to your employer the range of generic core skills that you have developed. Your PDP allows you to identify your personal development goals and evaluate your progress in achieving these. A PDP may be seen as a cyclical process as you identify an area for development, the action and resources required to meet your development, what evidence you will use to demonstrate achievement and an evaluation/reflection on your achievements so that further development needs may be identified. The cyclical process of a PDP is demonstrated in Figure 2.1.

As a PDP allows you to identify and demonstrate both personal and professional learning and development you may find that you use both short- and long-term goals. Subdividing long-term goals into shorter more manageable objectives will allow you to evaluate your achievements on a more regular basis as well as tackle something which appears ambitious and daunting in smaller chunks of activity which are achievable. This will ensure you gain a sense of achievement and motivation to achieve the bigger, longer-term goals.

Writing a PDP may appear daunting at first and the completion of a SWOT (Strengths, Weaknesses, Opportunities and Threats) analysis could be a good starting point. This will give you the opportunity to consider where you are in your career and from this you will be able to identify learning objectives to enhance your personal and professional development. You may choose to complete a SWOT analysis alone, with colleagues and/or with your tutor – there is no right or wrong approach. What is important is that you are realistic and that you consider why you have identified the areas that you have. This will help give meaning to your

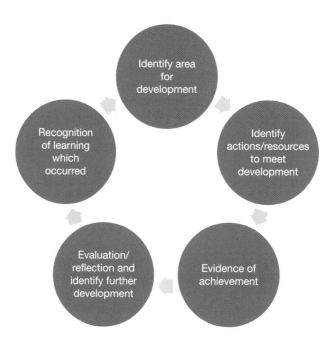

Figure 2.1 The cyclical process involved in PDP (Quality Assurance Agency (QAA) 2009).

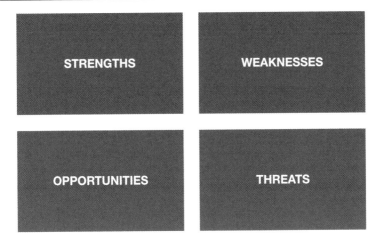

Figure 2.2 SWOT analysis.

SWOT analysis. Figure 2.2 shows a commonly used tool to allow you to keep your notes and thoughts from your analysis.

The list below gives you some of the criteria you may use to complete your SWOT analysis:

- **Strengths and weaknesses** – you may refer to knowledge, skills, expertise and experience.
- **Opportunities** – these may be personal or professional. For example by developing new knowledge and skills you will be a more confident, knowledgeable doer which will benefit your team and the individuals you support.
- **Threats** – these may include internal and external factors which may prevent you from completing your learning objectives for personal or professional development.

Once you have completed your SWOT analysis you are ready to commence planning and writing your PDP. To help you structure your PDP learning goals it is important that they follow SMART principles. This means that they are Specific, Measurable, Achievable, Realistic and Time-bound. Table 2.2 below gives an example of a PDP which has used SMART principles. You will note that two additional objectives, evidence of achievement and learning have been included. This is because you will need to demonstrate how your learning objective will be met and acknowledge your learning. It is important that you are aware of your learning, in terms of how you have developed both personally and professionally, but from this learning what further learning needs have you recognised? This is the cyclical nature of PDPs as discussed above and as demonstrated in Table 2.2.

ACTIVITY

Consider an aspect of your practice which you would like to develop.

Using a SWOT analysis as a starting point, complete a PDP using SMART principles.

Table 2.2 A completed PDP using SMART principles

Specific goal	To develop a nutritional information leaflet focused on the effects of having too much salt in your diet.
Measurable	A nutritional information leaflet will be developed.
Achievable	With the support of the nutritional specialist I will be able to design and develop an informative nutritional leaflet which focuses on the effects of too much salt in an individual's diet.
Realistic	I am undertaking a nutritional module at university and this leaflet will form part of the assessment for the module.
Time-bound	I will complete an informative nutritional leaflet in time for the module's assessment deadline.
Evidence of achievement	My leaflet was completed in time and I was awarded a pass grade.
Learning	This was an interesting exercise, I am not artistic and so I needed to learn how to convey my message in a visual format which was easy to access and understand for those who will read my leaflet.
	While searching for evidence to include in my leaflet I learnt a lot about healthy eating and I know how to learn more about the role of fat in an individual's diet.

To achieve your learning goal and recognise new learning it is important that you produce appropriate evidence to demonstrate that the learning has been achieved. You will need to be able to discuss how the evidence has allowed you to develop and what you have learnt as a result. The learning aspect of your development is critical as it supports you to enhance the care you give and allows you to embrace the concept of LLL. Like completing your SWOT analysis you may enlist your mentor/supervisor or tutor to help you identify appropriate sources of evidence or you could use the list in Figure 2.3 which provides some ideas to help you get started.

1   A reflective diary allows you to reflect on experiences from the workplace and helps you to make sense of what happened, what you might do differently if a similar experience occurred and what learning arose for you.
2   A survey from the workplace may demonstrate current practice prior to you implementing a change. For example a survey may demonstrate that patients are experiencing long waits to have their immunisation; you introduce the use of a numbering system and through a follow-up survey you are able to demonstrate that waiting times have been reduced and patient satisfaction improved.
3   A statement from a colleague which may outline an area of achievement. For example how you worked with a child who had a phobia of needles.
4   A copy of a poster, PowerPoint presentation or leaflet which you may have completed as part of your programme of learning and development.
5   Completed and signed competencies which are required for your programme or your job.

Remember you do not have to share all the sources of evidence you use to support your learning. For example you do not have to share your entire reflective diary – this is personal to

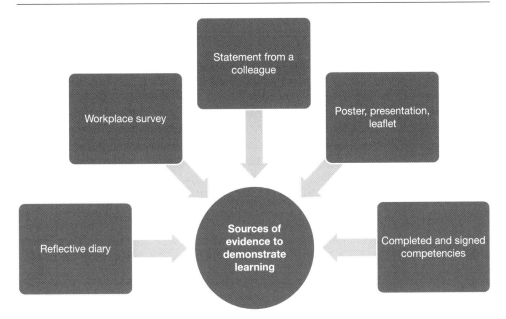

Figure 2.3 Sources of evidence for your portfolio.

you. What is important is that the evidence you choose is appropriate and relevant. However, what you must ensure is that you have considered the ethical issues of confidentiality so that an individual's identity is not revealed without their express permission. If anyone contributes to your evidence or assessments then you must tell them how you will use their information and who will have access to it. Any data from individuals or their notes should only be used for the purpose for which it was collected and is protected by the Data Protection Act (1998), so must be anonymous and not breach the rights of others.

Once you have identified the sources of evidence you are going to use to demonstrate your learning and development, the final stage of your PDP is to consider how you will evaluate your learning goals. This is necessary for a number of reasons:

- to ensure that you achieved the goals you set
- to identify formal and informal learning
- to identify any areas of improvement
- to consider whether any changes were required (was the learning goal too ambitious or could it have been more ambitious?)
- to outline future development needs.

Although it may feel out of order considering how you are going to evaluate your learning, it is important that you address this aspect in the design of your PDP to ensure your sources of evidence are appropriate. It is recommended that when you consider the evaluation aspect of your PDP you meet with the person who is going to support you in the process. This will give you the opportunity to discuss how frequently you will meet, if and how these meetings will be documented, whether you should have more than one mentor/supervisor and how you will demonstrate and evaluate your development – both for your programme of learning and for meeting your mentor/supervisor.

The role of your mentor/supervisor

WBL may, in the beginning, appear daunting as you enter into the unknown of working and learning. Perhaps you have not undertaken any formal study for a number of years and now you are being asked to identify and lead your learning. But rest assured you are not alone – you have your peers who are studying alongside you or working beside you, you have tutors who are there to support your learning and development journey and you will have identified or need to identify a workplace mentor/supervisor to support you.

There are many terms which describe this workplace support role but the term mentor/ supervisor will be used. This is because they may be required to assess learning in the workplace (mentor) through signing that you are competent in specific skills or they may supervise or facilitate your learning by identifying learning opportunities or help you make sense of your learning. Although your mentor/supervisor is responsible for supporting and facilitating your learning experience it is important that you take an active role in this relationship – remember that this is your learning and only you know what you do not know and what you would like, and need, to learn. The following suggestions might help you make the most of the learning opportunities which are available to you:

- Be clear about individual roles and responsibilities – what is your role as the learner and what is your mentor's/supervisor's role? This will ensure that expectations are clear from the outset.
- Find out the frequency and expectations of progress meetings and book these in. This will allow you to have planned regular meetings which can be difficult to arrange when the workplace is busy.
- Identify and agree learning opportunities at the outset. This will allow you to widen your experience, expose you to other learning opportunities and ensure that there is a clear plan to your learning and development. Have your learning outcomes available when you meet.
- Work with your mentor when you can and use this time to observe their behaviours and interactions with others – try and make sense of what they are doing and why, and ask questions after the interaction.
- Ask your mentor to alert you to learning opportunities that may arise in the workplace. This will help you to broaden your experiences and as in the point above try and make sense of the experience and ask questions after the event.
- Keep a list of questions which you want to ask your mentor/supervisor. This will allow you to use the time that you have together effectively and efficiently. But remember there are others in the workplace who may be able to answer these questions in a more timely fashion.
- Remember to support your mentor/supervisor in difficult situations by continuing to undertake your own workload and discuss the situation after the event when things are easier for them.

Whether you identified your own mentor/supervisor or were allocated a mentor/supervisor there may be occasions when the relationship does not meet your learning and development needs. It is important that you have a good working relationship with your mentor/supervisor to ensure you are able to meet your learning goals. Therefore, it is important that any difficulty is resolved in a timely and sensible manner and in many cases a quiet word to explain what you are finding difficult may be all that is required. Use assertive techniques to explain how you are feeling, for example 'I am not sure if I am using the correct approach'. This gives them the opportunity to consider your working relationship without them feeling criticised or defensive in their response. Unfortunately, on rare occasions, personalities clash and you may need to approach your workplace manager or tutor to help you resolve any differences. It may not be easy for you to take this approach and it will require tact, courage and assertive skills but remember that taking ownership of your learning is important and learning to work with others is part of integrating within a team and developing your skills of self-awareness.

If you are unable to resolve the issues you have with your mentor/supervisor and you are able to demonstrate evidence of addressing the situation then you will need to work with your employer and tutor to identify a new mentor/supervisor. There are a number of reasons why you might change your mentor/supervisor:

- There are minimal occasions when you are working with your mentor.
- Mismatched expectations of the purpose and outcome of your course.
- A desire to work with a different mentor/supervisor who has a different skillset/ workplace experience.
- Maternity leave, sickness absence or if your mentor/supervisor changes their place of work.

This section has helped you to make sense of WBL through the use of learning agreements and PDPs and the role of mentors/supervisors. The next section will consider how you may demonstrate your WBL through the use of a portfolio, reflection and reflexive practice.

Demonstrating your work-based learning

The use of a portfolio to demonstrate work-based learning

During your programme of learning and development you may be required to develop a portfolio to demonstrate how you achieved your learning goals. This may be at module level where the assignment is a portfolio of evidence demonstrating your learning and development with regard to specific learning outcomes – for example working with vulnerable adults. Or you may be required to keep a portfolio of evidence as part of your programme of learning and development. Whatever the reason for your portfolio development you must remember that you only need to share evidence that you want in the public domain, that the evidence you provide is appropriate and importantly that you demonstrate what learning has resulted. The spidergram in Figure 2.4 provides guidance on how your portfolio may be structured at module level but please note this is only guidance and your module tutor may require additional evidence.

- **Front sheet** – this is likely to include your name, learner/student number, module name and code.
- **Contents page** – this should list the contents of your portfolio and provide a clear structure for your tutor.
- **Module learning outcomes** – this will allow you to highlight which outcomes have been addressed in your portfolio and you could state how this was achieved and cross-reference to the section in which the evidence is included.

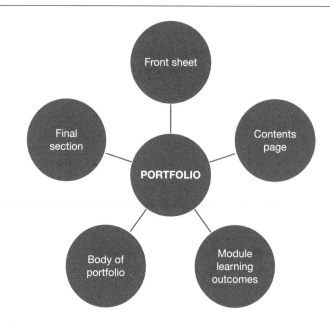

Figure 2.4 Portfolio content.

- **The body of your portfolio** – this may consist of one or more sections. The easiest way to achieve this would be to have a section for each learning outcome/goal, and it may include a SWOT analysis, PDP, competence achievement, certificates of attendance at study days, reflections on workplace experiences and evidence of reading which you have undertaken. It is important that the section has meaning to the reader and therefore you should provide an introduction to the section, link it to the learning outcome/s or learning goal/s that you are demonstrating, the evidence included and the learning that you have accomplished.
- **Final section** – you may choose to include a final section in which you provide an overview of your learning and development and outline future development needs.

If you are required to develop a portfolio as part of your programme of learning and development you may find that there are similarities to a portfolio which may be required at module level. As with a portfolio at module level it is important that the sections are clearly identifiable (using dividers may help), that the aim and purpose of the portfolio are included and there is clear evidence of learning and development. This may be linked to a module and how the learning from the module allowed you to enhance your workplace practice; it could be learning from interactions in the workplace with an individual that you are supporting; or it may be learning which has arisen from attending a mandatory training or study day. The following, therefore, is only a suggestion of how you might structure your portfolio:

- **A front sheet** – this should include your name and programme of study.
- **A contents page** – this should ensure ease of navigation through your portfolio.
- **Your curriculum vitae** (CV) – this will provide a summary of your learning and development and previous workplace experience.

- **Your job description** – this will allow you to link your learning to developing your workplace role.
- **SWOT analysis** – this will provide evidence of how you have developed and how your identified strengths, weaknesses, opportunities and threats link to your PDPs. It is recommended that you undertake a SWOT analysis and PDP at the commencement of your programme, at regular intervals during your programme and on completion. This will allow you to see your learning and development.
- **PDPs** – these will link to your SWOT analysis but may also link to your workplace appraisal and specific module learning.
- **Reflections** – reflections are a useful component of WBL as you make sense of your learning and identify future learning.
- **Competencies** – these will allow you to demonstrate how you have developed your knowledge and skills and practical development.
- **Written assignments** – these will allow you to demonstrate how you have progressed academically.
- **Additional evidence** – this may include certificates of attendance at in-house or external study days, evidence of reading, discussions or written statements from colleagues and individuals that you have supported.
- **Final section** – this could include an overview of your learning and development journey, the highs and lows and future learning and development requirements.

Whatever the requirement of your portfolio of evidence its purpose will be to bring together a range of evidence which supports and demonstrates your learning and development in, for and through work. It is your repository to fill as you deem appropriate, but make sure the information included is relevant and that you provide evidence of the impact of your learning, either professionally or personally. At the same time as providing concrete evidence of your workplace learning and development you may find yourself engaging in reflection which may be either in- or on-action (Kolb 1984), allowing you to explore your experiences and bring about changes in practice. Consequently, as you progress through your programme of learning and development you may find yourself engaging in reflexive practice – putting your theorising into practice.

Reflection

The Concise Oxford Dictionary (1999) defines reflection as 'serious thought or consideration; a considered idea, expressed in writing or speech'. However, for reflection to be effective you must not only think about the situation but give meaning to the situation so that you learn from the experience and move forward as a practitioner. Using reflection to learn not only allows you to consider experiences retrospectively but it also enables you to proactively plan your future learning based on what you know already and anticipating what may occur. Therefore, the use of reflection to inform your reflective practice (learning from experience to develop your practice) is seen as a cyclical process and is demonstrated in Figure 2.5.

Your reflection may be triggered by a number of drivers including your desire to understand workplace experiences in more depth; questions from your mentor which arise from observing your practice; identifying new learning needs and opportunities for learning and ultimately your personal and professional development. Schön (1983) identified two types of reflection – reflection-in-action and reflection-on-action.

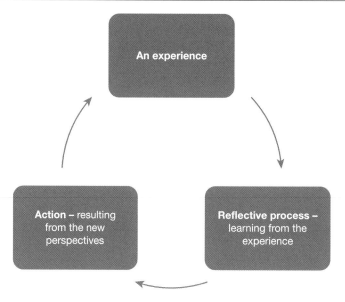

Figure 2.5 Cycle of reflective practice.

Reflection-in-action is the ability to think and theorise about practice while you are doing it. This form of reflection is often seen as an automatic activity which occurs subconsciously as you combine your knowledge, skills and practice as you practise and consequently it is not used deliberately. An example of when you might use reflection-in-action is when you are supporting an individual who is on bed rest to meet their own hygiene needs.

Reflection-on-action, unlike reflection-in-action, is a conscious activity where you make sense of an experience after it has occurred so that you are able to discover the knowledge which was used in the situation. On the whole this is a retrospective activity, for example sitting with an individual after they have administered their first dose of insulin to make sense of the situation.

For your reflection to have meaning and to support your learning it needs to be a structured process. Jasper (2003) advocated six fundamental stages associated with the reflective process (see Figure 2.6).

A number of structures and strategies have been developed to support the reflective process, known as frameworks. However, due to the confines of this chapter only the work of Driscoll (2007) and Gibb (1988) will be considered.

Driscoll developmental framework

Driscoll's framework consists of a linear or developmental approach offering trigger questions to develop your practice. It is based on Borton's (1970) educational framework which used three developmental questions:

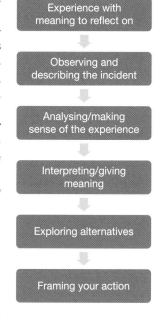

Figure 2.6 Structured reflective process, adapted from Jasper (2003).

- What?
- So what?
- Now what?

Driscoll's first question, 'What?' allows you to consider the context in which your reflection is occurring and to describe the event. This may be done verbally or in writing but the purpose of this action is to allow you to clarify the situation and perhaps see different perspectives. The second question, 'So what?' allows you to begin to analyse or make sense of the situation as you consider your learning emotionally, practically and theoretically. This process offers you the opportunity to explore your perceptions of the event and consider any changes which are required in your practice. This may be in terms of gaps in your knowledge and/or skills or how you approached the situation with regards to your attitude. The final question, 'Now what?' is a continuation of the second question and your analysis of the situation; allowing you to identify new learning or apply your learning to similar situations which you may encounter at a later date.

Gibb's reflective cycle

Gibb's reflective cycle (1988) is a staged and structured process which, through the use of cue questions, guides you through the reflective process and is demonstrated in Figure 2.7.

Gibb's reflective cycle allows you to describe the situation and place your experience in context. The second stage, unlike other models, allows you to explore your thoughts and feelings while the third stage provides the opportunity to consider aspects of the experience which went well and those which could be improved. This process allows you to begin to identify the knowledge and skills which you need to develop. Through the fourth stage you analyse the situation, what you know and what you do not know, allowing you to link theory to practice

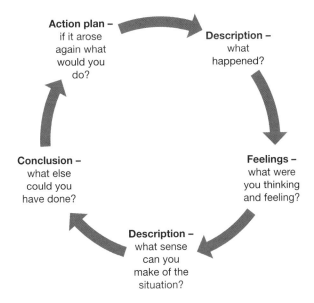

Figure 2.7 Gibb's reflective cycle, adapted from Gibb (1988).

and practice to theory. The fifth stage, the conclusion, allows you to consider strategies which were not used and whether they would have been applicable. This final stage requires you to formulate an action plan, to consider the way forward and how the knowledge and skills identified could be applied to future practice.

Whether you choose to use Driscoll or Gibb to structure your reflection and evidence your learning and development within your portfolio, the Activity below demonstrates how through reflection you can give meaning to situations and develop as a practitioner.

ACTIVITY – USING REFLECTION TO MAKE SENSE OF AN EXPERIENCE IN THE WORKPLACE

You may use this scenario as a basis for use with either Driscoll or Gibb's framework to see which you prefer.

I work on a care of the older person ward and it had been one of those busy early shifts where I did not have five minutes to think. I was looking after a bay of eight ladies with a staff nurse who was also in charge of the ward. The shift began well, the staff nurse and I worked as a team as we made sure everyone had breakfast and were supported, where required, in washing and dressing ready for the day ahead. As the staff nurse accompanied the doctors on the ward round I completed those observations which were required and spent time chatting to the ladies in the bay. While I was undertaking this activity I heard a commotion in the main corridor so I went to see what was happening.

It appeared that a lady from the next bay, who was frail and rather confused, had managed to get out of bed and slipped, breaking her hip. I realised that as a learner there was nothing which I could do to help but I wanted to observe the situation as part of my learning but I could not – I had to keep an eye on my bay. This was even more important as the staff nurse I was working with had to ensure that the lady who slipped received the appropriate care. I continued with the shift trying to meet individual needs but felt frustrated when the remit of my role meant that individuals had to wait for aspects of their care.

For some reason today's shift, unlike other shifts, had an impact on me. I found myself thinking about my role, what I was able to do and how the gaps in my role impacted on my patients and I found my thoughts drifting to the lady who had broken her hip. I realised that it was important that I continued to develop my practical skills and the theory to support my actions. This would allow me to make sense of such aspects as why I am undertaking observations which would allow me to consider the individual as a whole rather than just the task at hand. I realised that I knew little about confusion and the care of a broken hip, and I needed to develop this knowledge.

Spending time thinking about the shift and writing down what happened has helped me realise that I must focus my energy on developing the knowledge to underpin my care as this will enhance my practice and support my development as a practitioner.

Reflexive practice

Rolfe (1997) argues that it is the concept of reflection-in-action which forms a stage of expert practice which he terms reflexive practice. He believes that for reflexive practice to occur you need to incorporate theorising into and on practice. As a reflexive practitioner, therefore, you will need to concentrate on the task at hand, think about your actions and relate your theoretical knowledge to the task. According to Rolfe (1997) this way of learning will allow you to fuse your theoretical and practical learning into a unique theory which you can test and modify. As reflexive practice involves you fusing theory and practice you may find that this is not a process that you can relate to at the commencement of your programme of learning and development as you may find yourself practice rich and theory poor, similar to the scenario in the Activity above. Do not worry, you may find that you already reflect-on-action and the first step you need to undertake is to learn how to reflect-in-action before you engage in reflexive practice. What is important is that you engage at the stage which is most appropriate to your learning and development journey.

When you engage in reflexive practice it is about being honest with the choices you made and the actions which arose so that you can give meaning to your learning. You may find that working with your tutor or mentor/supervisor helps you progress from reflection to reflexivity as you engage in a critical dialogue focused on your experiences. Keeping a reflective diary or learning log may help you make sense of situations, experiences, feelings, concerns or issues which occur. Over time it is the critical engagement of these reflections which will allow you to undertake reflexive practice. It is the engagement with others which will provide you with the enlightenment you require to be a reflexive practitioner. The following questions based on the work of Johns and Freshwater (1998) might help you engage in reflexive practice:

- How does this experience connect/link with previous experiences which you have had?
- What would be the result of alternative actions for the individual that you are supporting, others and yourself?
- How do you now feel about the experience?
- Can you support yourself and others better as a result of the experience?
- How has it changed what you know?

Bringing these questions to a meeting with your mentor/supervisor might help you to engage in reflexive practice through a critical dialogue as you make sense of your experiences and the evidence required to support your actions.

This section has helped you to consider how you may demonstrate your WBL through the use of a portfolio, reflection and reflexive practice.

Chapter summary

- WBL is an integral part of developing skills and knowledge for the workplace.
- The principles of WBL and a range of definitions and aspects of WBL are explored.
- The importance of LLL, learning in the workplace and using reflexive practice to develop as an individual is established.
- Learning agreements and personal development plans are useful tools to focus on specific learning needs and to structure working with mentors/supervisors to achieve them.
- A range of approaches for providing evidence of, and demonstrating, learning and development are described, including the use of portfolios and reflection.

Further resources

Department of Health. Available at: www.dh.gov.uk/.
Lifelong Learning. Available at: www.lifelonglearning.gov.uk/.
Skills for Care. Available at: www.skillsforcare.gov.uk/.
Skills for Health. Available at: www.skillsforhealth.gov.uk/.

Further reading

Howatson-Jones, L. 2013. *Reflective Learning in Nursing Practice*. Exeter: Learning Matters.
Jackson, C. and Thurgate, C. 2011. *Workplace Learning in Health and Social Care*. Maidenhead: Open University Press.
Pearsall, J. (ed.). 1999. *The Concise Oxford English Dictionary*, 10th edn. Oxford: Oxford University Press.
Reed, S. 2011. *Successful Professional Portfolios for Nursing Students*. Exeter: Learning Matters.

References

Borton, T. 1970. *Reach, Touch and Teach*. London: Hutchinson.
Data Protection Act. 1998. London: HMSO.
Department for Children, Schools and Families (DfCSF). 2008. *The Work Related Learning Guide*. London: DfCSF.
Driscoll, J. 2007. *Practising Clinical Supervision: A Reflective Approach for Healthcare Professionals*, 2nd edn. Edinburgh: Balliere Tindall.
Eraut, M. 2004. *Developing Professional Knowledge and Competence*. London: Routledge.
Gibb, G. 1988. *Learning by Doing: A Guide to Teaching and Learning Methods*. Oxford: Further Education Unit.
Jasper, M. 2003. *Beginning Reflective Practice*. Cheltenham: Nelson Thornes.
Johns, C. and Freshwater, D. 1998. *Transforming Nursing through Reflective Practice*, 2nd edn. Oxford: Blackwell.
Kolb, D. 1984. *Experiential Learning: Experience as the Source of Learning and Development*. Englewood Cliffs, NJ: Prentice Hall.
Munroe, M., Holmshaw, J. and Brown, V. 2008. 'Review of Literature on the Impact of Learning Contracts on Teaching and Learning in Higher Education Institutions'. Unpublished report, Centre for Excellence in Work Based Learning, Middlesex University.
Quality Assurance Agency (QAA). 2009. *Personal Development Planning: Guidance for Institutional Policy and Practice in Higher Education*. London: QAA.
Raelin, J. 2008. *Work-based Learning: Bridging Knowledge and Action in the Workplace*. San Francisco, CA: Jossey-Bass.
Rhodes, G. and Shiel, G. 2007. 'Meeting the Needs of the Workplace and the Learner through Work-based Learning', *Journal of Workplace Learning*, 18(3), 173–87.
Rolfe, G. 1997. 'Beyond Expertise: Theory, Practice and the Reflexive Practitioner', *Journal of Clinical Nursing*, 6(2), 93–7.
Schön, D. 1983. *The Reflective Practitioner: How Professionals Think in Action*. London: Temple Smith.

Chapter 3

Communication

Mary Northrop and David Hingley

LEARNING OUTCOMES

By the end of this chapter you will be able to:

1   Understand the importance of effective communication in healthcare.
2   Consider the different issues when using different modes of communication.
3   Show understanding of how to adapt communication for different client groups.

Introduction

We communicate on a daily basis and access different modes of communication. However, we will all have experienced interactions which have gone well and others where there have been difficulties. In healthcare, good communication skills are vital to ensure that clients are included in their care and receive the right care. In 2010 the initial report from an inquiry into care at Mid Staffordshire Hospital was published in two volumes. The review was chaired by Robert Francis QC and covered the period 2005 to 2009. Communication was one of the issues raised and how this links to compassion, dignity and respect (Francis 2010). The report provides a clear message that communication in healthcare is essential but was not always effective. The report provided ten key areas where communication had broken down:

1   Lack of compassion for patients or lack of reassurance that staff care about individuals.
2   Lack of information about a patient's care or condition.
3   Lack of involvement in decisions.
4   Insensitive communication of information to patients.
5   Reluctance to give information.
6   Delays in giving information to patients and their families.
7   Failure of communication between staff.
8   Patients given the wrong information.
9   Failure to listen to patients and families.
10 Lack of engagement.

In his report, Francis refers to the draft *Essence of Care 2010: Benchmarks for Communication* (published by the Department of Health in 2010). The *Essence of Care 2010* document sets thirteen benchmarks to ensure good practice, which include: effective inter-personal skills, creating opportunities for communication, assessing communication needs and information sharing.

ACTIVITY

Looking at benchmarks 2 and 3 below:

- Opportunity for communication
- Assessment of communication needs

Consider how these are met in your own area of practice. Are there any recommendations that you could make to improve how these are addressed?

You will find it useful to look at the full benchmark from the *Essence of Care* document available from the Department of Health (2010).

Definitions of communication

There are a number of definitions of communication in the literature. *Essence of Care 2010: Benchmarks for Communication* (Department of Health 2010) provides a useful working definition stating that communication is:

> a process that involves a meaningful exchange between at least two people to convey facts, needs, opinions, thoughts, feelings or other information through both verbal and non-verbal means including face-to-face exchanges and the written word.
>
> (Department of Health 2010: 7)

The definition suggests that a meaningful exchange needs to take place in order for communication to occur. Burnard and Gill (2008) highlight the tendency to think that communication is about words, whether spoken or written. However, they suggest that communication is much wider and includes the symbols we use, giving the examples of Christians who wear a cross, the clothes that we wear and our accents. They argue that 'we cannot not communicate' (Burnard and Gill 2008: 31).

ACTIVITY

Think of two people who you know and consider what they may communicate through the way they dress.

You may have chosen people who subscribe to a specific way of dress due to belonging to a particular group which shares a specific set of values and beliefs. For example, in teenage culture individuals may choose to be seen as a Goth or an Emotional (EMO) and therefore conform to the dress code of that group and its values. You may have chosen someone who wears a uniform that conveys certain values and expectations, for example a policeman or a fireman.

Methods of communication

There are a number of methods of communication that may be used; some will use electronic devices, and others will be face to face, or rely on verbal communication. Others will use written text which may be synchronous (received and replied to immediately) or non-synchronous (seen and replied to at a later date).

ACTIVITY

Think of the ways you have communicated throughout the day and list them in the first column. In the second column consider why you used that method.

Method of communication	Why method is used

For example in one day I used the following:

Method of communication	Why method is used
Email	Geographical distance and not a complex issue
Telephone	Geographical distance. More complex issue which requires two-way synchronous conversation
Face to face	Person in the same building
Face to face	Teaching students
Skype (Internet)	Family member who lives in another country. Free and synchronous conversation and able to see the other person
Phone text message	To arrange a time to talk on the phone with a family member who works shifts including evenings and weekends
Wearing smart clothes	To indicate working in a professional role
Wearing casual clothes	To indicate no longer at work and moved into social role

All the above were used for different reasons, including the form in which the initial contact took place, but also the content of the communication and why it needs to take place. Whether the method is face to face, written, synchronous or asynchronous the purpose of the communication will be to transfer a message from one person to another. Therefore we need to consider a number of factors: the type of message, who the message is from and who it is going to, and the medium in which the message is being transferred.

Modes of communication

Communication is complex, with a number of factors coming together that individuals need to sort through and make sense of. When looking at effective communication there are a number of ways in which communication is delivered, all of which have different components, depending on whether communication is face to face or via technology, written or spoken. The following sections look at the different components for the different methods. Underpinning all of these are the social and cultural influences, the relationship between those taking part and individual attitudes and values.

Face-to-face communication

The way in which we deliver messages includes the words we use, our body language and how we speak. Figure 3.1 provides an overview of the factors that link to face-to-face communication.

Verbal

The language we speak often brings with it underpinning cultural and social factors which influence meaning and how we communicate. There are also variations in the way the same

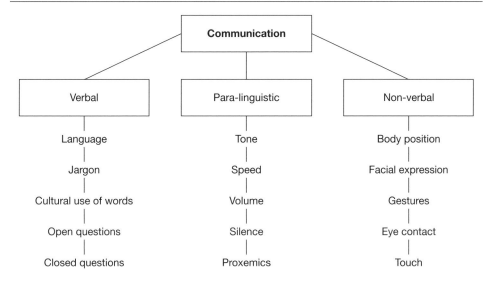

Figure 3.1 Face-to-face communication.

language may be used across the society. For example, words may have different meanings and may be used differently which can lead to misinterpretation, or there may be collo-quial words which are region specific i.e. shoes worn for physical education may be called plimsolls, pumps or rubbers.

Types of questions

When working in healthcare you need to collect information about clients as part of the assessment processes. There are different forms of questions which are useful dependent on the type of information required:

*   Closed questions: useful for factual information which does not require elaboration i.e. name, age, address etc.
*   Open questions: when you need elaboration, details, opinions or sharing of experiences. There are a number of types of open questions:

    *   Probing: questions that aim to get a better understanding of what is happening.
    *   Clarifying: questions that check that the receiver has understood what was said.
    *   Leading: when there is a need to move the person to a specific topic.

Phatic communication

In both everyday life and in healthcare we use certain types of interactions in order to build a relationship or to show that we are open to a conversation. Burnard and Gill (2008) define phatic communication as:

Phatic communication relates to all the aspects of conversation which are 'content free'. When we say 'Hello, how are you?' we are engaging in phatic communication: we are not enquiring about the other person's health, but merely indicating that we are friendly and open to conversation.

(Burnard and Gill 2008: 164)

This type of content is often termed small talk but is seen as pivotal to spoken word communication and the formation of interpersonal relationships. Phatic communication is part of the social aspect of communication which places the person at ease. It signifies that we are available to talk and gives the other person a chance to consider whether they want to maintain the interaction. Burnard and Gill (2008) suggest that much of our spoken communication uses phatic communication to pad out conversations. Using phatic communication is important and acts as an icebreaker to develop interaction and is part of everyday life. Bach and Grant (2009) suggest phatic communication aids in forming interpersonal relationships through creating a sense of connection. Phatic communication can be seen as the precursor to establishing a relationship and building trust. The content is not important but the act of communicating is. For example, when working with clients diagnosed with depression it may take a while for them to feel comfortable in disclosing their feelings. By having short interactions which show interest but do not pressure the individual this can mean that when they are ready to talk they feel able to trust you.

ACTIVITY

Reflect on a recent conversation with a client, friend or family member.

What sort of questions did you ask?

Did you use phatic communication and if so how and why?

Para-verbal communication

The above term refers to how we deliver the language component of the face-to-face interaction. This includes tone, volume and speed and what these signify to the receiver and what is implied by the sender. For example, your manager may ask you to come to the office as they need to speak to you. The tone of voice and how different syllables are pronounced will aid the receiver in deciding whether the request means the conversation is likely to be positive or negative. The speed may indicate that someone is excited or nervous, whereas volume may also indicate excitement or indicate a hearing problem. Another aspect of para-verbal communication is proxemics. Most people feel uncomfortable when people we do not know get too close. There are some exceptions where we may tolerate this, for example if travelling on a packed train or at a concert or sporting event.

Burnard and Gill (2008) highlight that in different cultures there may be more variation, with Latin countries tending to stand closer together whereas in some Asian countries they stand further apart and touch may be prohibited in public places.

Hall (1966, cited by DeVito 2013) identified four spatial distances: intimate, personal, social and public.

- Intimate space – between 0 to 18 inches – close family and friends.
- Personal (casual) – 1½ to 4 feet – informal conversations with friends and acquaintances.
- Social – 4 to 12 feet – more impersonal professional transactions.
- Public – 12 to 25+ feet – making speeches and addressing large groups at formal gatherings.

Non-verbal communication

Non-verbal communication comes in many forms and communicates messages to others whether intended or not. Goffman (1959) introduced the concept of social actors in that we are constantly on stage and observed by others. For example, at some time you may have

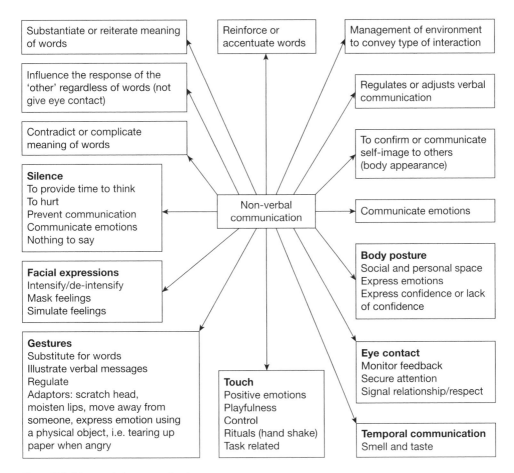

Figure 3.2 Non-verbal communication.

walked into a post or tripped over – the first thing we check is if anyone was watching, then we check for injuries. People form opinions of others before they talk to them and in some cases before they see them. Chapter 5: Valuing people brings in how stereotypes can influence our behaviour and attitudes towards others. Non-verbal communication through dress and expression of emotions can confirm or question our perception of others. The mind map in Figure 3.2 demonstrates how non-verbal communication is used and types of non-verbal communication. The list is not exhaustive and you will think of other examples.

Electronic communication methods

There are a range of electronic communication methods that aid in healthcare delivery but also bring with them different problems and potential barriers to effective communication.

ACTIVITY

Make a list of the different activities where you use electronic communication in both healthcare and everyday life.

What are the positives and what are the drawbacks?

Electronic communication	Positives	Drawbacks

Telephone communication

The telephone is used widely in healthcare delivery for making appointments, triage, and health promotion and to coordinate day-to-day activities both for work and home life. Telephones are used to follow up clients in the community following hospital procedures, to text test results, and between healthcare professionals for referrals or organising services and equipment. For healthcare workers in the community they ensure they can communicate with colleagues and monitor each other's whereabouts. There are a number of advantages with conversations being synchronous and therefore clarification can be sought if meaning is not clear. Disadvantages are the lack of physical proximity if the individual is upset and the lack of visual cues to aid understanding.

There are a number of considerations, some of which overlap with the use of other electronic communication. Confidentiality and ensuring privacy is important as conversations may be overheard and therefore client information may be shared unintentionally. A second consideration is whether it is polite to answer the phone when in a client's home as this may suggest that they are not your priority. It is also important to check the identity of the person at the end of the phone to ensure it is appropriate to give them information. As healthcare workers we need to build good relationships with clients and their relatives and carers without breaking confidences and respecting individuals' rights.

Email

Email can be an effective form of communication if used well. As it is asynchronous communication there can be a gap between sending and getting a reply and this may need to be taken into account if there is a degree of urgency. There is also a lack of visual and auditory cues for the receiver to understand the feelings that may be behind the communication. This may lead to misinterpretation, particularly if the sender is trying to be witty or sarcastic but the receiver does not interpret the message in this way. How the email is written can also give the reader an impression of the sender. For example, the use of text language may be appropriate between friends but not between a student and tutor or employer and employee. It is important to consider the relationship with the email recipient and whether email is the best form of communication for the message.

ACTIVITY

Using Figure 3.3 below, consider your own use of emails and how you could be more effective in using this form of communication.

Do
- Consider whether email is the best method of communication for the message content
- Keep email messages short and to the point
- Reread message before you send it or get someone else to read, is it clear or open to misinterpretation?
- Consider relationship with who sending email to and word appropriately
- Remember manners and niceties
- Let people know if you are getting emails you do not need

Do not
- Send messages that are hard to understand
- Copy people in to emails who do not need to be copied in
- Respond to an email when you are not sure who sent it
- Forward email chains to other participants. Contributors may not wish their communication to be seen by others without giving permission

Emails

Email security and confidentiality
- Are there any legal and data protection issues?
- Are you breaching confidentiality?
- What is the organisation's policy on using emails?
- Ensure correct person is receiving the information
- How sensitive is the information? Is email appropriate?
- Set up separate email accounts for work, family and friends and for websites used for shopping or offers as this reduces spam emails
- Set up Junk filters to protect your inbox
- Report any suspicious emails to the IT services at work or where you are studying
- Be aware of phishing emails: any email asking for a password to access accounts is suspicious and needs to be reported

Good practice
- Check message is going to the right recipients
- If more than one recipient, make clear what you want each one to do. Or is it better to do separate emails?
- Use sections and numbering/bullet points
- Put important information first, particularly any deadlines
- Use subject line to state what the message is about
- Start a new email chain if bringing in different recipients
- Make sure if you use emoticons person getting them knows what they mean
- If you are unsure whether to send an email, don't. It may be better to use the telephone or see the individual
- If you receive an email that has been sent out using a mailing list, consider if you need to reply to everyone or just to the sender

Figure 3.3 Email communication, adapted from Talktalk (n.d.). Do's and don'ts and good practice, adapted from Emailogic workshop on How to get better results from your email (Emailogic n.d.).

Principles of communication

Active listening

Communication is not just about sending the message but also receiving messages. One of the skills that is often overlooked is that of listening. We can all think of instances where we have heard what someone is communicating but take it at face value rather than really listening. This is usually after we have moved on from the person and we have a sense of 'Did I really understand what they meant?'

The functions of listening are:

*   To focus specifically upon the messages being communicated by the other person.
*   To obtain a full, accurate understanding of the other person's communication.
*   To convey interest, concern and attention.
*   To encourage full, open and honest expression.
*   To develop an 'other-centred' approach during an interaction (Hargie *et al.* 1994).

A number of techniques are recommended to check whether the message heard has not only been understood but also that the sender of the message feels comfortable and the communication is occurring as equals. The first approach is adapting to the language and terms used by the client or reflecting. For example, if the client uses the term 'belly' adopt the same term rather than using 'abdomen' or 'stomach' (Quilter, Wheeler and Windt 1993, cited by Hargie *et al.* 1994). The second approach is to paraphrase or summarise the content in order to check with the client whether you have understood what they are saying, allowing them to correct any misunderstandings. Paraphrasing is rewording or restating a phrase. Summarising does not reword but draws out what the receiver perceived as the main points in the sender's message. Listening includes the use of non-verbal communication. This may be unconscious – you will find that when you sit with a group of people similar postures tend to occur, e.g. legs crossed. By consciously adopting a similar body posture the client may feel more relaxed. This needs to be done with caution as obvious copying may make the client think you are making fun of them. Egan (2007) provides a mnemonic to follow to show active listening. Emphasis is on using non-verbal communication to demonstrate that the speaker has the attention of the listener.

S – Sit squarely in relation to the other person
O – Maintain an open position and do not cross arms or legs
L – Lean slightly towards the other person
E – Maintain reasonable and comfortable eye contact
R – Relax

ACTIVITY

With a partner try the following exercises:

1   The speaker talks for one minute about a topic of their choice. The listener uses some of the actions below:

    •   Stare at the floor
    •   Look at the space to the right of the person
    •   Check your phone
    •   Stand up and stretch
    •   Fiddle with your hair
    •   Turn away from the speaker
    •   Cross and uncross your legs or swing your legs

2   The speaker talks for another minute on a subject of their choice. The listener uses SOLER and verbal and non-verbal prompts.

Reflect on the exercise.

How did you both feel during each of the exercises?

What will you consider when listening to clients or others?

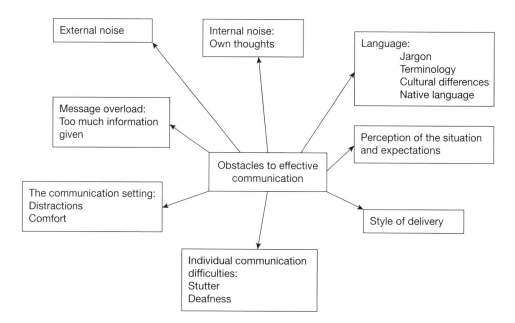

Figure 3.4 Communication barriers.

Barriers to communication

Effective communication is something we all try and achieve but do not always succeed. There are a number of barriers that can affect the ability to both communicate and hear the message (see Figure 3.4).

For example, you may have come across an individual who delivers communication effectively and it is not until later that you realise they were lying. The opposite also happens where we do not take the individual seriously and get caught up on certain characteristics. Dunn and Goodnight (2011) give the example of focusing on how many times the person uses a certain phrase rather than the rest of the content. One of my lecturers would always use the phrase 'assess the situation' and this became a focus to guess how long it would take in a session before he used the phrase. A common problem in healthcare is the use of terms (jargon) which may not be understood by others. The onus is on the professional to adapt their language to the audience but without becoming too simplistic and further alienating the receiver. In classroom settings there may be a need to develop a vocabulary linked to the subject, for example when learning anatomy and physiology, ethics or research as they include a range of terminology that allows us to undertake a health and social care role.

STUDENT TIP

I keep a notebook handy so that when I come across new terms I jot them down and then look them up.

The next obstacle, message overload, refers to being given too much information or too much detail resulting in the receiver not understanding or hearing the important part of the message or becoming confused.

ACTIVITY

Look at the information you provide to clients new to your service/department or information you received as a client.

• Is the information easy to understand?
• Is there too much information?
• What techniques could be used to help clients understand the information?

You might consider a number of means that could be used to communicate the information. Welcome packs can be used to enable clients to look at information again. Another technique is to deliver the information in smaller chunks over a period of time, ensuring the essential information is given first. DeVito (2013) describes the primacy effect, where the individual is more likely to remember what came first, and the recency effect, where the last information is remembered or exerts the most interest. Both of these highlight that information in the middle is not always remembered.

The setting can also send different messages as to how formal or relaxed the interaction is. For example, sitting at a desk is more formal than sitting in chairs without the table as a barrier. Settings can be used to indicate power relations. In healthcare, clients admitted to hospital may feel powerless as the environment is the domain of health professionals. Conversely, healthcare professionals visiting clients in their own homes have to recognise that they are in the clients' territory.

The perception of the situation and our expectations may be influenced by previous experiences. Children may have experienced pain on a previous visit to the doctor and therefore may be reluctant to visit the doctor's surgery. Incorrect knowledge or lack of knowledge can also be a barrier. My daughter injured her arm and needed to have an X-ray. She was reluctant to go in and the radiographer and I were getting frustrated as we could not understand why. We finally asked her; she thought that if her arm was broken it would have to be cut off. She had been watching a television show about animal hospitals and had seen a cat having its foot amputated following a fracture.

Communication and culture

Underpinning communication whether verbal, non-verbal or electronic are different conventions in relation to the culture of the individuals communicating. Cultural differences are not limited to different ethnic groups and may include age, social groups and religion. Within healthcare, effective communication includes considering how culture and belief systems may impact on the sending and receiving of messages and we may have to modify or adapt our approach to meet this. Common examples of communication differences are the use of gestures, where hand gestures may have different meanings. Other examples include the use of eye contact; in some cultures (Hispanic, Asian and Middle Eastern) eye contact is avoided as it is deemed rude.

ACTIVITY

Make a list of different gestures that may be used in the UK and explore their meaning in other countries.

Burnard and Gill (2008) provide a more detailed explanation of how culture may impact on health delivery and how as individuals we can become more culturally aware. They advise that there are six steps to developing cultural awareness:

1   Information – finding out about different cultures either through searching the Web or asking the client or appropriate others.
2   Empathy – developing empathy with the client by seeing the world as they see it and putting aside your own view of the world.
3   Open-minded – become open-minded and override the part of us that sees things as right or wrong and become more aware of what we are closed-minded about.
4   Interest in other people – listening and taking a genuine interest in the other person.
5   Willingness to learn – being open to new learning and prepared to question and read.
6   Lack of prejudice – acknowledge the prejudices you hold and consider them from the opposing viewpoint.

The overriding issue when communicating with others is to be aware of cultural aspects, but establish with the individual what their beliefs and values are and how these link to their healthcare. By doing this, individualised care will be delivered based on individual needs rather than based on assumptions about what is best for the individual which may be formed through stereotypes or beliefs.

Communicating with clients

Within healthcare we meet clients of different ages, different cultures and with different life experiences, attitudes and values. Some clients may have health issues or genetic conditions that may impact on their ability to interact and these need to be taken into account. The underpinning principle is to treat people as individuals rather than forming stereotypes of how clients need to be communicated with because they fit into a specific category, e.g. learning disability and deaf. We need to establish which forms of communication are appropriate, and what actions can be taken to ensure active communication and to develop a toolkit of skills that can adapt to individual situations.

An example from a hospital setting illustrates the seriousness of not communicating clearly:

ACTIVITY

A client had been admitted into hospital and was told by the nurse that they would not be there long. As the individual was not sure what was wrong with them, they interpreted this as meaning they were dying. The nurse had meant they were going home.

Consider how you would have handled this situation differently.

This is an example of how the context comes to the fore in communication and also of individuals' different knowledge and understanding.

The mind map in Figure 3.5 describes a number of terms used to describe problems with speech and language, both oral and written.

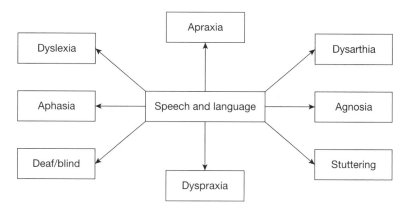

Figure 3.5 Speech and language problems.

ACTIVITY

Look up the terms that you do not know. Find out tips and hints for effective communication and services available.

There are a number of resources available that suggest good practice when communicating with clients. MENCAP's website provides a brief guide for communicating with clients with learning disabilities and provides ten top tips:

1 Find a good place in which to communicate.
2 Ask open questions.
3 Check with the person that they understand what you are saying.
4 If the person wants to take you somewhere to show you something, go with them.
5 Watch the person.
6 Learn from experience.
7 Try drawing.
8 Take your time, don't rush your communication.
9 Use gestures and facial expressions.
10 Be aware that some people find it easier to use real objects to communicate but photos and pictures can help too. (Source: MENCAP 2010)

The above points are also useful for any interpersonal communication and emphasise the need for clients to be given time to respond and also to be listened to, rather than being ignored, with carers or relatives asked how they are feeling. The guide highlights a number of tools available to aid with communication including: Signalong, Makaton, Talking Mats and Widgit.

The Alzheimer's Society (2013) also provides a fact sheet for communicating with clients with dementia which advocates a range of good practices. These include the importance of gaining eye contact and using a calm tone to prevent startling or scaring the individual and the need to include the individual in social groups to prevent isolation.

VERA – a framework for compassionate communication

VERA is an acronym intended to help staff frame interactions with clients whose communication is impaired (Blackhall *et al*. 2011). It suggests a four-stage process that helps to guide professionals to engage in compassionate, person-centred care.

VERA attempts to overcome a view that because a person is confused, any behaviour is also confused and therefore has no meaning. Compassionate care means finding a way to communicate with a person in a meaningful way, and this starts with validation of the client, their world and their experience.

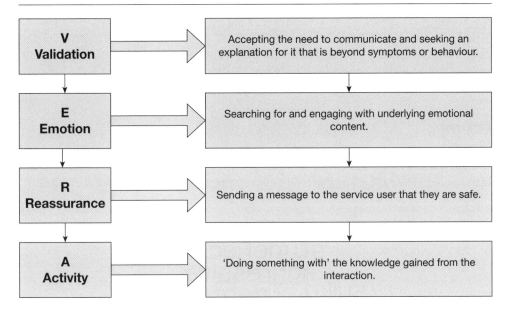

Figure 3.6 VERA acronym.

Validation

Validation is acceptance of the need to communicate with others. In everyday life, we accept that when people, speak, laugh, cry, groan, grunt or whisper they are indicating to the world a desire to communicate with another. This does not change just because someone develops symptoms that prevent clear expression. Validation involves acknowledgement that any behaviour is an attempt to communicate, and compassionate care means that these attempts should be acknowledged, leading to communication in return. Sometimes, when people lose the ability to communicate directly, they may express themselves indirectly by engaging in behaviour that is hard for us to understand. Some people who show signs of confusion may refuse to eat, or rearrange furniture, pace up and down, try to leave home or the care environment, or even play with or smear faeces. These behaviours are both confused (on the part of the service user) and confusing for professionals to understand since they seem beyond the norms of human experience. However, accepting these unusual behaviours as something other than symptoms of mental decline and instead seeing them as means of communication, makes them easier to deal with.

Once this basic validating stance is accepted, it is possible to develop validation further. If a person uses words, noises or behaviours that attract our attention, and we accept communication is occurring, we can begin to find a way to communicate back by seeking to develop a meaning that is associated with the attempt to communicate. This involves applying both self-knowledge and professional interpretation to the attempt to communicate. A client who walks up and down a ward asking for the way out may be expressing a desire to return to somewhere they can recognise; people who spend all day pushing furniture around may be communicating a desire to be occupied; screaming or crying may not be simply symptoms of confusion, but may be a sign of physical or emotional pain. With someone who has periods of lucidity, we may explain what we think and ask for confirmation. Where such an opportunity for the service user to explain does not exist, we may merely reflect back to the person what we observe them doing to let them know that we accept them and are noticing them. Where a person is so closed down that they do not respond to verbal communication, we may just validate a person by standing or sitting close, and using our body language sensitively to letting them know that they exist for us.

Emotion

In all situations, where a level of consciousness remains, communication is underpinned by expression of emotion. The way in which people express emotions is very complex, and language has evolved in a way that reflects this complexity. This is illustrated in Figure 3.7.

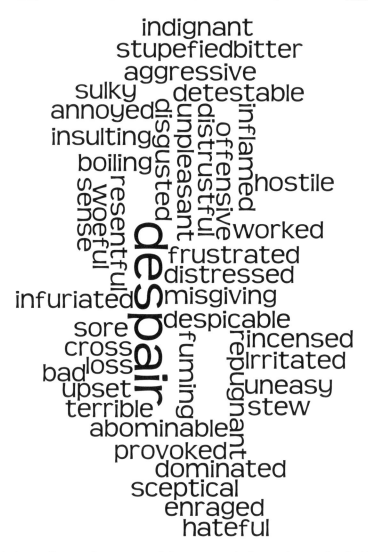

Figure 3.7 Understanding emotions – some of the many words that can be associated with anger

Whether or not it is difficult to connect verbally, trying to understand someone and demonstrating compassion is achievable if we are able to engage emotionally with a person. This process means attempting to understand the emotional message being conveyed by 'tuning in' to it and responding appropriately.

Reading people's emotions is a complicated process that combines subjective and objective activities. We can objectively observe a number of behaviours that commonly indicate a feeling. A facial grimace might indicate pain, a smile may indicate happiness, and a frown may show disapproval. However, our interpretation of these visual cues is both subjective and objective, learned through observing others and the way they show their feelings, and by feeling things for ourselves. In infancy we quickly learn to differentiate friendly and unfriendly faces and the sound of safe and unsafe voices; the process of reading the emotional state of another person helps to keep us away from potential dangers. We learn that an angry person needs a different type of response than a happy one, and we adjust our own behaviour accordingly. As we grow we gather experiences that create deeper feelings within us, and we learn their nature and their effect; sometimes we discover personal feelings that are so significant to us we find ways to avoid feeling them or seek them out more frequently. We also learn that interpreting visual clues is not always enough: tears do not necessarily mean pain, a grimace, as well as a frown, can mean disapproval, and sometimes people smile when they feel like crying. Facial clues combine with tone of voice, body language, familiarity with the person, cultural methods of expression, and the situational context, and these interpretations help us to make judgements about how we should react to another person's emotional state. In short, we use expressions of emotion to communicate and seek out appropriate responses from others. A compassionate and non-judgemental response to an emotion indicates that you are trying to connect with the other person; it shows that their feelings are recognisable to another human being and suggests that the person is not alone.

Reassurance

Reassurance is another response that helps us to connect with a person and has, at its heart, an intention to convey the message that a person is safe while in your care. People who find themselves needing to be looked after, regardless of whether they are confused or not, can feel vulnerable and need to know that those who are meant to care for them have the intention of doing so. Reassurance takes many forms, and is shown through facial expression, body language, adjusting the physical space between you, a carefully considered reassuring touch, holding someone's hand, a hug or a verbal statement. Deciding how to offer reassurance to someone is a matter of careful judgement about what is appropriate, but whatever approach is decided upon the intention is to indicate 'you are safe in our hands' or that 'things can be better than this'. When communication is very confused, the intention of a reassuring action is to let the person know that you have heard, recognised and acknowledged a universal need to feel safe.

Activity

Validating, attending to emotions and offering reassurance are routinely considered part of many approaches to therapy and offer a basic approach to behaving therapeutically with service users, but healthcare practitioners are charged with meeting people's needs when they are unable to do that for themselves. It is for that reason that we include activity as the last step in this process. Communication is an act in itself, but by paying attention to the client through validation, attending to emotions, reassuring them and by carefully observing their responses to us we learn more about what is, and what is not, helpful to them in terms of our communication with them. If one client becomes less agitated for a little while because of the way one member of the care team communicates with them, then the activity would involve doing that more frequently, which means sharing the approach with other members of the team so that they can use the same means of communicating. We may learn, through using VERA, that a service user finds it helpful to keep occupied at certain times of day, and that to improve their experience they need to be given tasks they enjoy doing, or we may learn that we need to take more time to actively reflect on the success or failure of our attempts to help.

The acronym VERA combines three basic communication techniques with a directive to ensure that action emerges as a result of communicating with people. It reflects what many good practitioners do instinctively when working with those in our care and provides a structured way in which to remember the process. The framework is intended to help health-care practitioners remember to ensure that compassion and engagement is at the heart of interactions with clients.

Applying communication skills

Planning an interaction can assist with establishing effective communication. It is not possible to predict how the other person responds or interprets the message and therefore active listening and checking needs to be part of the toolkit. Building a therapeutic relationship needs time and effort in order for trust to be developed. Using who, why, where, when, what and how can aid in planning interactions (Table 3.1).

Table 3.1 Planning communication

WHO	Who are you communicating with? Are there any specific factors that need to be clarified or taken into account? E.g. age, culture, any conditions or genetic disorders that may influence how you communicate?
WHY	What is the purpose of the communication? Is it to gather or give information? Are you trying to understand how the client is feeling or their understanding of what is happening?
WHERE	What is the setting? Do you need to change it? E.g. move the furniture, change the lighting or move to a more appropriate setting to ensure privacy? If you cannot move, how can you modify the communication to ensure privacy?
WHEN	When is the conversation taking place? Is it a good time for the client and taking place across an appropriate time span?
WHAT	What are you communicating and what skills do you need to use? What is the client communicating to you? Are you both interpreting the interaction in the same way?
HOW	What method(s) of communication are being used and are they appropriate for the client?

Models of communication

This chapter has outlined the complexity of communication and how a number of factors come together in any interaction. Communication models can be used to aid effective communication and will take into account the methods and barriers to communication. Most will include the following:

- a sender – who initiates the exchange
- a message – the way the information is to be exchanged
- a medium – the way of passing the message
- a receiver – the person who receives the message
- barriers – factors that affect the delivery of the message.

The models consist of: a linear approach to communication which emphasises sending and receiving, an interactional approach where the receiver responds and sends a message back to the sender, or a transactional approach which includes both people within the interaction communicating simultaneously (DeVito 2013; Beebe *et al.* 2014). More detailed models introduce the context of the communication and factors that can affect the delivery of the message, for example the Circular Transactional Framework of Communication (Bach and Grant 2009). Other models focus on intercultural communication (DeVito 2013). Both transactional and cultural models take into account the individual's self-concept and self-awareness and how these influence how we communicate. Figure 3.8 provides a model of communication which encompasses the range of factors discussed in this chapter. It includes individual characteristics and contextual aspects of communication. In addition it highlights that communication is not always between two individuals but there may be multiple recipients and therefore multiple respondents, and that individuals may communicate to third parties who may feed back to the original sender.

Reflecting on communication

To develop our own skills, reflecting on our experiences and interactions can highlight areas of good practice and areas where skill development is needed, and can point towards appropriate training. As already stated, communication is complex and therefore we need a toolkit of skills to be able to adapt within different situations and with different individuals. There are a number of reflective models available which help to structure reflection whether looking at communication or other aspects of our performance. Reflection can focus on situations that went well and those that did not go so well. O'Toole (2012) provides a specific framework for reflecting on communication when problems occurred.

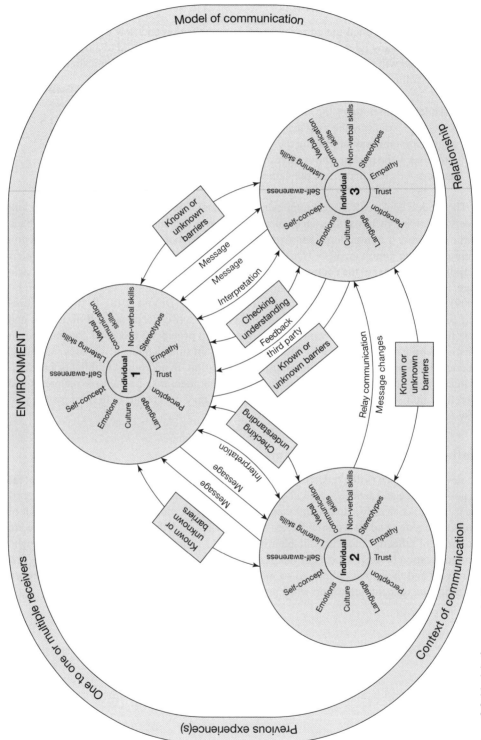

Figure 3.8 Model of communication.

ACTIVITY

The table below sets out O'Toole's questions.

Answer the questions based on a recent interaction.

What did you learn from doing the exercise?

After answering the questions below, consider what the EFFECTIVE COMMUNICATION was during the situation, what could be developed and how?

Questions
What was the purpose of the communicative interaction?
What was I feeling before the interaction?
Was I preoccupied?
Was I focused?
Do I have a fundamental bias relating to this person or situation?
Do I have a past negative history when communicating with the person or in similar situations? If so why?
• When did this interaction start to go wrong? • What was the trigger? • Something that was said? • Something that happened before? • Something the person was already feeling? • Non-verbal? • From who?
How do I feel in response to this event?
What is the cause(s) of these emotions?
What could I have done differently?
What do I do now?
What do I need to do in relation to the other person?
What do I need to do within myself to ensure positive interactions in the future? (Adapted from O'Toole 2012: 47)

Chapter summary

This chapter has provided an outline of communication principles, models and techniques to consider for effective communication.

• Communication is a complex process which needs to take into account both the sender(s) and receiver(s) involved in the interaction and the method(s) of communication.
• Effective communication involves active listening and using techniques to ensure understanding.
• Developing communication skills will aid in the ability to adapt to different clients, situations and settings.

Further resources

MENCAP. Available at: www.mencap.org.uk.
Alzheimer's Society. Available at: www.alzheimers.org.uk.

Further Reading

Kraszewski, S. and McEwen, A., eds. 2010. *Communication Skills for Adult Nurses*. Maidenhead: McGraw Hill.

References

Alzheimer's Society. 2013. *Factsheet 500LP Communicating* [online]. Available at: www.alzheimers. org.uk/site/scripts/download_info.php?fileID=1789 [Accessed 18 November 2014].

Bach, S. and Grant, A. 2009. *Communication & Interpersonal Skills for Nurses*. Exeter: Learning Matters.

Beebe, S. A., Beebe, S. J. and Redmond, M. V. 2014. *Interpersonal Communication: Relating to Others*, 7th edn. Boston, MA: Pearson.

Blackhall, A., Hawkes, D., Hingley, D. and Wood, S. 2011. 'VERA Framework: Communicating with People Who Have Dementia', *Nursing Standard* 26(10): 35–9.

Burnard, P. and Gill, P. 2008. *Culture, Communication and Nursing*. Harlow: Pearson Education.

Department of Health. 2010. *Essence of Care 2010: Benchmarks for the Fundamental Aspects of Care – Benchmarks for Communication* [online]. London: HMSO. Available at: www.gov.uk/government/ uploads/system/uploads/attachment_data/file/216695/dh_119973.pdf [Accessed 18 November 2014].

DeVito, J. 2013. *The Interpersonal Communication Book*, 13th edn. Boston, MA: Pearson.

Dunn, D. and Goodnight, L. J. 2011. *Communication: Embracing Difference*, 4th edn. Boston, MA: Pearson.

Egan, G. 2007. *The Skilled Helper*, 8th edn. Belmont, CA: Thomson.

Emailogic, n.d. *Emailogic Reference Book: How to Get Better Results from Your Email*. Quedgeley: Emailogic.

Francis, R. 2010. *Independent Inquiry into Care Provided by Mid-Staffordshire NHS Foundation Trust* January 2005–March 2009, Volume 1 [online]. Available at: www.midstaffsinquiry.com/assets/docs/ Inquiry_Report-Vol1.pdf [Accessed 7 June 2013].

Goffman, E. 1959 (reprinted 1990). *The Presentation of Self in Everyday Life*. London: Penguin Books.

Hargie, O., Saunders, C. and Dickson, D. 1994. *Social Skills in Interpersonal Communication*, 3rd edn. London: Routledge.

MENCAP. 2010. *Communicating with People with a Learning Disability: A Guide* [online]. Available at: www.mencap.org.uk/sites/default/files/documents/Communicating%20with%20people_updated. pdf [Accessed 18 November 2014].

O'Toole, G. 2012. *Communication: Core Interpersonal Skills for Health Professionals*, 2nd edn. Chatsworth: Churchill Livingstone.

Talktalk, n.d. 'Top Tips for Staying Safe Online: Email Do's and Don'ts' [online]. Available at: http:// help2.talktalk.co.uk/top-tips-staying-safe-online [Accessed 6 January 2015].

Chapter 4

Working in teams

Jayne Crow and Iain John Keenan

LEARNING OUTCOMES

By the end of this chapter you will be able to:

1   Appreciate the importance of effective team working.
2   Understand the importance of effective leadership.
3   Develop the skills to communicate and work effectively with others.

Introduction

When you are part of a workplace team that is working well it can be a joy and when you have colleagues in your team who are good 'team players' it is likely that you recognise them as such and really appreciate them. This chapter does not have all the answers to create effective and happy team working (no one does!). However, it aims to help you reflect on the teams you work in, identify what works and what doesn't work in communication behaviour and importantly consider the ways in which you can enhance your own contribution to help the team function better for the benefit of both staff and service users. When you have worked through this chapter you may wish to explore the subject further by undertaking the exercises produced by Flying Start NHS (2015) which will further develop your team working skills.

Teams differ in many ways. Some are formed for a short time with a particular goal in mind while others are long-standing with long-term goals. The membership of some teams remains stable whilst in others the membership is more fluid. Some teams may consist of staff from different professional backgrounds and specialties and there may also be considerable difference between team members in terms of culture, ethnicity and academic attainment. Leadership within all teams should strive to bridge differences, recognise the strengths and weaknesses of each team member and work to achieve a collaborative and productive working environment for all.

ACTIVITY – TYPES OF TEAMS

Take a moment to think of the various teams you work in and list them in the left-hand column below. It is important to consider the purpose and goal of any team you are part of, so jot down this information in the right-hand column.

Team	Team purpose and goal

Understanding relationships within teams

Within every team there is a hierarchy or 'order' that exists either explicitly (clearly defined roles and responsibilities) or covertly (defined by personalities). Thus there is inevitably a use of power within teams and this may or may not be used benevolently. Team members may be empowered by their colleagues or sometimes power may be misused. It may also be fought for and conflict can arise as a result. Identifying the power and hierarchy within teams is important. Understanding it and working towards ensuring that it is constructive and practical will help towards fostering positive collaborative working relationships. Your working life is peppered with different working relationships (Engleberg and Wynn 2013). Understanding these relationships and the dynamics that exist within them can help you to improve your team working skills and leadership. Look at Figure 4.1 and you will see a variety of different relationships that can exist within a team environment.

People to whom you report

Think of people that you directly report to. This could be a manager, supervisor or senior staff member. What works well within this relationship? What problems do you encounter within this relationship? It may be that if you consider the issue of power within this relationship it may appear uneven in that the person you report to seems to have it all. They get to tell you what to do and when to do it. One of the most frequent problems in this relationship is the feeling of disempowerment and the perception that you are not being heard. You might think that your views don't count and that it is a one-way relationship. It doesn't have to be that way.

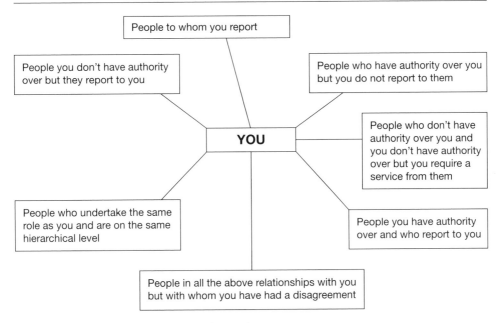

Figure 4.1 Some possible power relationships within teams.

People who have authority over you but you do not report to them

There may be people who have authority over you but to whom you do not directly report. They may be in charge of certain aspects of a role or have a different professional responsibility and occupy a senior position to you. These relationships can be very important to you. If handled inappropriately you may sometimes feel patronised and as if there is a struggle to gain control. Sometimes you may feel that your opinion is not considered or that it is overlooked. Again, it does not have to be this way.

People who do not have authority over you and you don't have authority over but you require a service from them

Relationships such as this are common in health and social care and can arise when we need to refer service users to other services, transfer their care or when staff from other professional agencies come to see our service users. You may feel that you can communicate well within this type of relationship or you may feel you struggle to be heard and get your views across.

People you don't have authority over but they report to you

We all have people that may report to us. This could be students, carers and even relatives. Listening is a key skill in our interactions with this group of people. If they feel they cannot approach you, you may miss out on vital information. However, sometimes such people may be labelled as 'demanding' of our time which is reflected in our non-verbal behaviour to them (see Chapter 5: Valuing people) and causes frustration for both parties. Awareness of these communication dynamics may help you to manage these encounters more effectively.

People who undertake the same role as you and are on the same hierarchical level

These relationships have the potential to cause a lot of competition (but also foster some of the best team working) as we continually compare and contrast our work and output with these colleagues. We have a tendency to judge these relationships in terms of the other person '*pulling their weight*'. When we feel we are contributing more or less equally, camaraderie may build which makes team working enjoyable and fulfilling. However, if we feel we contribute more to the team than these people, resentment and anger can take hold and this may start to show in our interactions with them. They may not perceive the situation in the same way!

People you have authority over and who report to you

When we have authority over colleagues it is most important that we are self-aware and reflect on the way in which we interact with them. Overly 'bossy' or disrespectful behaviour is, of course, likely to be resented by those lower down in a hierarchy and taking into account how our communications are received may help us communicate more effectively and gain willing cooperation from those who report to us. To be liked by others is a common human need. To what degree we feel that need varies from person to person. This need can potentially make these types of relationships difficult. We may worry about delegating in fear that the other person will form adverse judgments about us. If we are worried about delegating then we tend to take on the roles ourselves – often overworking ourselves and causing increased anxiety.

People in all the above relationships with whom you have had a disagreement

It is very rare, in any working environment, that we will not 'fall out' with someone at some point. Sometimes there are clear reasons apparent to both parties, sometimes only one party may be clear as to the reasons. We need to be clear that behaviour directed towards another person that is harmful, derogatory, excluding or abusive is deemed as bullying and there are strict policies in all organisations to tackle this. Bullying aside, there are still low-level disagreements that rarely get resolved and lead to long-term resentment and disharmony within a team. Staff may choose to work in isolation rather than with the person they have fallen out with. They check rotas or work allocations to see if they are due to work with that person and change if they are. All these unresolved broken relationships have a huge impact on the team, as sides are taken, and ultimately it is the service user who suffers. Individuals need to recognise the damage that is caused by these broken relationships and seek resolutions.

Reflection and developing empathy with colleagues

One of the key skills that you will need in all the above relationships is empathy. You need to imagine yourself in the shoes of your colleagues and reflect on what they are thinking and feeling. For example, you may feel powerless in the relationship but maybe they do too. Or you may feel that they do not listen to you but maybe they feel the same way.

This approach is not a panacea for all problems in teams but it is a good start and may open a route for constructive dialogue between team members.

Communication within teams

ACTIVITY

Consider the many different types of communication behaviours that take place between individuals within teams. Add your ideas to the spider diagram. We have started you off with a couple of ideas:

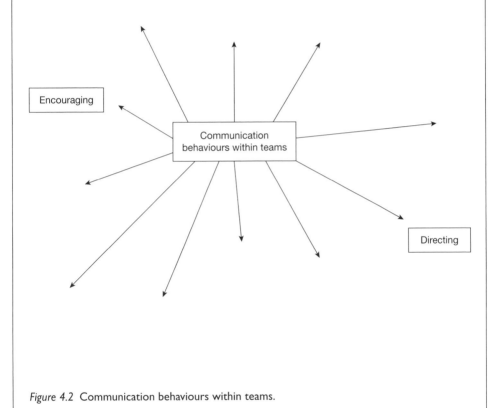

Figure 4.2 Communication behaviours within teams.

Here is a list of types of communication behaviours that you may have included:

Challenging
Influencing
Persuading
Informing
Praising
Advising
Enquiring/seeking information.

There may well be some less desirable ones too! For example:

Point scoring
Bossing
Humiliating
Embarrassing.

As you will have gathered, the types of communication behaviours within teams are many and varied and some are more conducive to good team working than others. In the next part of this chapter we will concentrate on ways to help you contribute to good communication in your team.

Strategies for improving communication in teams

One of the most common causes of friction within teams and between teams is the tendency for each of us to become defensive when we perceive that someone is criticising us. It may be that the other party does not intend to criticise, what matters is that we jump to the conclusion that the remark is an attack and we go into 'defence' mode.

Scenario:
Person A: This has not been done properly.
Person B: Well that is not my fault it was like that when I arrived.

Sometimes we decide that attack is the best form of defence!

Person A: This has not been done properly.
Person B: Well it was your job to see that it was done right.

It is easy to see how this type of exchange can turn into a cycle of mutual blame and recrimination.

Person A: This has not been done properly.
Person B: Well it was your job to see that it was done right.
Person A: Actually it is your fault for not checking when you first arrived.
Person B: I can't be checking everything just because you are not doing your job!

Exchanges like this do damage to teamwork (even if they are thought or said behind each other's back). In fact they usually do very little to improve the situation and often the task that has not been done properly becomes lost in the bitter personal exchange rather than being the focus of a conversation about improving the situation. Both sides have probably stopped listening to anything the other has to say.

Non-defensive communication

We are all human and no one is saying that we can all communicate perfectly with each other all the time, but here is a strategy that you can try to make sure you minimise defensiveness on your own part and maybe even stop the downward spiral in such situations. The strategy is called non-defensive communication.

There are many different versions of non-defensive communication presented by a myriad of different authors which you can explore in the further reading suggestions. However, many will include the five main communication behaviours involved in non-defensive communication that we present below as worthy of your consideration. They can be utilised separately but are probably most effective if employed together. Below, you will find the five behaviours applied to the example exchange outlined above between PERSONS A and B.

- **Step back**. If you are PERSON B take a moment to think before you snap back an answer. If you are angry, recognise the fact and if possible wait until you calm down before responding. This will make it easier to do the following:
- **Empathise**. Try to put yourself in PERSON A's shoes. How are they feeling and why? Understanding their point of view makes it easier to respond positively.
- **Depersonalise**. Try not to take the comment as a personal attack. In this example it may be a statement of fact that 'the task has not been done properly'. You may even agree that it has not been done correctly. Concentrate on this aspect of the communication rather than any personal affront.
- **Disclose**. Sometimes people don't realise the effect their remarks have on us. In this example, PERSON A may not realise that we (PERSON B) pride ourselves on carrying out such tasks well and that their remark will wound our sense of professionalism. 'Disclosing' means pointing out gently how you feel when they made this remark. This should not be another chance to blame them but more an explanation of how you feel:

  Person A: You have not done that properly.
  Person B: I feel very upset when you say that.

- **Enquire**. Rather than snap back defensively ask for more information that will lead toward finding a solution:

  Person A: This has not been done properly.
  Person B: How often does this happen? Is there some way of improving the way this is done?

So there are steps you can take to become less defensive and they are worth trying. However, I can hear you saying, 'What about PERSON A?' Perhaps they should look at the effect of their initial remark. You are right. Giving criticism in the most effective way takes some thought too.

Offering constructive criticism

ACTIVITY

Below are two comments on a written report. Decide which comment is the most useful and why?

A: 'The report you have written is hopeless.'
B: 'The introduction of your report sets the scene well but the second part needs more detail about the incident and particularly about the consequences. It would be useful to include dates and times.'

It is likely that you said B was of more use than A. This is because A is simply critical whereas B contains 'constructive criticism'.

A tells us the report is not good enough but gives no indication of why or what we should do about it. It leaves us disheartened and/or angry.

B also tells us the report is not good enough but points out what we have done well and gives a clear indication as to what we should do to improve it. It leaves us less annoyed and more equipped to make the required improvements.

So when you are offering judgement on a colleague's work, whether it is written or practical, make sure your criticism is constructive. You will generally get a better response.

Avoiding blame culture

Giving constructive criticism is just one way of trying to change behaviour and it is behaviour worth cultivating. The examples given above show the effect of individuals 'blaming' each other rather than tackling the issue at hand. This type of behaviour may happen across whole organisations and even between organisations and can lead to what is often termed a 'blame culture'. Huge amounts of time and energy may be put into identification of a 'guilty party' and mutual recriminations. It may be useful to know where things went wrong so that they can be put right but unfortunately in a 'blame culture' people are more likely to cover up their mistakes than own them and learn from them.

However, there is often a wider problem of a 'blame culture' in many workplaces and one that has been highlighted in several reports on the NHS. *The Berwick Review into Patient Safety Report* (Department of Health 2013a) made it quite clear that a shift in leadership behaviour across the NHS was required from behaviour that used blame as a tool in trying to improve care.

Influencing other people's behaviour in teams

Our most powerful way of changing someone else's behaviour is to change our own.

Therefore it is worth trying the following:

- **Reflexivity** – this is the ability to look at your own behaviour and the motivation and attitudes that underpin it. Asking what we did and why may help us empathise with and understand the actions of others.
- **Listening** – don't jump to conclusions about what someone is saying. Actively listen to them and perhaps seek clarification before reacting.
- **Praising** – no matter what our role, we all thrive on praise. All too often we let good work by others slip by without comment but are quick to criticise or point out when things go wrong. So make a point of praising good work when you see it.
- **Challenging** – since the NHS Constitution (Department of Health 2013b) we have a 'Duty of Candour' so we are obliged to challenge poor practice if we see it. However this needs to be done in a way that maintains the dignity of the colleague we are challenging. Remember that we are more likely to change a person's behaviour if they understand the challenge and trust our motivation for raising the issue.
- **Supporting** – feeling part of a team can be most rewarding and satisfaction can be gained from helping out colleagues and accepting help from them when needed. Building reciprocal support systems within teams builds cooperation and trust.

Role modelling

Role modelling is another powerful way of influencing teamwork. Most of us can think of someone we have worked with whose work we have admired. It may be they had a particular practical skill or handled a difficult situation successfully or demonstrated particularly good communication skills. They may or may not have been aware that they were acting as an example for us. Whatever it was and whenever it happened we made a mental note to emulate them and to try to act in the same way when it was our turn to be in that situation. This is an example of role modelling in action. Bear in mind that within a team you can learn in this way from your colleagues but equally you can act as a role model too. Keep this in mind and try to be a positive role model to anyone who crosses your path.

Whistleblowing

'Whistleblowing' is when a worker reports suspected wrongdoing at work. Officially this is called 'making a disclosure in the public interest' (Gov.UK 2014).

It is probable that if you work in health or social care for any length of time you will see a lot of good practice but it is sadly also the case that at some point you will meet with poor practice and maybe even dangerous or illegal practice. It is at this point that your professionalism will be tested and you are obliged to act to stop or prevent further wrongdoing even though this may be difficult for a variety of reasons. For example, if the wrongdoing involves your team and colleagues you may feel you are betraying your colleagues in some way or you may fear retribution from them or from the organisation. These are very understandable concerns but they will not excuse a lack of action on your part. Elsewhere in this book we have discussed the need to act as an advocate for the patient when necessary and the Francis Report (Francis 2013) has all too clearly identified the dire consequences of ignoring and/or covering up wrongdoing. There will be line management and local formal channels that you should utilise to stop and prevent future wrongdoing where possible and your organisation will have its own whistleblowing policy, but if these fail you or you are in any doubt as to what you should do it is important to seek independent and unbiased advice as to how to proceed. This can be easily obtained at the Whistleblowing Helpline where advice is free, confidential and anonymous.

Keeping quiet and hoping that someone else will tackle the issue is not an option.

Tribalism related to teams

In our everyday lives we become part of many groups. Groups like this come in all forms and sizes. Some are formal, some are informal. Some are work related, some leisure related and some geographically based. Many of these groups would consider themselves to be teams. Writers on social interaction have been known to describe these groups as 'tribes' in order to help us understand how they influence our behaviour and how the groups may interact.

Below are examples of 'tribes' in this sense of the word:

- The 'Residents of a particular road or block of flats' tribe.
- The 'Parents who wait for their children outside the gate of a certain school at 3.30 pm every school day' tribe.
- The 'Participants of the Thursday evening aerobics class' tribe.

- The 'Rehabilitation Unit staff' tribe.
- The 'Public Health Foundation degree' tribe.
- The 'Accident and Emergency' tribe.
- The 'Night staff' tribe.

ACTIVITY

What tribes are you in? Write down as many tribes as you can think of that you feel you belong to. Then underline those related to your work.

You will notice that you can be a member of many different 'tribes' at the same time. For the purposes of this chapter we will focus on work-related tribes which may take the form of teams but may be much looser.

As a student you may move between workplaces and will therefore be temporary members of a variety of work tribes. Each tribe will have its own ways of working and maybe even its own language in the form of particular jargon and abbreviations. When a new member of staff joins the workplace they have to learn to 'fit in' with 'the tribe'. Along with learning what they have to do in their role in this new environment they learn the customs and practices of the 'tribe'. They learn the way the tribe works and the relationships within the tribe and between this tribe and others they come into contact with. This will often include generally agreed stereotypes (see Chapter 5: Valuing people), maybe positive but often negative, of these other tribes. Some of this learning takes place through watching and listening and some by direct instruction and 'tips' given by longer-standing members of the tribe. This is a process of 'socialisation' into the tribe. During this process the new staff member takes on many of the behaviours and attitudes of the 'tribe'. As can be seen in the case study below this can have both useful and harmful effects.

CASE STUDY

Staff at Health Centre A (TRIBE A) generally dislike the staff at Health Centre B (TRIBE B) even though they have never met any of the staff and only ever speak to one or two receptionists there on the telephone. They have a very negative stereotype of Health Centre B as a whole and when it is mentioned there is general negativity and criticism in all their comments. They usually warn new staff or students joining their own Health Centre, that Health Centre B is difficult to deal with and offers an inferior service.

Whenever a member of Health Centre A staff has to ring Health Centre B they are already prepared for a poor response and often go into the conversation 'ready for a battle'.

Staff at Health Centre B feel exactly the same about Health Centre A staff and behave in the same way.

ACTIVITY

Write down a list of the probable consequences of the situation in the case study above.

Table 4.1 Positive and negative aspects of being in a 'tribe'

Positive aspects of being in a tribe	Negative aspects of being in a tribe
It increases camaraderie – it feels good to be included.	Stereotypes members of other tribes.
Seems easier – each member can adopt tribe behaviours and tribe likes and dislikes without thinking for themselves.	Being stereotyped yourself by the members of the other tribe.
It seems to help with group cohesion to have a common 'enemy' in the form of another 'tribe'.	Cease to see the individuals in the other 'tribe' or to try to get to know them as individuals.
	Promotes a lack of understanding of each other's role.
	MOST IMPORTANTLY: hinders or closes down communication between the 'tribes'.
	Reflects badly on both 'tribes' when the animosity is noticed by service users.

It is likely that communication between the two health centres will be affected in the following ways:

- Self-fulfilling prophecy. Staff from each health centre will be unwelcoming and unhelpful in response to any communication from the other. Each will see the other as acting in their usual predictable way.
- Defensive communication (see above).
- Minimal communication between the health centres. Staff from each will avoid contact with the other.
- Poor service user service/possible dangerous miscommunication. Information that should be shared will not be communicated between the health centres and this will disadvantage their patients.
- Service users will pick up on the negativity relating to each team and it is likely to undermine their trust in both.

So as you can see, tribalism is by no means the benign influence in teams that it may at first seem. Table 4.1 outlines the positive and negative aspects of being in a 'tribe' and as you can see there are many pitfalls. Being aware of these and working against the negative influences will enhance the way your team interacts with other teams.

Collaboration

Health and social care these days is generally a complex undertaking and a person's care will rarely be undertaken by one person or profession. If you have ever been on the receiving end of health and social care you will know only too well the importance of collaboration between all the individual professionals, teams, departments and organisations involved in your care. Failure in communication between these parties is one of the most common causes of complaints, and failure of the professionals to communicate and collaborate effectively with the patient and/or their relatives often renders care ineffective or even dangerous (see Chapter 3: Communication for a related discussion of this subject).

Leadership in teams

> There is no 'I' in 'Team' but there is in 'Leadership'.

So far we have considered working in teams and identified some key components and strategies to consider. Uses of power and authority have been mentioned but now we turn our attention to focus on leadership issues.

Within any team, effective leadership is required for that team to have a clear sense of purpose and direction. Too often we believe that leadership is someone else's responsibility and we think that other people are better placed to lead. Whilst we have recognised that to be successful at work we must be members of a team, we rarely recognise the need for ourselves to lead and take up a leadership role within those teams. We tend to think of managers and senior staff as the leaders but in fact we all have leadership within us. We all play a part in guiding and directing the work of others and we can all directly affect the work of others through our actions and words. It is rarely the service users who directly cause us to become frustrated with our working lives but the action, or inaction, of the people we work with. With this in mind we need to understand that if we are to successfully care for our service users we have to build strong and effective teams and we have to develop and encourage effective leadership from all team members (Engleberg and Wynn 2013).

Leadership and management

Whilst there are expectations that managers lead, not all managers are effective leaders and not all effective leaders are actually managers. Good effective leadership has become a key theme in recent years, highlighted specifically within the report of Robert Francis QC (2013). In the report in Chapter 24, Leadership in healthcare it specifically states:

> Good leadership must be visible, receptive, insightful and outward looking. Leadership and managerial skills are not the same but both are required. Leadership skills are required to be shared at all levels in an organisation, from board to ward, and all staff must be empowered to use their own judgement in providing the best possible care for patients.
>
> (Francis 2013, Vol. 3: 1545)

It is clear from the report that poor leadership can lead to poor care and that good, effective leadership is at the heart of proactive, responsive and collaborative care.

ACTIVITY – LEADERSHIP SKILLS

Effective leaders possess key attributes. These attributes are clearly evident in their practice; in the way they communicate and through the decisions they take.

Here is a list of positive and negative skills and attributes. See if you can identify which are which and place them in the correct column.

Knowledgeable	*Vindictive*	*Consistent*	*Dishonest*
Selfish	*Honest*	*Hypocritical*	*Indecisive*
Recognises own limitations	*Supportive*	*Favouritism*	*Flexible*
Blaming			

Positive attributes	Negative attributes

How did you do? The table below shows our answers.

Positive attributes	Negative attributes
Knowledgeable	Indecisive
Recognises own limitations	Favouritism
Honest	Selfish
Supportive	Vindictive
Flexible	Hypocritical
Consistent	Dishonest
	Blaming

Bearing in mind what we said earlier in this chapter about role modelling, think of two people who you have worked with, one who you consider to be a good leader and one who you consider a poor leader. Consider whether any of the attributes listed above contribute to the quality of their leadership. The list of positive attributes of an effective leader is obviously longer than that listed above. What other attributes do you think the person you identified as an effective leaders possesses? List them in the table below.

Positive skills and attributes

Of all the attributes that we listed, including those you have added, how many do you think that you possess?

REFLECTION POINT

Make lists of the attributes you have and the ones you think you need to acquire.

What will you need to do to develop these attributes?

Look at the exercises in Chapter 5: Valuing people and you will see the similarities between the skills needed by us all to value people generally and those needed for good and effective leadership.

It is incumbent upon us all to develop these attributes by constant self-awareness and self-reflection and the more responsibility we assume in our professional life the more we need to develop and role model these attributes.

Recognising burnout in our colleagues

It would not be right to complete this chapter without mentioning the necessity of health and social care professionals to extend their caring attitude and behaviour to their colleagues.

Working in a team should mean that the members of the team act in a generally supportive way towards their colleagues in order to give the best possible service to the service user. This is enshrined in many codes of professional conduct including that of the NMC (2015). This will often mean looking out for our colleagues and being aware of whether they are showing signs of extreme or long-standing stress. There is a considerable literature on the possible stressful effect of long-term caring known as 'burnout'.

ACTIVITY

Which of the following is a definition of burnout?

A. A complete mental breakdown.
B. A condition suffered by long-serving staff who have become bored with their job.
C. An emotional condition marked by tiredness, loss of interest, or frustration that interferes with job performance. Burnout is usually regarded as the result of prolonged stress.

The correct answer is C.

ACTIVITY

Which of the following are possible manifestations of burnout? Circle your answers:

a generally negative attitude

difficulty focusing on work

depression

being fatigued all of the time

becoming irritable easily

problems with concentration

a general emotional detachment from your patients and colleagues

high blood pressure

chronic headaches

gastrointestinal problems

back pain

All of the above and many other symptoms may be signs of burnout so it can be a difficult condition to identify both in ourselves and in our colleagues.

Being alert to negative changes in your colleagues' behaviour and/or to the symptoms listed above may enable you to alert them to your concerns and may even prevent deterioration in the service the team provides to the service user.

We are in the caring professions and a team will work better if we extend this caring to our team members.

Chapter summary

- You are likely to belong to many different types of team with different purposes and goals.
- Within teams the hierarchy and relationships will vary but the way in which we utilise our power within teams will influence the effectiveness of the team.
- We all influence the effective working of our team by our use of communication skills and strategies.
- Non-defensive communication, the giving of constructive feedback and the use of positive communication are skills worth practising and can enhance team working.
- Blame culture and the adverse effects of 'tribalism' are counterproductive in teams.
- Effective collaboration between professionals, teams and organisations is essential to the provision of good health and social care.
- Leadership is not just a skill for managers. We can all take some leadership responsibility within our team.
- Good communication behaviour is a key to both good team membership and to good leadership.

• Looking out for the welfare of both patients and colleagues is the responsibility of all team members.

Further resources

The Leadership Academy. Available at: www.leadershipacademy.nhs.uk/resources/healthcare-leadership-model/ [Accessed 10 January 2015].
Skills for Health. Available at: www.skillsforhealth.org.uk/ [Accessed 10 January 2015].

Further reading

Potter, B. 2004. *Overcoming Job Burnout: How to Renew Enthusiasm for Work*. Oakland, IL: Ronin.
Thompson, N. 2009. *People Skills*, 3rd edn. Aldershot: Palgrave Macmillan.
Worth, R. 2009. *Communication Skills*, 3rd edn. New York: Ferguson.

References

Department of Health. 2013a. *The Berwick Review into Patient Safety Report*. London: HMSO.
Department of Health. 2013b. *The NHS Constitution* [online]. London. HMSO. Available at: www.gov.uk/government/publications/the-nhs-constitution-for-england [Accessed 10 January 2015].
Engleberg, I. N. and Wynn, D. R. 2013. *Think Communication*, 2nd edn. London: Pearson.
Flying Start NHS. 2015. *Teamworking* [online]. Available at: www.flyingstart.scot.nhs.uk/learning-programmes/teamwork/teamworking/ [Accessed 10 January 2015].
Francis, R. 2013. *Report of the Mid Staffordshire NHS Foundation Trust Public Inquiry* [online]. Available at: www.midstaffspublicinquiry.com/report [Accessed 10 January 2015].
Gov.UK. 2014. *Whistleblowing* [online]. Available at www.gov.uk [Accessed 10 January 2015].
NMC. 2015. *The Code: Standards of Conduct, Performance and Ethics for Nurses and Midwives* [online]. London: NMC. Available at: www.nmc-uk.org [Accessed 23 April 2015].
Whistleblowing Helpline. Available at: www.wbhelpline.org.uk [Accessed 10 January 2015].

Chapter 5

Valuing people: Fostering dignity and respect

Vicki Elliott and Jayne Crow

LEARNING OUTCOMES

By the end of this chapter you will be able to:

1 Explore the concepts of dignity, respect, culture, ethics, diversity, discrimination and prejudice.
2 Explore your own values and attitudes.
3 Reflect on how these impact on your practice in health and social care.

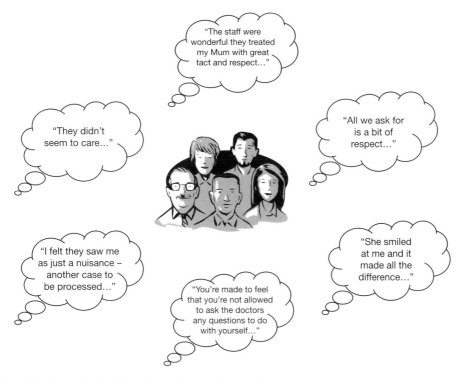

Figure 5.1 Your attitude affects the service user's experience.

Introduction

One of the most frequent sources of both complaint and praise from NHS patients concerns staff 'attitude' to them. It really matters to people not only what happens to them in the care system but the way in which people behave towards them and the attitudes they convey by that behaviour.

REFLECTION POINT

Are you able to identify with these experiences?

Think about a time when you were affected by someone's attitude to you.

How did it make you feel?

How could it have been avoided?

Valuing people as individuals and caring for them as such is essential to anyone working in the health and social care arena. This respectful attitude is not an optional extra but is at the very core of the helping professions. In this chapter we will look in more detail at this issue and at the ways in which we can enhance this aspect of the service we give. We will consider the reasons why we do not always succeed in delivering something that we and the public think is so easy.

This involves reflecting on our own thoughts and feelings and consequent behaviour. Whatever your job title, stage of training, status or role, valuing people and fostering dignity and respect will always need self-awareness to keep it at the top of everyone's agenda where it belongs.

The essence of this chapter is to explore some of the key concepts which influence how we care for the individual in health and social care and how we relate to our colleagues. Understanding the ethical principles; challenging our attitudes to discrimination, stereotyping and prejudice; and enhancing our knowledge of diversity and cultural difference will ultimately impact on the way we practice, our individual learning and our own development. This understanding will also impact on the way in which we make decisions and address conflicts, dilemmas and tensions. This chapter is about how we treat others and how we expect to be treated by others.

Values, attitudes and culture

The way in which others perceive our behaviour is often related to our attitude and how we communicate. Our attitude towards something expresses how it makes us feel and this can influence the way we behave in a particular situation.

Whether you have direct patient contact or not, health and social care practice involves making choices about how to deal with other people and therefore involves values. This is true of all professions, and indeed all human activities. Your personal values also affect the way in which you do your job so it is important to understand what your values are and where they come from.

What do we mean by 'values'?

Our values relate to things which are important to us, things which have significance or worth. A value system is a term that refers to a set of principles, standards or beliefs, relating to things of ultimate importance.

The word can be used in a number of ways. Value is often seen as a measure of the financial worth of a commodity such as the price of gold. This is usually higher than the price of silver and therefore gold is considered to be more valuable. You may be familiar with Oscar Wilde's (2012) phrase 'knowing the price of everything but the value of nothing' which suggests that valuing something by its financial worth alone is misplaced. Value can also refer to something that we appreciate in terms of what it means to us personally, for instance 'I value your company'. What we are saying here is that the time you spent with me made a difference and I consider that to be important. Values held by groups of people are often culturally or politically based, for instance, Christian values, Islamic values or liberal values. Just as personal values differ, so do cultural values. They may be such things as family loyalty, freedom, justice or religious observance but which of these is considered the most important may vary between cultural groups.

Culture can be a challenge to valuing people, just as cultural awareness can promote respect. Knowledge, understanding and communication can break down barriers but there is a need for participation and commitment from both sides. Cultural awareness can no longer be defined by country as we now live in a multicultural society, so in order to create this awareness there is a need to develop cultural sensitivity.

How are our values and attitudes formed?

Values and attitudes are shaped by experience which may be a personal experience or an observed experience.

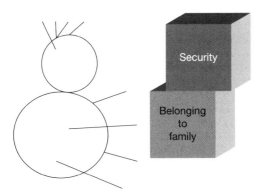

Our values begin to develop with influences from our family, our culture and our upbringing

Figure 5.2 Our family and upbringing are the foundations for our values.

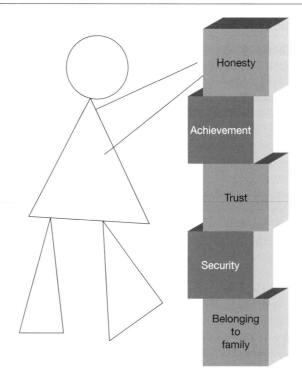

Figure 5.3 We develop our own value system through education and experience.

ACTIVITY – IDENTIFYING YOUR CORE VALUES

Consider the list of commonly held values in the table below.

Are these values important to you?

Are there any you would add or delete?

In the third column try to place each value in order of its importance to you.

Discuss your choices with friends and family. Reflect upon the similarities and differences.

Values	Add/delete	Prioritise
Belonging to family		
Trustworthiness		
Honesty		
Integrity		
Fairness		
Compassion		

Confidentiality		
Courtesy		
Friendship		
Loyalty		
Autonomy		
Freedom		

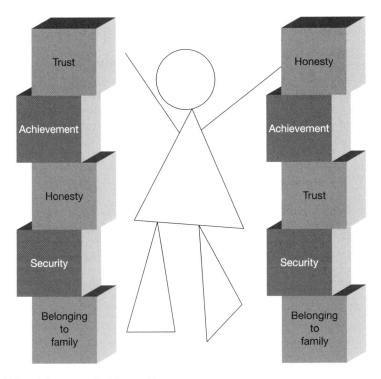

Figure 5.4 Values inform our decision-making.

The order in which we place our values may change depending on the situation we find ourselves in (see Figure 5.4). When faced with a dilemma we need to decide between different courses of action and although it is useful to know the facts, our choice will be based on our personal preferences. These choices are known as value-based judgements.

ACTIVITY

In the following scenarios you are presented with a series of choices. Think about how you would decide what choice to make in each case, and ask yourself what set of values you would base your choice upon:

1   You are buying a new school uniform for your son. You have a choice between two ranges of similar quality: one is more expensive because the company pays a good price to the factory workers, the other is cheaper because the company pays the minimum rate possible to the workers. Which range do you choose from?

2   You are a manager of a small department with three staff. One of your staff, Anne, is very able and efficient, works hard, contributes ideas and has a sparkling personality. The other two are inexperienced and although enthusiastic need their colleague to organise their activities and keep them on task. There are a series of minor thefts within the neighbouring departments and you discover that Anne is responsible. You have a significant project to complete and Anne is the key to the department's success. How do you handle the situation?

These scenarios demonstrate how the order in which we prioritise our values may change depending on the situation we are faced with. In scenario 1, are you willing to forego the ability to make another purchase in order to support your value of fairness to the factory workers? In scenario 2, if you believe that theft is a serious crime it implies that honesty is high up in your hierarchy of values. In this situation does that override the value you place on meeting targets and achieving a good outcome for your employer? Our actions have consequences in terms of how people regard us. Does what others think about you also have a place in your value system?

The way you handle this incident will have consequences for the future, particularly if you decide not to act. Does this mean that by compromising your values in this dilemma your values would change?

It is clear that our values may be challenged in certain situations and the hierarchy of values may change. Our actions are influenced by our values and facing a dilemma can make us examine and reassess our personally held values.

In any given situation, therefore, we need to decide which principle or standard is the most important. Here are some values and approaches about the appropriate way to treat service users:

• promoting anti-discriminatory practice
• maintaining confidentiality of information
• promoting and supporting individuals' rights to dignity, independence and safety
• acknowledging individuals' personal beliefs and identity
• protecting individuals from abuse
• promoting effective communication and relationships
• providing individualised care
• keeping them safe from harm.

This value system applies equally to the patients we serve and the staff we work alongside.

The importance of valuing people

Muir Gray (2006) suggests that the patient or client is moving through a disease journey, a healthcare journey and an emotional journey. How they face their journey and the choices they make depend upon the information they are given, but also on their personal values and beliefs. Listening to and acknowledging the service user's point of view can help us understand their experience and show that we value them as individuals. Each patient or client is a unique individual, not a medical condition nor social care problem.

Dignity

Whether you are in a clinical role or not it is important to have an understanding of what dignity means in practice, both in terms of how service users are cared for and how you relate to each other in the working environment. Understanding what dignity means to you will enable you to promote it.

Defining the term

The definition of dignity used by the Social Care Institute for Excellence (SCIE) (2010) is:

> A state or manner worthy of esteem or respect; and (by extension) self-respect. Dignity in care therefore means the kind of care, in any setting which supports and promotes, and does not undermine, a person's self-respect regardless of any difference. . .
>
> (PRIAE/Help the Aged 2001)

It is generally assumed that the concept of dignity is understood by all healthcare staff and furthermore that they know what is necessary to promote it within their services. The word 'dignity' is rooted in the Latin *dignitas* meaning the state of being worthy of honour or respect. This is a simple and succinct definition but dignity is one of those concepts which can be better understood when reflecting on what makes people feel undignified, vulnerable, humiliated, and inadequate or undervalued.

ACTIVITY

Explore what the terms dignity and respect mean to you as a healthcare user.

Think of an occasion when you felt that your dignity was compromised or that you were disrespected. How did that make you feel?

Think of an occasion when you felt your dignity was upheld. How did that make you feel?

Reflect on incidences in your workplace when you or your colleagues may have upheld the dignity of OR disrespected a fellow worker. How did that make you feel?

Your responses to these questions are likely to fall into two categories. First, dignity is a feature of our behaviour and the way in which we treat each other. You may have noted comments such as 'She was treated with dignity' or 'He was made to feel undervalued'. Second, dignity is linked to our self-esteem and our perception of our self-worth. Your comments may include examples such as 'I felt respected and important' or 'I felt humiliated and embarrassed'.

We have established that dignity can be challenging to define but each of us expects to be treated with dignity and can describe situations when that has not happened. In addition dignity can also describe an individual's behaviour, for instance, 'She reacted in a dignified manner'. It is important to remember that even when a patient or client acts in an undignified manner it is our duty to treat them with dignity.

ACTIVITY

With reference to the previous activity, are you able to identify some of the reasons why it can be challenging to treat individuals with dignity and respect?

Many of the challenges faced in treating people with dignity and respect relate to our awareness and understanding. Acknowledging that individuals have differing expectations of care, differing values and attitudes, differing backgrounds and cultural beliefs is a good foundation for enhancing our ability to treat others with dignity and respect. Other barriers could include challenging behaviour, a workplace culture of disrespect, or a busy or unrealistic workload.

The right to be treated with dignity and respect was established in the Declaration on the Promotion of Patient Rights in Europe (World Health Organization 1994) and this informs professional codes of practice in the NHS. There is an assumption that we have a moral duty to respect those in our care, our colleagues and in fact all people we come into contact with.

What is respect?

The Concise Oxford Dictionary (Stevenson and Waite 2011) defines the word 'respect' as 'paying attention to; honouring; avoid damaging; treating with consideration and not offending'. Respect may be considered to describe how dignity works in practice. Therefore, dignity is promoted by the level of respect given to, but not limited to, such things as an individual's values, beliefs, rights and freedoms, capabilities and limitations, culture, preferences and self-esteem.

The importance of respecting dignity

In health and social care environments the service user may find themselves in a vulnerable position and fear losing their dignity. When they need to access these services they are often unwell and may be asked to expose intimate parts of their bodies or find their feelings under scrutiny. It is precisely because of this lack of privacy and the intrusive nature of some services that users are acutely aware of their dignity and it is important that this is recognised and protected by all health and social care workers. The level at which people perceive their self-esteem is related to their well-being so ensuring service users are treated with dignity and respect is essential to good-quality care and service delivery.

Fuller (2008: 6) warns that:

> People routinely violate others' dignity in large and small ways, throughout the world. When people's dignity is not respected, negative feelings and unhealthy consequences result, for individuals and society.

This is exactly what the CEO of Patient Opinion, Paul Hodgkin, meant when he said that '. . . every member of staff has it in their power to improve the experience of their patients. . .' (2011). Our values such as upholding dignity, honesty, kindness and trust can be converted into acts which respect dignity such as listening, empathising and compassion.

ACTIVITY

Think of three things you could do to show respect for someone's dignity. Try to carry them out within the next week.

Reflect on how it made you feel and what impact you think it may have had on the individuals involved.

Ethics

The relationship the health and social care practitioner has with the service user is a privileged one and is based on a specific ethical code of behaviour.

An introduction to ethics

Ethics is the study of moral behaviour. It is concerned with questions of right and wrong and helps us to understand what is good and what is bad. It is a system of moral principles concerned with how people ought to act, what is good for society and how individuals lead a good life.

In some texts morals and ethics are treated as synonymous but there is a basic difference. Morals are personal principles, based on our values, whereas ethics define a social system of generally accepted standards of behaviour. A person's moral code may change with new experiences but is centred on what an individual believes to be right or wrong. The ethics he or she practises can be dependent on other factors such as current Codes of Conduct and tend to be more stable.

It is important to study ethics in the health and social care context so that we can provide appropriate care and protect the sick and the vulnerable. It is also important that we understand ethical principles when applied to making decisions, particularly in instances which rely on the individuals' personal integrity.

The purpose of studying ethics is so that we are able to identify what is regarded as right and wrong in our professional roles. This will enable us to apply ethical principles to understand and prevent tragedies happening to people to whom we have a responsibility to care for and protect.

We all have a responsibility to speak out and not assume that someone else, particularly someone higher up the ladder, will identify the problem and deal with it.

The majority of health and social care staff interact with each other, patients, clients, relatives and many others. This means that they are often in a position to make decisions about care or treatment and as such are in a position of power in which they have the potential to do good or harm.

> So far, about morals, I know only that what is moral is what you feel good after and what is immoral is what you feel bad after. . .
>
> (Hemingway 1932: 2)

This discussion of ethics is very relevant to working in teams and it is important to consider these issues when reading Chapter 4: Working in teams.

Ethical theories

Ethical theories are based on ethical principles. People usually base their individual choice of ethical theory upon their life experiences. Here we will consider two ethical theories, namely Deontology and Utilitarianism, and four ethical principles.

Deontology

The deontological theory states that people should adhere to their obligations and duties regardless of the consequences. It is derived from the work of Immanuel Kant (1724–1804) and means that a person will follow his or her obligations to another individual or society because upholding one's duty is what is considered the right thing to do. For instance, a deontologist will always keep his promises to a friend and will always follow the law no matter what the outcome is. A person who follows this theory will produce very consistent decisions since they will be based on the individual's set duties.

Deontology provides a basis for special duties and obligations to specific people, such as patients within one's care but is sometimes difficult to follow and can be inflexible.

VIGNETTE

Consider the following scenario: you and your colleagues are caring for a patient with dementia. Her husband visits every day at the same time to spend some time with her. One day he doesn't arrive and you discover that he has passed away. The patient continually asks where her husband is. What do you tell her?

As we discuss ethical theories and principles in the remainder of the chapter we will consider how we can use these to reach an ethically correct decision.

What would the deontologist do? It is generally accepted that telling the truth is the right thing to do. Faced with this dilemma a deontologist would tell the truth regardless of the consequences. This would mean telling the truth to the patient every time she asked causing her to experience distress and sadness on a continual basis.

Utilitarianism

The utilitarian theory is based on the ability to predict the consequences of an action and is also known as consequentialism. To a utilitarian, the choice that results in the greatest benefit to the most people is the choice that is ethically correct. It is often paraphrased as the theory that proposes to achieve 'the greatest good for the greatest number'. Utilitarian theory is based on the work of Jeremy Bentham (1748–1832) and John Stuart Mill (1808–73).

One branch of utilitarianism takes account of fairness to reach a decision; however, this is not always the case. This means that a decision may be made which does not benefit an individual but benefits the majority of the others involved.

What would the utilitarian do? In this scenario the utilitarian would consider past experiences of similar situations and also the implications for all involved – for example the patient, the staff, and the friends and relatives. The decision is made regardless of personal values or a sense of duty. The utilitarian may decide that it is in the interest of the majority to tell the patient an untruth which will cause less distress. On the other hand, whilst the staff may see the benefits of this they may feel uncomfortable about telling a lie.

Ethical principles

Ethical theories and principles provide guidance for the choices we make. Each theory emphasises different points, such as following one's duty to others or predicting the outcome in order to reach an ethically correct decision. Ethical principles are the common goals that each theory tries to achieve in order to be successful. In 1977 Beauchamp and Childress proposed four moral principles that guide ethical practice in healthcare (Beauchamp and Childress 2013). They are beneficence, non-maleficence, respect for autonomy, and justice. The four are considered to be of equal importance.

Beneficence

The principle of beneficence guides the ethical theory to do what is good. This principle is related to the principle of utility, which states that we should attempt to generate the largest ratio of good over evil possible in the world. It states that ethical theories should strive to achieve the greatest amount of good because people benefit from the most good. An example of 'doing good' is found in the practice of medicine in which the health of an individual is improved by treatment from a healthcare practitioner.

Non-maleficence

This is the obligation to avoid causing harm. It is similar to beneficence, but deals with situations in which neither choice is beneficial. It states that a person should choose to do the least harm possible and to do harm to the fewest people. One could also reasonably argue that people have a greater responsibility to 'do no harm' than to take steps to benefit others.

Autonomy

This principle states that people should have control over, and be able to make decisions about, their own lives. Individuals deserve respect because only they have had those exact life experiences and understand their emotions, motivations and body in such an intimate manner. There are, however, two ways of looking at the respect for autonomy. Acting in a paternalistic manner towards a patient means that you would curtail their autonomy by making decisions about them that you feel are in their best interests or for their own good. This may be appropriate if the patient is vulnerable as it removes the stress of making their own decisions. It is nevertheless important to be aware that the values of the carer and the patient may differ. Alternatively the libertarian view prioritises the patient's choices regardless of whether or not they may suffer harm.

Justice

The ethical principle of justice states that ethical theories should prescribe actions that are fair to those involved. An ethical decision that contains justice within it has a consistent logical basis that supports the decision. For example, a policeman is allowed to speed on the highway if he must arrive at the scene of a crime as quickly as possible in order to prevent a person from getting hurt. Although the policeman would normally have to obey the speed limit, he is allowed to speed in this unique situation because it is justified under the extenuating circumstances.

Consider the scenario again. If we aim to do good in this situation and avoid harm, our decision may be to tell a lie so that we avoid distressing the patient. Furthermore, if we act in a paternalistic way we may decide that not telling the truth would benefit this patient although we would be denying her autonomy. Would this action be fair to her? This scenario demonstrates how challenging it can be to make an ethically right decision but also offers a framework by which we can consider the merit of the range of options available.

Ethical theories and principles applied to decision-making

The process we follow in making a decision can be guided by a combination of these ethical principles and theories. It is worth noting that individuals may reach different conclusions in any given situation depending on the merit they afford these concepts and also their personal values. Nevertheless, these ideas give us an informal structure to guide the many decisions we must make and to help us to reach the ethically correct decision.

Diversity and equality

When we think of discrimination and equality we often think of minority or vulnerable groups. In truth anyone can be discriminated against and discrimination can take many forms. People can be discriminated against, or negatively stereotyped, for many reasons including age (ageism), race (racism) and gender (sexism).

As Vincent points out:

> Ageism, like racism or sexism, refers to both prejudice and discrimination; the first being an attitude, the second a behaviour.
>
> (2000: 148, cited by Payne 2006)

More importantly it can be difficult to establish the basis of the discriminatory actions.

Diversity is considered to be the variety that occurs in every aspect of humanity, involving both visible and invisible characteristics.

ACTIVITY

Think about diversity in your own life, particularly in your working environment.
   Here are some examples of diversity:

- Different ages
- Ethnicity
- Different languages
- Cultures and religions
- Sexual orientation
- Economic and social backgrounds
- Different lifestyles
- Differently able (disabled), learning styles.

Take a few minutes to think about the diversities you encounter in your daily life.

One of the most prized assets of being a human being is our individuality. Each one of us wants to be recognised for our individual identity and personality and to be seen as independent and worthwhile in our own right. In this instance we value difference.

ACTIVITY

Think about your friends and consider each one in turn. Try to identify how you relate to them in different ways and how you would quantify their attributes. Perhaps one is a good listener and another is the one with whom you would choose to share a fun evening in town.
   Not only are these the things that make us different from one another but they are clearly diverse attributes that should be valued. This does not mean that one should be more valuable than another, although this may be the case at a specific point in time depending on your circumstances.
   As healthcare practitioners we have a responsibility to value diversity within our team. Of course we should treat others with tolerance and respect but we should also accept that others have a right to their opinions.
   Now **consider** the people you interact with on a daily basis:

- What are their differences? Try to identify their attributes and their weaknesses.
- What are the special qualities they contribute to the team?
- Are their opinions valued?

Include yourself in this reflection. What are your differences, attributes and weaknesses? Are these valued by your friends and in your workplace?
   This exercise is important to undertake when looking at your work within teams and the nature of leadership so do make sure you read Chapter 4 and make the connections.

Equality is about creating a fairer society, where everyone can participate and has the opportunity to fulfil their potential. Although sometimes used interchangeably, equality and diversity are not the same. They are however interdependent. We have already established that diversity is the acknowledgement and respect of differences within and between groups of people. Equality is the framework that enables opportunity, access, participation and contribution that is fair and inclusive.

Equality does not mean treating everyone the same. Just as people are different their needs are different. This is clearly apparent in the healthcare environment where you will encounter a huge range of diverse people with diverse needs. What is important is that the same principles of fairness are applied to all individuals. Therefore equality implies that they should be treated fairly. Failure to respect another's right to equality puts them at a disadvantage. This can happen because of ignorance or naivety.

Consider your own knowledge and how this can be improved to ensure that you treat everyone equally.

Prejudice is prejudging or making a decision about a person or group of people without sufficient knowledge. Prejudicial thinking is frequently based on stereotypes. A prejudice can be positive, but is most often a negative attitude.

Prejudices are often accompanied by ignorance, fear or hatred. Prejudices are formed by a complex psychological process that begins with attachment to a close circle of acquaintances or an 'in-group' such as a family. Prejudice is often aimed at people who are not part of the 'in-group'.

Social scientists believe children begin to acquire prejudices and stereotypes as toddlers without really understanding their significance. Early in life, most children acquire a full set of biases that can be observed in verbal slurs, ethnic jokes and acts of discrimination (Tenner 2013).

Once learned, stereotypes and prejudices can be difficult to change, even when evidence fails to support them or points to the contrary. People tend to embrace anecdotes that reinforce their biases, but disregard experience that contradicts them.

Discrimination

Prejudice and discrimination can exist in isolation but there is often a close link between the two. Discrimination is behaviour that treats people unequally because of their group memberships. Discriminatory behaviour, ranging from slights to hate crimes, often begins with negative stereotypes and prejudices.

Most of us, probably all of us, would like to believe that we do not hold prejudices and we do not discriminate. In fact we all hold some prejudices and it is important that we recognise them and where possible eliminate them. When this is not possible we should aim to develop strategies to avoid our prejudices resulting in discriminatory actions.

Stereotyping is an exaggerated belief, image or distorted truth about a person or group – a generalisation that allows for little or no individual differences or social variation. Thus assumptions are made about a group of people, based on one or more characteristics, and present barriers to understanding. Stereotypes can be positive or negative and are based on images in mass media, or reputations passed on by parents, peers and other members of society.

Why do people stereotype? They are seeking order in a complex world; it is quick and easy; it tells us what to expect and how to behave and it helps us feel part of the 'in-group'.

In healthcare the consequences of stereotyping can be significant. It may result in treating patients differently according to stereotype and not need, making incorrect assumptions, and failing to recognise the individual.

National character is the notion that nations are rooted in their history and culture, distinct patterns of consumption, personality and self-expression. It is not uncommon to hear somebody refer to an individual, an action or a product (a film perhaps) as 'typically English' or 'typically Scottish' or 'typically Italian'. Most of us would have some idea of what was implied by these statements.

Bias is perpetuated by conformity with in-group attitudes and socialisation by the culture at large. Mass media routinely take advantage of stereotypes as shorthand to paint a mood, scene or character. The elderly, for example, are routinely portrayed as being frail and forgetful, whilst younger people are often shown as vibrant and able.

Stereotypes can also be conveyed by omission in popular culture, as when TV shows present an all-white world. Psychologists theorise that bias conveyed by the media helps to explain why children can adopt hidden prejudices

Labelling is defined as 'expectations we hold about other people's behaviour, attitudes, beliefs and character'. Labelling may result in a self-fulfilling prophesy (that is, if we expect things to happen they will) and it is linked to the existence of stereotypes.

ACTIVITY – PERSONAL ACTION PLAN

Try answering the following questions:

1 How will the things I have learnt in this chapter change the way I think and act towards others who are different to me?
2 What has this chapter helped me to learn about myself with regard to:

- my beliefs
- my attitudes
- my values
- my knowledge of others
- my behaviour; my use of language
- my responsibilities
- the way I see the world?

3 How do I need to change in order to become:

- fairer
- more sensitive
- more understanding
- less prejudicial
- less discriminatory
- better able to deal with people according to their needs?

Chapter summary

- Valuing people is at the very core of the helping professions.
- Values and attitudes are shaped by upbringing and experience and may change depending on the situation we find ourselves in.
- A value system applies equally to the patients we serve and the staff we work alongside.
- Dignity in care supports and promotes a person's self-respect regardless of any difference.
- Ethics is concerned with questions of right and wrong and helps us to understand what is good and bad.
- Ethical theory can be useful in helping us to understand the decision-making process when faced with a dilemma.
- Diversity and equality are concerned with recognising individuality and creating fairness for all.

Further resources

www.dhcarenetworks.org.uk/dignity – this website gives you access to a lot of information and resources that can help you enhance dignity and respect in your workplace. It is a forum for good ideas and best practice. You can also sign up as a 'Dignity Champion' and become part of the Dignity campaign.

www.ccpdignity.com/introduction – Skills for Care Introduction to the seven common core principles to support dignity in social care.

www.skillsforhealth.org.uk – on this website you can find the National Dignity Council Report on the Common Core Principle of Dignity.

Further reading

Duncan, P. 2010. *Values, Ethics and Health Care*. London: Sage Publications.

Mason-Whitehead, E., McIntosh, A., Bryan, A. and Mason, T., eds. 2008. *Key Concepts in Nursing*. London: Sage Publications.

Tschudin, V. 2007. *Ethics in Nursing: The Caring Relationship*, 3rd edn. Edinburgh. Butterworth-Heinemann.

References

Beauchamp, T. and Childress, J. 2013. *Principles of Biomedical Ethics*. Oxford: Oxford University Press.

Fuller, R. W. 2008. *Dignity for All*. Williston, VT: Berrett-Koehler.

Hemingway, E. 1932. *Death in the Afternoon*. New York: Charles Scribner's Sons.

Hodgkin, P. 2011. *NHS Staff Are Rude, Negative and Lacking in Compassion* [online]. Available at: www.locallyhealthy.co.uk/story/nhs-staff-are-rude-negative-and-lacking-compassion [Accessed 21 July 2013].

Muir Gray, J. A. 2006. *The Resourceful Patient*. Oxford: eRosetta Press.

Payne, G., ed. 2006. *Social Divisions*, 2nd edn. Basingstoke: Macmillan.

PRIAE/Help the Aged. 2001. *Dignity on the Ward: Towards Dignity: Acting on the Lessons from Hospital Experiences of Black and Minority Ethnic Older People: A Report from Policy Research Institute on Ageing and Ethnicity for the Dignity on the Ward Campaign* [pdf]. *PRIAE* [online]. Available at: www.priae.org/index [Accessed 7 January 2015].

Social Care Institute for Excellence (SCIE). 2010. *Dignity in Care* [online]. Available at: www.scie.org.uk/publications/guides/guide15/selectedresearch/whatdignitymeans.asp [Accessed 7 January 2015].

Stevenson, A. and Waite, M., eds. 2011. *Concise Oxford Dictionary*, 12th edn. Oxford: Oxford University Press.

Wilde, O. 2012. *The Picture of Dorian Gray*. London. Penguin Classics.

World Health Organization. 1994. *Declaration on the Promotion of Patients' Rights in Europe* [online]. World Health Organization. Available at: www.who.int/genomics/public/eu_declaration1994.pdf [Accessed 11 November 2014].

Tenner, M. D. 2013. *240 Ways to Close the Achievement Gap: Talking Points for Salvaging the Lives of African-American and Latino Students*, 2nd edn. St Paul, MN: Gold Boot Publishing.

Chapter 6

Healthcare delivery

Mary Northrop

LEARNING OUTCOMES

By the end of this chapter you will be able to:

1 Explain how healthcare policy is developed and the factors that influence that development.
2 Show understanding of how policy is implemented in the healthcare setting.
3 Outline the structure of healthcare delivery in the UK.
4 Gain understanding of how healthcare delivery is monitored and regulated.

Introduction

This chapter focuses on how healthcare is delivered within the UK and the factors that influence what care is given, for whom and why. It provides an overview of what healthcare policy is and how this is developed based on an understanding of the health problems and welfare needs of the UK and how services are delivered to meet the needs of the society. The first part of the chapter looks at factors that influence what healthcare is provided and how these are used to plan future services. The second part of the chapter looks at healthcare policy and how it is developed and who makes those decisions and why. The third part will look at the current structure of healthcare delivery in England and how this is monitored.

Factors influencing healthcare delivery

There are a number of factors that influence the type of healthcare available within a specific society. These include the size and make-up of the population (demographics), the types of illness and causes of death (morbidity and mortality), the infrastructure (including type of employment, income and access to healthcare) and the healthcare beliefs dominant within the society.

Demographics

Demographics includes features of a society: age, gender, ethnicity, where people live, and the number of births and deaths. The make-up of the population impacts on the services needed and allows for planning for future needs. In order to do this both national and local statistics need to be taken into account.

ACTIVITY

What healthcare services would you need to consider if we have a major increase in births in the UK?

What other services need to be taken into account that are not healthcare, but link to future health for individuals?

You may have included the need for more obstetricians, midwives, health visitors and maternity beds. In addition, we would need more nurseries, playschools and eventually school places and therefore more childcare workers and teachers. We may also need to look at available housing and financial assistance for those with low incomes. Eventually we would have to look at the impact on employment and what happens when these children reach retirement age and how pensions will be provided. However, we also need to know both national and local statistics, as national statistics will tell us how many children are being born each year but local statistics may show that there are more children being born in some areas than others. If we increased school places across the UK this would result in some areas spending money on services that would not be used.

This demonstrates how demographic changes could impact on the services provided and why being able to predict what services are needed and where is important. The Office of National Statistics (ONS) provides current statistics for the UK – these include age, gender and ethnicity mix, number of births and deaths (including the main causes of death) – and compares them to previous statistics. For example, at the time of writing, there were 698,512 live births in England and Wales in 2013, a decrease of 4.3 per cent from 729,674 in 2012 (ONS 2014a) and there were 506,790 deaths in England and Wales compared to 499,331 in 2012 (ONS 2014b). Of these deaths, 48 per cent were men and 52 per cent were women. The statistics predict that for people born in 2013 one in three babies will live up to 100 years of age, with men living on average until 90 years of age and women 94 years of age. However, these statistics only show numbers of births and deaths and not who died, why, nor the age ranges. They do show that more people were born than died that year which would mean an increase in the population numbers overall. However, demographics also take into account immigration and emigration. If more people leave the country than enter, or vice versa, this will also have an impact on the overall numbers. If we want to know more about why people die (mortality rates) and why they are ill (morbidity) we move into the area of epidemiology.

Epidemiology

Healthcare delivery looks at the health problems that are common within the country and globally. In order to plan for healthcare there is a need to understand what services are potentially needed both now and in the future. These statistics will then influence healthcare policy which sets out how care should be delivered and by whom and forms part of wider social policy that helps societies to organise and deliver services within a given society. Epidemiology is the study of patterns of diseases and other causes of healthcare problems. It is used to estimate the number of occurrences of illnesses, to find out what causes different health issues and what can be done to prevent or minimise the spread of diseases (see Chapter 10: Improving public health).

For most illnesses there will be an expected number of cases each year. Epidemiologists look at if there is an increase in cases and whether this is due to changes in the virus which would require new types of vaccination or because vaccinations have not been taken up, or other factors that may have impacted on control of the virus. If a new illness occurs in a society, research can identify the cause and how the illness is spread and it may be possible to develop vaccinations to reduce the incidence and protect the population. Healthcare policies can then be put into place to address the causes and educate healthcare professionals so they can target individuals at risk. With this information the Department of Health can look at what are the main needs for the population, who is affected and whether there is a need to introduce a social policy to try and meet this need.

Social policy

Social policy is concerned with the organisation and delivery of social and welfare services and is a term used to describe any policy that regulates the above and includes how resources will be allocated to provide the service. Social policy is traditionally concerned with five main areas:

- Income maintenance – unemployment benefit, child allowance.
- Health services – NHS, private care etc.
- Education – provision of schooling and National Curriculum.
- Social services – care provision in the community and safeguarding (see Chapter 12: Safeguarding individuals and families).
- Housing – policies on new builds, maintenance of existing housing stock.

These areas were developed from the Victorian era and were in response to what was seen as the 'five giant evils of society' which were: poverty, ignorance, disease, squalor and idleness ('Report on Social Insurance and Allied Services' Sir William Beveridge Foundation n.d.). Social policy development is influenced by politics and economics. It focuses on welfare and well-being and targets needs or problems in the society. The function of social policy is to meet needs and/or prevent poverty, to promote equality of opportunity and compensate for any diswelfares (when individuals are disadvantaged by welfare policy implementation; Spicker *et al.* 2006) that may have occurred.

The way in which welfare is defined and delivered will differ depending on the country and underlying politics, economics and beliefs about health, education and the degree of support that should be provided. These will influence how much welfare is provided and what kind of welfare. In order to provide welfare a range of institutions may be involved including the family, the community, state intervention, voluntary and charitable organisations and international organisations.

ACTIVITY

Identify welfare services that you and/or your family have accessed.

All of us will have benefitted from welfare services provided within the UK, this may include free schooling, dental care, access to a general practitioner, income support or assistance with housing.

There are a number of systems that deliver welfare which were described by Titmuss (1955, cited by Hudson 2013):

- Social welfare – provision by government.
- Occupational welfare – provision by employers.
- Fiscal welfare – provision by taxation.
- Private welfare – provision by private sector.
- Voluntary welfare – charities.
- Informal welfare – provision in the home by the family.

In England, social welfare provided by the state is underpinned by fiscal welfare as we pay for the NHS and other services through taxation. The extent to which services are provided will differ across countries and in some instances between different areas. In some countries there is limited state provision and healthcare is mainly through private sector delivery and paid for by insurance premiums (for example the USA). In some areas there is limited healthcare provision and the burden of care is placed on informal welfare or voluntary welfare.

Social policy legislation in England can be traced back to Elizabethan times when the first major Poor Law was passed in 1601 (Bloy 2002). This placed responsibility on the local parish to provide a set sum of money for the poor and created 'overseers' to manage this and provide work for the poor. Policies change over time; for example, it was once against the law to attempt suicide but since the Suicide Act 1961 (Legislation.gov.uk n.d), it is now no longer a criminal offence, but related to mental health. However, it is still a criminal offence to assist someone else to commit suicide and this carries a maximum sentence of 14 years. Similarly, historically mental health patients had few if any rights if they were perceived to be a risk to themselves or others. Several parliamentary acts have subsequently changed how these individuals are treated by society as a whole. For example you could compare the Mental Health Act 1959 with the 1983 Act.

In this context a policy is a statement of intent and/or a course of action. Social policy is therefore concerned with the following:

- The way a service or an area of social life is structured and functions.
- The delivery of services.
- The actions of those working to deliver the service.
- The way that resources are allocated.

The NHS Act 1946 addressed all of the above, as it laid down how healthcare would be delivered in our society. The service changed from a mixture of private, charity and state hospitals to a National Health Service. The service was to be free at the point of delivery and to be available for all. It set down what services were to be delivered and by whom. Funding of the service was established through the taxation system.

Social policy may relate to a specific area of provision or across the scope of provision. For example Choosing Health (Department of Health 2004) addressed health initiatives that included local councils, health services, schools, food companies and the leisure industry.

If we compare policies in England with other countries there may be similarities but also major differences. Most European countries have policies that address the five areas above. Political influence, attitudes to welfare, the economy and other factors will all influence the type of provision. In addition, people will benefit in different ways from the provision available. Many may only access certain services while others may use the welfare system extensively.

ACTIVITY

Find out the amount of paternity leave entitlement in England and two other European countries.

1   What are the similarities?
2   What are the differences?
3   Why do you think the length of leave has increased in England?
4   Who benefits from the policy?
5   Are any people excluded from the policy, if so why?

Some of the information you gathered will show different lengths of paternity leave and leave may be shared between both parents. Usually there are economic costs for the employer and employee. In some instances employers cannot bear the cost (or are not prepared to) or individuals will not qualify due to the type of work they do or the length of time in employment. For example, if you work in the local shop or if you are self-employed taking leave would not be a viable option.

Development of social policy

When looking at policy an understanding of why the policy is needed and how it came into being is essential. Furthermore, there is a need to evaluate whether the policy is meeting either the need of the target group and/or addressing social inequalities. Banting (1979) highlighted the stages that occur in deciding whether a policy is needed and, if so, what the policy will include and why (Figure 6.1).

One of the criticisms of implementing new policies was that they were often not evaluated to see if they had worked. Evaluation is now the next stage and is carried out within set timeframes to see if the initiatives set in place are working or need revising. The above criteria would also be used if the health problem was related to lifestyle or behaviour that leads to higher demand on health services. For example, since the National Audit Office (2001) reported on the increase in people who are overweight and obese, a number of policies have been brought in to try and solve the problem. These included policies on food labelling, school food and monitoring children's weight and local council requirements to provide healthy walks, cycling routes and outdoor play areas.

When a policy is created it can become mandatory through becoming an Act of Parliament and therefore the policy has to be implemented. For example the Health and Social Care Act 2008 (Department of Health 2008) set out the requirements for the management of infection control within healthcare delivery. Failure to meet the requirements is punishable by law and

Awareness of the problem
What is the problem that may or may not need addressing?
A number of people present to health services with the same symptoms but they
do not correspond with any known illnesses

If only a small
number of
people are
affected and/or
the symptoms
are manageable
no new policy
may be
required

Degree of importance attached
This includes looking at:
The seriousness of the symptoms
How many people are affected?
What happens if we do nothing?

If high
numbers are
affected
and/or people
are dying
from the
illness a
policy may
be required

Definition of the problem
Research is required to understand what the
problem is.
What is the cause and why is it happening?
How is the illness spread? Does this illness
exist elsewhere? Who is it affecting?
What are the possible treatments/management?

Consideration of alternatives
Having researched the problem, what options do we have for
managing it? Are there a number of options available? What is
the cost of the alternatives? Do the current services available meet
the need?

Choice between the alternatives
The choice of what option(s) is made and put into policy. This may
be a number of different approaches and may require new
services to be developed, staff training, new drugs or vaccinations

Figure 6.1 Decision process for developing a social policy (adapted from Banting 1979).

could include fines or imprisonment. In order for a policy to become an Act of Parliament there are a number of stages:

STAGES FOR THE PASSING OF AN ACT OF PARLIAMENT

- Recognition of the need to produce a new law or change an existing law.
- Creation of a draft Bill in consultation with appropriate individuals and groups i.e. voluntary organisations, pressure groups and professional bodies.
- Green Papers may be produced which set out draft proposals and are sent out for consultation prior to finalising the draft Bill.
- White Papers set out the proposals for legislative change and are sent out for consultation.
- The draft Bill is considered by a departmental select committee which may consist of members from both the House of Commons and the House of Lords. This is pre-legislative scrutiny and allows for changes before the Bill is presented to the House of Commons and/or House of Lords.
- The Bill can be presented through either the House of Lords or House of Commons initially.
- First reading: the title of the Bill is presented to the House.
- Second reading: the Bill is sent to the members of the House for review and to raise any concerns. Individuals put their name on a 'Speakers List'. The Bill is then debated within the House and interested parties present their views. This can take a few hours or a few days.
- After the second reading the Bill moves to the committee stage. Before the committee meets, tables of amendments are produced. At the committee sessions each line is examined and amendments from the second reading are made following discussion.
- The Bill is resent out in the form of a report to all members usually 14 days after the committee stage. Members can then review and suggest further changes.
- Any amendments are made and then the Bill enters the third and final reading and is the last opportunity for any changes.
- The Bill is then sent to the House of Lords if it originated in the House of Commons or vice versa. It then goes through the same process.
- The Bill may then ping-pong between the two Houses if there are further changes required. If the exact wording is agreed then the Bill is put forward for Royal Assent.
- Following Royal Assent the Bill becomes a Law and may be introduced immediately or following a commencement order by a government Minister. The commencement order may involve partial implementation with parts of the Act being put in place at a later date.
- The implementation of an Act is carried out by the relevant government department (Source: Parliament n.d).

Other policies are for guidance purposes and there are no legal sanctions if they are not adhered to. However, in healthcare it is expected that these will be followed, and the National

Institute for Health and Care Excellence (NICE) provides a range of guidance for healthcare practitioners (see Chapters 7 and 9 for further discussion of the role of NICE). NICE sets quality standards related to aspects of care, an example being the guidance on *End of Life Care for Adults* (NICE 2011) which was updated on 31 October 2013, following the phasing out of the Liverpool Care Pathway. The standard was set in consultation with a range of groups and organisations and endorsed as good practice by seventeen organisations including: the Association for Palliative Medicine of Great Britain and Ireland, the Association of Hospice and Palliative Care Chaplains, Macmillan, brainstrust and the Patients Association.

Healthcare policy

Healthcare policy is specifically aimed at the provision of healthcare needs and focuses on both preventative measures and implementing appropriate care for the population. The policies therefore cover a broad range of issues and can address major healthcare initiatives or focus on a specific aspect of service provision. National policies will influence how local services are delivered including: who does what, best practice, and how care may be delivered. Day-to-day care activities will be underpinned by local policies which have been created in order to meet national policies. For example safe practice when moving and handling both objects and patients is governed by a number of policies including: Lifting Operations and Lifting Equipment Regulations 1998 (LOLER) (Health and Safety Executive n.d.a), Reporting of Injuries, Diseases and Dangerous Occurrences Regulations 2013 (RIDDOR) (Health and Safety Executive n.d.b) and Manual Handling Operations Regulations 1992 (Health and Safety Executive 2004) (amended 2004). The three policies provide guidance for employers and employees around the safe use of equipment, the reporting of any injuries and guidance on best practice to avoid injury. These were introduced due to the high rate of back injuries in both healthcare and other workplaces. The above policies are all mandatory and have to be met.

Policies that provide guidance for healthcare delivery can focus on the management of specific health conditions. These stem from statistics on the main causes of ill health in the UK and those that cost the most in relation to treatment and higher mortality rates. An example of current policy addresses the incidence of obesity in the UK. Following the National Audit Office report in 2001, on the expected levels of obesity and overweight people, a number of strategies have been introduced that include prevention of obesity and the management of obesity. Previously obesity had been identified as a lifestyle factor that was linked to other conditions such as diabetes (type 2), coronary heart disease and some cancers. In 2001, *Tackling Obesity in England* (National Audit Office 2001) stated that rates of obesity in both women and men had tripled since 1980. Incidence in women was 21 per cent, and 17 per cent of men were now obese. One-third of men and half of women were classified as being overweight and around half a billion pounds was spent on healthcare related to obesity management. In addition 18 million sick days a year and 30,000 deaths a year were associated with obesity. Obese individuals were on average dying nine years earlier than those without weight problems. The problem of obesity is complex and a number of factors needed to be taken into account: diet, exercise, other lifestyle factors, mental health and other underpinning health problems. The policies put into place addressed a range of these and the best ways in which to tackle the problem. Table 6.1 outlines some of the reports and policies and what they aimed to achieve.

Table 6.1 Reports and policies and what they hope to achieve

Policy/reports	Content
Chief Medical Officer (2004) *At Least Five a Week: Evidence on the Impact of Physical Activity and Its Relationship to Health*	Call to action to increase levels of physical activity across age groups. Reported on a range of research linked to the benefits of exercise and the reduction in a range of health problems. Suggested a number of strategies at local council level, schools and primary care. These included prescriptions for exercise.
Department of Health, Physical Activity, Health Improvement and Protection (2011) *Start Active, Stay Active: A Report on Physical Activity for Health from the Four Home Countries' Chief Medical Officers*	Superseded the above report. Set out what constitutes physical activity and benefits. Guidelines included: • Children under 5 to be active for 3 hours a day (spread over the day). • Children over 5 to be intensely active for a minimum of 60 minutes per day and active for several hours a day. • Adults (19–64) and older adults (65+) should aim to be active daily. Over a week, activity should add up to at least 150 minutes (2½ hours) of moderate intensity activity in bouts of 10 minutes or more. To include activities that improve muscle strength at least twice a week. Guidelines to be used by health professionals and local authorities. Suggested actions included setting up cycling clubs.
National Audit Office (2006) *Tackling Child Obesity – First Steps*	Aim: To halt, by 2010, the year-on-year increase in obesity among children under 11 in the context of a broader strategy to tackle obesity in the population as a whole (2006: 9). Key programmes include: • DfES revision of school meals nutritional standards. • School sports strategy. • Local Authority development of play facilities.
Government Office for Science (2007) *Foresight – Tackling Obesities: Future Choices*	Looked at projected impact of obesity and states: • Most adults in the UK are already overweight. Modern living ensures every generation is heavier than the last – 'Passive Obesity'. • By 2050 60% of men and 50% of women could be clinically obese. • Without action, obesity-related diseases are estimated to cost society £49.9 billion per year. • The obesity epidemic cannot be prevented by individual action alone and demands a societal approach. • Tackling obesity requires far greater change than anything tried so far, and at multiple levels: personal, family, community and national. • Preventing obesity is a societal challenge, similar to climate change. It requires partnership between government, science, business and civil society (2007: 3).
Marmot Review (2010) *Fair Society, Healthy Lives*	Major public health document which looked at inequalities. Stated six areas for policy development: • Give every child the best start in life. • Enable all children, young people and adults to maximise their capabilities and have control over their lives. • Create fair employment and good work for all. • Ensure a healthy standard of living for all. • Create and develop healthy and sustainable places and communities. • Strengthen the role and impact of ill-health prevention.

Policy/reports	Content
Cross-Government Obesity Unit, Department of Health and Department of Children, Schools and Families (2008) *Healthy Weight, Healthy Lives: A Cross-Government Strategy for England*	Main policy document which set out a broad range of strategies and level of funding to introduce initiatives. The strategies stated covered a broad range of services and worked with a number of organisations. Many of these have been initiated. These included: • Working with families to improve diet and levels of physical activity of children. • Healthy Towns initiatives. • Food advertising and reduction of fast food outlets near schools and parks. • Working with technology producers to encourage computer games that are more active. • Working with employers to improve food choices and other activities.
NICE (2014) *Obesity: Identification, Assessment and Management of Overweight and Obesity in Children, Young People and Adults*	Sets out the current guidance on management of obesity for health professionals including different interventions and when to implement them.

The sample of documents in Table 6.1 highlights the range of research and approaches being undertaken to tackle the obesity epidemic in England and the rest of the UK. Other reports and strategies are available from a global perspective from the World Health Organization (WHO) which recognise obesity as a worldwide health issue.

ACTIVITY

Pick a national policy relevant to your own area of work or interest.

What are the main aims of the policy?

How does it link to your area of work?

For example you could choose to look at an infection control policy and how measures are put in place. Alternatively you could look at public health policies about smoking, sexual health etc. and what is in place to try to reduce incidences and associated health problems.

Healthcare delivery

Within the UK, healthcare is delivered via a number of sources and we will have accessed a number of these. For example, most of us have visited a GP, pharmacy and a dentist. The majority of healthcare is provided within the home by families and friends. If you have a cold you may look after yourself or a family member may give advice or care. This is known as informal care and includes long-term care provided by relatives and volunteers.

Formal care includes accessing relevant professionals and services which may be provided by the state (the NHS), the independent sector (private provision), charitable organisations (for example, a hospice) and social enterprises (organisations set up to meet communities and life chances).

ACTIVITY

List the formal care provision that you and your family have accessed.

You may have consulted with a pharmacist to provide over-the-counter medication, the GP or a walk-in centre, accident and emergency possibly via the ambulance service, outpatient services, hospital inpatient services, dentists, ophthalmologists and physiotherapy. In order to receive treatment sooner you may have paid for private consultations or care.

With the introduction of Choose and Book in 2004 (Health and Social Care Information Centre (hscic) n.d.), individuals were able to choose where they would attend for appointments and inpatient care from a list of available services. The system included choosing appointment times and allowed GPs to see where the care was available and the ratings of those services. Patients could then decide on what service to access. The new NHS e-Referral Service, which will replace Choose and Book, is being launched in 2015 with the aim to have paperless referrals and a paperless NHS by 2018 (Health and Social Care Information Centre (hscic) n.d.).

It is the role of the Clinical Commissioning Groups (CCGs) to decide what services are needed in a locality, through the collation of demographic and epidemiology statistics and knowledge of the demand for services for the year before, and then who will deliver them. Requests for tenders are sent out to interested parties and the CCG decides which tenders to accept and sign a contract with. The CCG works to the NHS budget set by Parliament and devolved to them. In 2013/14 the total budget was £95.6 billion, with £65.6 billion allocated to local authorities and CCGs. £25.4 billion was allocated to specialist services and £1.8 billion to Public Health services for screening, immunisation and Health Visiting services (NHS England 2015).

The way in which the NHS is structured changes over time. At the time of writing, the current structure can be found on the NHS England website at www.nhs.uk/NHSEngland/thenhs/about/Documents/nhs-system-overview.pdf.

Figure 6.2 shows people and communities as at the centre of NHS provision and the services available. Other bodies and organisations set up to monitor or regulate services are provided in the outer boxes. Figure 6.2 lists some of these, the Department of Health is the main government department associated with healthcare delivery, but joint policies with the Department of Education particularly around child health are common. Quality issues come under the remit of the Care Quality Commission (CQC) and are discussed in Chapter 7.

Two of the agencies mentioned have a role in the development of healthcare services. MONITOR is responsible for advising NHS Trusts that wish to become Foundation Trusts and if successful they then regulate and evaluate their performance. The NHS Trust Development Authority is responsible for supporting those trusts that do not have Foundation status and monitoring quality and delivery of services. They also look at governance and risk management and have the authority to appoint chairs and other board members at the request of the Secretary of State (National Trust Development Authority n.d.).

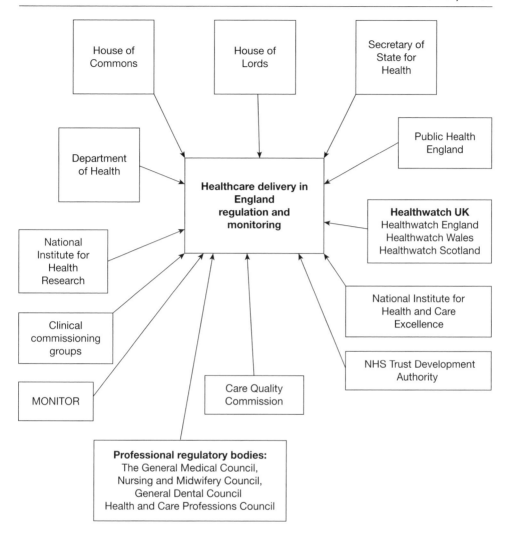

Figure 6.2 Healthcare delivery in England.

Day-to-day running of healthcare delivery: National Health Service

The NHS is responsible for the majority of healthcare delivery in the UK. Day-to-day delivery takes place in both the community and inpatient services. The current provision includes:

- **Social Enterprises** – a number of NHS Trusts which delivered Care in the Community became Social Enterprises and contract with the NHS to provide services including District Nurses, Continence Management and Hospital At Home.
- **Foundation Trusts** – are not-for-profit, public benefit corporations. They include over half of NHS hospitals including mental health and ambulance services. They are able to decide on their own services and are not directed by the government. People in the local community have a say on the services and they are managed through a board of governors.

- **NHS Trusts** – are directed by government to provide health services. These include acute hospital care, community care (where they have opted not to become a social enterprise) mental health and specialist services. They were expected to obtain Foundation status by the end of 2014, at the time of writing this target had not been reached and over 99 trusts were still in existence (NHS England 2013a).
- **General practitioners** – are independent from the NHS and are contracted to provide a range of services by CCGs. Their role includes consultations, usually in a GP surgery, and some home visits and some GPs will do minor surgery. They are also involved in health screening and health promotion and receive extra income through meeting set targets (NHS England 2013b). They act as gatekeepers for other services, for example GPs confirm if you are pregnant and then you can access maternity services.

Roles within healthcare delivery

There are a wide variety of roles within healthcare delivery across hospital and community provision, including professional and support roles. Figure 6.3 includes some of these:
   Two of these roles are:

- **Pharmacists** – pharmacists can work within hospital services and in the community. Their role includes providing advice on medicine management to doctors and nurse prescribers and monitoring prescriptions for the public. Community pharmacists also advise the public on appropriate over the counter medications. Their role has broadened to include prescribing for a specified number of conditions (after further training) and providing advice on medicine management for individuals with long-term conditions (NHS Careers n.d.a).
- **Dentists** – the role of the dentist varies, with some working as specialists within hospital services and employed on contracts with the NHS. This involves surgical roles and others. General dentists are self-employed and work in the community. They may provide private or NHS care (through NHS contracts) and are paid according to a set scale dependent on the type and amount of treatment (NHS Careers n.d.b).

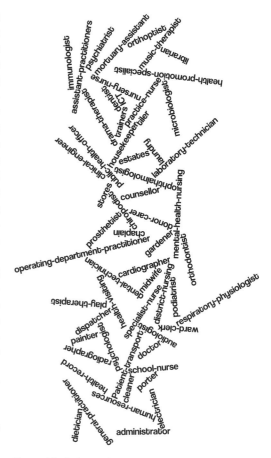

Figure 6.3 Roles within healthcare delivery.

> ## ACTIVITY
>
> Explore some of the job roles that you are unfamiliar with or that you are unsure of
> what the role is in relation to the service you work in (or intend to work in).

Public and patient involvement in healthcare delivery

If you were to look back at a structure diagram of healthcare delivery prior to 2000 you would
notice that these consisted of the organisations involved and emphasised the management
structure. From 2000 onwards more emphasis was placed on including patients and public
within the structure and this is reflected in the current structure diagram with patients and
public in the centre of healthcare delivery. The Health and Social Care Act 2001 section 11
set out the requirement that any changes in service delivery would involve consultation and
the involvement of the public. A number of bodies were set up to aid in this process: Patient
and Public Involvement in Health Forums, Overview and Scrutiny Committees, and Patient
Advice and Liaison Services (House of Commons Health Committee 2007).

- **Patient and Public Involvement in Health Forums** (PPIfs) consisted of volunteers
  drawn from the public who formed forums attached to each of the NHS Trusts. Trusts
  were expected to liaise with the group concerning the delivery of current services and any
  possible changes. The members of the forum could arrange to visit areas and held meetings with the public to inform them about changes and also to hear any concerns. The
  forums were managed by the Commission for Patient and Public Involvement in Health
  and reported back any issues. These were disbanded in 2008 and Local Involvement
  Networks were introduced (see below).
- **Overview and Scrutiny Committees** formed part of the county councils' role to ensure
  public health needs were being met. They could investigate any changes in service which
  they felt would have a detrimental effect on the population's health. If PPIfs had any
  concerns they could inform the commission who would pass these to the county council.
- **Patient Advice and Liaison Services** (PALs) were introduced to deal with patients'
  issues and concerns. They are based within NHS Trusts but are not employed by them.
  Their role was to aid with patients' concerns and complaints and offer impartial advice.
  They monitor and record the concerns and if a significant number of complaints were
  received they informed the PPIfs who could then look into these.
- **Local Involvement Networks** (LINks), took over from PPIfs in 2008. They had the
  same remit but brought together representatives from voluntary groups and user-led
  services. They also worked with Overview and Scrutiny Committees and PALs. They
  were attached to local authorities rather than trusts with funding from the Department
  of Health (NHS England 2007). Within the current healthcare structure LINks have also
  been disbanded and the role is part of Healthwatch England (see Figure 6.4).

It remains a statutory obligation that any changes in healthcare delivery have to include
public consultation. In addition, the Department of Health has implemented consultation
events for any major policy proposals since 2004 when this was part of developing Choosing
Health (Department of Health 2004). Figure 6.4 outlines the current legislation and organisations involved in ensuring that patients and public continue to be involved in decision making,
either in relation to their own care or health initiatives that impact on populations.

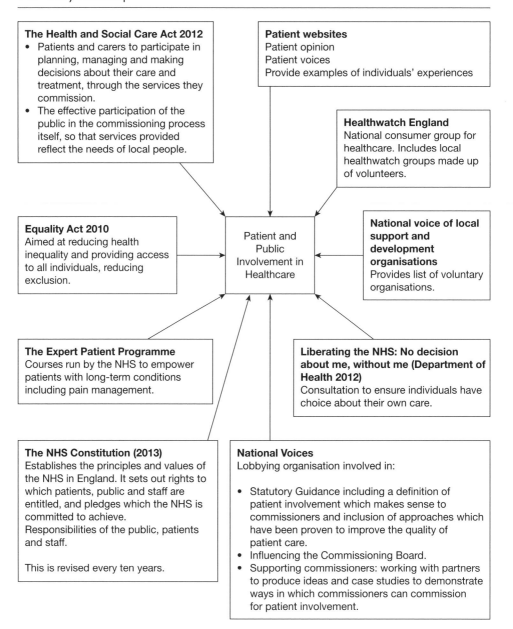

The Health and Social Care Act 2012
• Patients and carers to participate in planning, managing and making decisions about their care and treatment, through the services they commission.
• The effective participation of the public in the commissioning process itself, so that services provided reflect the needs of local people.

Patient websites
Patient opinion
Patient voices
Provide examples of individuals' experiences

Healthwatch England
National consumer group for healthcare. Includes local healthwatch groups made up of volunteers.

Equality Act 2010
Aimed at reducing health inequality and providing access to all individuals, reducing exclusion.

Patient and Public Involvement in Healthcare

National voice of local support and development organisations
Provides list of voluntary organisations.

The Expert Patient Programme
Courses run by the NHS to empower patients with long-term conditions including pain management.

Liberating the NHS: No decision about me, without me (Department of Health 2012)
Consultation to ensure individuals have choice about their own care.

The NHS Constitution (2013)
Establishes the principles and values of the NHS in England. It sets out rights to which patients, public and staff are entitled, and pledges which the NHS is committed to achieve.
Responsibilities of the public, patients and staff.

This is revised every ten years.

National Voices
Lobbying organisation involved in:

• Statutory Guidance including a definition of patient involvement which makes sense to commissioners and inclusion of approaches which have been proven to improve the quality of patient care.
• Influencing the Commissioning Board.
• Supporting commissioners: working with partners to produce ideas and case studies to demonstrate ways in which commissioners can commission for patient involvement.

Figure 6.4 Patient and public involvement in healthcare.

Chapter summary

This chapter has explored why we have social policies, and how they are developed, and provides examples of a range of policies that link to healthcare practice.

•   The delivery of healthcare includes consideration of a number of factors including demographics and epidemiology and also how healthcare is structured.

- Social policy is developed to meet the needs of a society and may be in the form of mandatory legislation or guidance.
- There are a number of organisations involved in delivering, monitoring and regulating healthcare delivery.
- Patient and public involvement needs to be at the forefront of healthcare delivery.

Further resources

Department of Health. Available at: www.gov.uk/government/organisations/department-of-health.
Healthwatch UK. Available at: www.healthwatch.co.uk/.
Houses of Parliament. Available at: www.parliament.uk/.
NHS Choices. Available at: www.nhs.uk/.
NHS England. Available at: www.england.nhs.uk/.
National Institute for Health and Care Excellence. Available at: www.nice.org.uk/.
National Voices. Available at: www.nationalvoices.org.uk/patient-involvement.
Patient Opinion. Available at: www.patientopinion.org.uk/.
World Health Organization (WHO). Available at: www.who.int/.

References

Banting, K. G. 1979. *Poverty, Politics and Policy: Britain in the 1960s*. London: Macmillan Press.
Bloy, M. 2002. *The 1601 Elizabethan Poor Law* [online]. Available at: www.victorianweb.org/history/poorlaw/elizpl.html [Accessed 6 January 2015].
Chief Medical Officer. 2004. *At Least Five a Week: Evidence on the Impact of Physical Activity and its Relationship to Health* [online]. Available at: http://webarchive.nationalarchives.gov.uk/20130107105354/www.dh.gov.uk/prod_consum_dh/groups/dh_digitalassets/@dh/@en/documents/digitalasset/dh_4080981.pdf [Accessed 2 January 2015].
Cross-Government Obesity Unit, Department of Health and Department of Children, Schools and Families. 2008. *Healthy Weight, Healthy Lives: A Cross-Government Strategy for England* [online]. Available at: http://webarchive.nationalarchives.gov.uk/20100407220245/www.dh.gov.uk/prod_consum_dh/groups/dh_digitalassets/documents/digitalasset/dh_084024.pdf [Accessed 2 January 2015].
Department of Health. 2004. *Choosing Health: Making Healthier Choices Easier* [online]. Available at: http://webarchive.nationalarchives.gov.uk/20130107105354/www.dh.gov.uk/prod_consum_dh/groups/dh_digitalassets/@dh/@en/@ps/documents/digitalasset/dh_133489.pdf [Accessed 10 November 2014].
Department of Health. 2008. *Health and Social Care Act 2008* [online]. Available at: http://webarchive.nationalarchives.gov.uk/+/www.dh.gov.uk/en/Publicationsandstatistics/Legislation/Actsandbills/HealthandSocialCareBill/DH_080604 [Accessed 10 November 2014].
Department of Health, Physical Activity, Health Improvement and Protection. 2011. *Start Active, Stay Active: A Report on Physical Activity for Health from the Four Home Countries' Chief Medical Officers* [online]. Available at: http://webarchive.nationalarchives.gov.uk/20130107105354/http://dh.gov.uk/prod_consum_dh/groups/dh_digitalassets/documents/digitalasset/dh_128210.pdf [Accessed 2 January 2015].
Government Office for Science. 2007. *Foresight – Tackling Obesities: Future Choices – Summary of Key Messages* [online]. Available at: www.gov.uk/government/uploads/system/uploads/attachment_data/file/287943/07-1469x-tackling-obesities-future-choices-summary.pdf [Accessed 2 January 2015].
Health and Safety Executive, n.d.a. *Lifting Operations and Lifting Equipment Regulations 1998* [online] Available at: www.hse.gov.uk/work-equipment-machinery/loler.htm [Accessed 2 January 2015].
Health and Safety Executive, n.d.b. *Reporting of Injuries, Diseases and Dangerous Occurrences*

Regulations 2013 (RIDDOR) [online]. Available at: www.hse.gov.uk/healthservices/riddor.htm [Accessed 2 January 2015].

Health and Safety Executive. 2004. *Manual Handling: Manual Handling Operations Regulations 1992 (as amended) Guidance on Regulations*, 3rd edn. London: HMSO [online]. Available at: www.hse.gov.uk/pubns/priced/l23.pdf [Accessed 2 January 2015].

Health and Social Care Information Centre (hscic). n.d. *NHS e-Referral Service Vision* [online]. Available at: http://systems.hscic.gov.uk/ers [Accessed 1 January 2015].

House of Commons Health Committee. 2007. *Patient and Public Involvement in the NHS: Third Report of Session 2006–07 Volume I* [online]. Available at: www.publications.parliament.uk/pa/cm200607/cmselect/cmhealth/278/278i.pdf [Accessed 2 January 2015].

Hudson, J. 2013. 'Welfare', in Dwyer, P. and Shaw, S., eds, *An Introduction to Social Policy*. London: Sage Publications, Ch. 1, pp. 3–13 [online]. Available at: www.uk.sagepub.com/upm-data/55173_Dwyer.pdf [Accessed 10 November 2014].

Legislation.gov.uk. n.d. Suicide Act 1961 [online]. Available at: www.legislation.gov.uk/ukpga/Eliz2/9-10/60 [Accessed 6 January 2015].

Marmot Review. 2010. *Fair Society, Healthy Lives – Executive Summary* [online]. Available at: www.instituteofhealthequity.org/projects/fair-society-healthy-lives-the-marmot-review [Accessed 2 January 2015].

National Audit Office. 2001. *Tackling Obesity in England* [online]. Available at: www.nao.org.uk/wp-content/uploads/2001/02/0001220.pdf [Accessed 2 January 2015].

National Audit Office. 2006. *Tackling Child Obesity – First Steps, Executive Summary* [online]. Available at: www.nao.org.uk/wp-content/uploads/2006/02/0506801es.pdf [Accessed 2 January 2015].

NHS Careers, n.d.a. *Pharmacist* [online]. Available at: www.nhscareers.nhs.uk/explore-by-career/pharmacy/pharmacist/ [Accessed 1 January 2015].

NHS Careers, n.d.b. *What Types of Dentists Are There?* [online]. Available at: www.nhscareers.nhs.uk/explore-by-career/dental-team/careers-in-the-dental-team/dentist/what-types-of-dentists-are-there/ [Accessed 1 January 2015].

NHS England. 2007. *Local Involvement Networks Explained* [online]. Available at: www.nhs.uk/NHSEngland/aboutnhs/Documents/Link%20easy%20read.pdf [Accessed 2 January 2015].

NHS England. 2013a. *The NHS in England* [online]. Available at: www.nhs.uk/NHSEngland/thenhs/about/Pages/authoritiesandtrusts.aspx [Accessed 1 January 2015].

NHS England. 2013b. *NHS General Practitioners (GPs)* [online]. Available at: www.nhs.uk/NHSEngland/AboutNHSservices/doctors/Pages/NHSGPs.aspx [Accessed 1 January 2015].

NHS England. 2015. *NHS Allocations for 2013/14* [online] available at www.england.nhs.uk/allocations-2013-14/ [Accessed 1 January 2015].

National Trust Development Authority, n.d. *About* [online]. Available at: www.ntda.nhs.uk/about/ [Accessed 1 January 2015].

NICE. 2011. *Quality Standard for End of Life Care for Adults (revised 31 October 2013) QS13* [online]. Available at: www.nice.org.uk/guidance/qs13/resources/guidance-quality-standard-for-end-of-life-care-for-adults-pdf [Accessed 1 January 2015].

NICE. 2014. *Obesity: Identification, Assessment and Management of Overweight and Obesity in Children, Young People and Adults – NICE Clinical Guideline 189* [online]. Available at: www.nice.org.uk/guidance/cg189/resources/guidance-obesity-identification-assessment-and-management-of-overweight-and-obesity-in-children-young-people-and-adults-pdf [Accessed 2 January 2015].

Office of National Statistics. 2014a. *Births in England and Wales 2013* [online]. Available at: www.ons.gov.uk/ons/rel/vsob1/birth-summary-tables--england-and-wales/2013/stb-births-in-england-and-wales-2013.html [Accessed 1 December 2014].

Office of National Statistics. 2014b. *Deaths in England and Wales 2013* [online]. Available at: www.ons.gov.uk/ons/rel/vsob1/death-reg-sum-tables/2013/info-deaths-2013.html [Accessed 1 December 2014].

Parliament, n.d. *Draft Bills* [online]. Available at: www.parliament.uk/about/how/laws/draft/ [Accessed 1 January 2015].

Sir William Beveridge Foundation. n.d. *Sir William Beveridge* [online]. Available at: www.beveridge-foundation.org/sir-william-beveridge/ [Accessed 10 November 2014].

Spicker, P., Alvarez Leguzamon, S. and Gordon, D. 2006. *Poverty: An International Glossary*, 2nd edn. London: Zed Books.

Chapter 7

Quality in healthcare

Sarah Kraszewski

LEARNING OUTCOMES

By the end of this chapter you will be able to:

1 Explore the use of the term 'quality' within a healthcare context.
2 Understand what is meant by 'clinical governance'.
3 Understand how to carry out an audit.
4 Consider patient safety in the healthcare context and how to maintain a safe working environment.

Introduction

> *Prevention is better than cure.*
>
> Erasmus (n.d.)

How do we define 'quality' in the healthcare arena? Do we mean that a procedure was successfully undertaken? Do we mean that the patient was happy with the outcome, or merely that the patient survived the procedure or indeed that the procedure was successfully carried out but the patient died? Can we define quality through monitoring and measurement against a standard? In this chapter we will explore the concepts of quality in healthcare, clinical governance, patient safety and their application in the daily practice of healthcare.

ACTIVITY

What does 'quality' mean to you? Consider it in terms of an everyday activity such as going to the hairdresser, shopping, visiting the dentist or buying a new car.

What do you expect, not only in terms of the product, but also in terms of the service you encounter?

What is quality assurance?

Quality assurance is a term often used in daily life, whether it is in relation to the manufacture of goods (for example medical devices, medicines or car parts) or referring to a service provided (for example an interaction with a shop assistant or a doctor's receptionist). Quality can mean different things to different people. A client attending your service for care may be concerned about accessibility (can they travel there easily, can they park, do you see them on time, do they feel comfortable, are the staff friendly and caring, is anyone concerned about their pain?). A surgeon might be more concerned about the technical excellence of his procedure and the use of evidence-based practice to achieve a technically successful procedure. A manager may look at it from a financial perspective in terms of providing cost-effective care from a finite pot of money (Lee *et al.* 2013). In order to be able to start thinking about how we measure quality, we need to think about *standards*.

The approaches to quality that we now accept as everyday practice emerged in the 1980s and 1990s as a result of a government white paper called *Working for Patients* (Department of Health 1989). Weerakkody (2012) describes a situation where clinicians asked themselves if they were doing the 'right thing'. They realised that no one could really say what the right thing was because there were no standards, and so everyone was doing their 'own thing'. From these situations and musings, the frameworks of clinical governance and clinical audit emerged, the setting of standards and the rise of evidence-based practice. To be able to measure something, you need to have set a standard to measure against.

Quality assurance, therefore, involves a series of procedures and administrative activities that set standards and targets for a product, service or goal to be fulfilled, and a means of measuring the activities against the standard, with a feedback mechanism to detect and prevent errors. It can also include a commitment by the healthcare staff to work towards excellence in all they do.

Quality assurance programmes

A quality assurance programme can be grouped into three levels:

The World Health Organization (WHO) (2006) suggests that when discussed from a systems-based approach, there are six dimensions of quality.

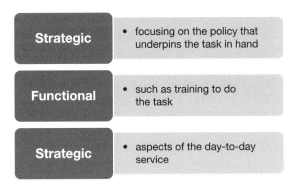

Figure 7.1 Quality assurance programme levels, adapted from WHO (2006).

That healthcare should be:

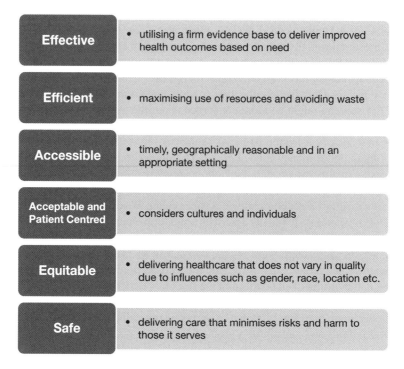

Figure 7.2 Quality dimensions, adapted from WHO (2006).

Strategies for quality can only be designed and implemented with the engagement of the healthcare providers, service users and communities involved (WHO 2006).

Leatherman and Sutherland (2003, cited by Lee *et al*. 2103) offer six domains for the measurement of quality in healthcare delivery:

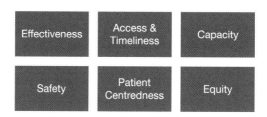

Figure 7.3 Quality measurement domains, adapted from Leatherman and Sutherland (2003).

This model provides a client-focused approach and offers opportunities to audit the quality of care within a service. Many approaches to measurement can involve the collection of metrics that may be irrelevant to the patient's quality of care as it does not focus on their personal, individual or family experience. Consider the following example in terms of the model above:

CASE STUDY

George, aged 52, underwent mitral valve repair (heart surgery) at a specialist hospital. Four months later, on a Thursday, he developed flu-like symptoms and atrial fibrillation (an irregular heartbeat) and was admitted to his local hospital for observation and tests to rule out the potentially serious complication of endocarditis (infection in the heart valves). George was self-caring, fully mobile and less than impressed at being admitted. The consultant prescribed a medication to control his heartbeat on Friday afternoon. The ward staff didn't give the medication until they were reminded by another doctor on Saturday afternoon who noticed the omission on the chart. The drug was administered and George's heartbeat resumed a regular rhythm within a couple of hours. A healthcare assistant (HCA) then arrived to check his charts. Without engaging to ask how he was feeling or about his response to the drug, she proceeded to pick up a checklist and go though it: 'Your bed is low enough so you can't get caught under it?', 'Are your pressure areas intact?', 'Are you fully continent?'... George stopped her and pointed out that he was dressed and fully mobile and didn't think these questions applied to him but that what she needed to note on his chart was that his heart was now in sinus rhythm (normal heartbeat). The HCA was confused by this and asked how George could know as he wasn't on a monitor – he patiently pointed out that he had taken his own pulse.

REFLECTION POINT

How do you use patient charts and checklists in practice?

Think about how these need to be interpreted in view of the patient you are caring for.

Large organisations often have checklists and collate metrics to record and measure particular aspects of care. The example above might be interpreted as a 'nursing by numbers' approach as there was no individual assessment of the client's needs or situation (*patient centredness*). The aspects the HCA was interested in, for her list, were not relevant to this particular man and detracted her attention from providing high-quality care and ensuring a good experience for George, who felt that his personal needs (i.e. an interest in monitoring the condition for which he had been admitted), were not being addressed. Evidently the organisation wanted to collate statistics on the prevalence of pressure ulcers for national targets (*effectiveness, safety*) and to ensure patient safety through ensuring staff checked bed height regularly (*safety*), but this led to an unsatisfactory encounter for this particular patient and is a poor indicator for the quality of care (Mayer *et al.* 2009, cited by Lee *et al.* 2013). Furthermore, the late administration of the medication raises quality and safety concerns (*effectiveness, safety, capacity* and *timeliness*). Measuring quality in care needs to span all the domains and the focus should be on the client and the impact that the quality of care has upon him/her and his/her family. The experiences of the client before and during treatment are of huge significance as these are often the times where they are suffering the most (Lee *et al.* 2013).

It is common practice in healthcare environments to collect health metrics as part of standardised care but it is very easy to lose the individual person amongst a myriad of goals and targets, as demonstrated above. This can result in confusion and a poor experience for both client and healthcare workers (Haslam *et al.* 2008, cited by Lee *et al.* 2013).

Lee *et al.* (2013) propose three key aspects for defining quality from the client's perspective: experience, healthcare and subjective well-being. They do so because so many of the existing measures utilised do not address the clients' experience and sense of well-being. Individual metrics can help to design services and measure particular events and are an important aspect of maintaining quality in healthcare, but the effect of a healthcare intervention on a person's quality of life is so much more difficult to measure.

Further thoughts about quality

Quality for any activity in healthcare means getting it right the first time and every time to ensure the best possible outcomes, patient satisfaction, staff retention and sound financial outcomes. The challenge in today's healthcare services is to improve the quality of healthcare, improve patient outcomes, increase patient satisfaction but also cut costs – all at the same time. All healthcare organisations are working with limited budgets and financial efficiency is essential. What we spend on one service inevitably means another service will have less. However, poor-quality healthcare can be costly and aside from resulting in poor satisfaction for patients, it can also result in a huge cost in terms of human suffering, mental and physical distress, staff dissatisfaction and stress and financial implications if extended stays and compensation are factors.

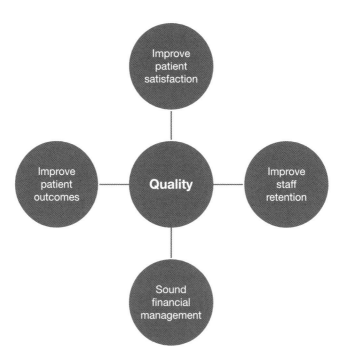

Figure 7.4 Quality objectives.

Consider the following case:

CASE STUDY

A young man who was quadraplegic, deaf and had severe learning disabilities died from asphyxiation after his head became trapped in the metal railings of his bed in a district general hospital. His mother had requested safety bumpers for his bed but they were not fitted. On transfer to a new ward, new staff were not made aware that the young man was deaf, one-to-one care was discontinued and his bed was still not appropriately equipped for his needs. Two days later he was found dead with his head caught in the cot sides. The hospital trust was prosecuted by the Health and Safety Executive for failure to ensure a patient's safety and the verdict listed many failings and was referred for sentencing at the Crown Court where an unlimited fine could be imposed (Leigh Day 2010).

ACTIVITY

What could the staff on the wards have done differently to ensure the young man was provided with safe care?

Think about some examples of safe, good-quality care and how it can be achieved.

Does good-quality care always need to cost more?

What are the financial implications of poor-quality care?

REFLECTION POINT

Reflect on the human and financial cost of the above scenario.

You might want to consider it in terms of the patient, his family, the staff and the hospital.

Quality itself can be considered a free entity, but the cost behind it can come from either non-conformance (which can be human and financial) or by observing conformity, which requires monitoring and evaluation for improvement. Planning (preventative) and appraisal (monitoring/doing) costs are both concerned with preventing errors from affecting patient care. There is an old saying 'prevention is better than cure' (Erasmus n.d.). The cost of preventing poor-quality care is much less than the situation that can evolve as the result of poor-quality care in both financial terms and that of the resulting human misery.

REFLECTION POINT

Consider your role in practice. How do you know what the standard is that you are expected to achieve?

Quality assurance agencies: the CQC

Perhaps the most well-known quality assurance agency in the context of healthcare is the Commission for Quality in Healthcare (CQC). The CQC's stated role is to monitor whether hospitals, GPs, dentists, care homes and services in peoples own homes are meeting national standards. The CQC undertakes visits and rates an organisation against specific criteria which results in one of three verdicts:

- met all standards
- not met all standards
- enforcement action

The reports are published on the CQC's website and are open to public scrutiny. There have been many high-profile cases in recent years, involving hospitals and care homes where improvements have been required. The most high-profile in recent years has been the Mid Staffordshire NHS Trust which led to the Francis Report (Francis 2013) and consequently far-reaching recommendations for reforms in terms of quality in healthcare services.

ACTIVITY

Access a copy of the Francis Report 2013 at www.midstaffspublicinquiry.com/report and read the executive summary.

What can you as an individual do, in your organisation and in your daily work, to ensure that patients receive safe and appropriate care?

Understanding clinical governance

> Clinical governance is a system through which NHS organisations are accountable for continuously improving the quality of their services and safeguarding high standards of care by creating an environment in which excellence in clinical care will flourish.
>
> (Scally and Donaldson 1998: 61)

Clinical governance is an organisational approach to quality and can be described as an overarching umbrella under which a range of activities and actions that maintain and enhance high-quality care are managed. It is underpinned by the concepts of quality and accountability and sits on the premise that the business operates in accordance with agreed principles, standards and rules. It is a proactive way of ensuring that the risk of errors is minimised and that a learning culture is embedded so that mistakes are learned from. Its origins can be traced back to a government white paper *A First Class Service* in 1998 (Department of Health 1998) and as part of the developments that adopted the evidence-based practice approach and development of a standards-based culture. The overall drive is to continuously improve quality.

The National Institute for Health and Clinical Excellence (now the National Institute for Health and Care Excellence) (NICE) was born out of the drive to continuously improve quality, as were other quality assurance initiatives such as the Quality and Outcomes Framework (QOF) in primary care (Jacks-Fowler 2011).

The traditional areas of clinical governance are:

- Risk management
- Openness
- Education and training
- Clinical audit
- Clinical effectiveness
- Research and development.

Furthermore, within these headings there are a number of components of clinical governance. These include:

- Quality improvement.
- Leadership.
- Dissemination of good practice, ideas and innovation.
- Clinical risk reduction.
- Detection of adverse events.
- Learning lessons from complaints.
- Addressing poor clinical performance.
- Professional development programmes.
- High-quality data and record keeping.

These pillars and components interlink and overlap. Clinical governance should be viewed as an integrated process. Successful approaches to clinical governance require an open, learning culture where quality is paramount and the patient is the most important person. Team working and training are key, as is the aim for perfection, whilst remembering there is always scope for improvement.

The audit cycle

Definition of clinical audit – 'Clinical audit is a quality improvement process that seeks to improve patient care and outcomes through systematic review of care against explicit criteria and the implementation of change' (NICE 2002).

A central feature of quality improvement is clinical audit. It provides a process whereby teams can review:

- The quality of care given to patients with common conditions or characteristics.
- The update and efficacy of screening or health promotion activities – for example breast screening or immunisation.
- Significant events – for example how has the infrastructure supporting a routine activity contributed to a significant event?

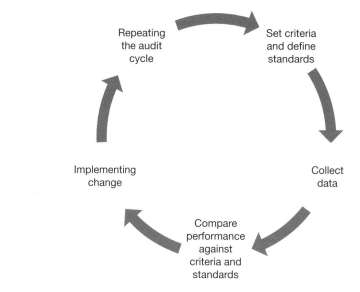

Figure 7.5 The audit cycle.

Clinical audit is a tool that can be used to systematically address quality improvement and can be used to drive up standards. High-profile cases such as the public inquiry into children's heart surgery at the Bristol Royal Infirmary between 1984 and 1995 give a clear indication of the role of audit (Department of Health 2002) and more recently in 2013 Professor Bruce Keogh, Medical Director of NHS England led a review team to look at 14 hospitals (Keogh 2013) with higher than average death rates. In Primary Care, funding is linked to the QOF which is the annual incentive and reward scheme for achieving a set of targets.

ACTIVITY

What does 'audit' and 'clinical audit' mean to you? Try to write a definition that relates to your service.

What aspects of quality could you audit in your service?

Clinical audit is a process used to review performance against agreed standards. This then leads to a comparison, a plan to drive up quality, followed by further audit to test the quality of the changes made. The aim is to continually drive up standards, and is different from other types of audit, such as financial audit. It is also important to note the difference between research and clinical audit. Whilst there are some common features, research is about the creation of new knowledge, whilst clinical audit ensures this knowledge is being utilised correctly (UBHT 2005).

Undertaking a clinical audit

To undertake a clinical audit, the following stages need to be considered:

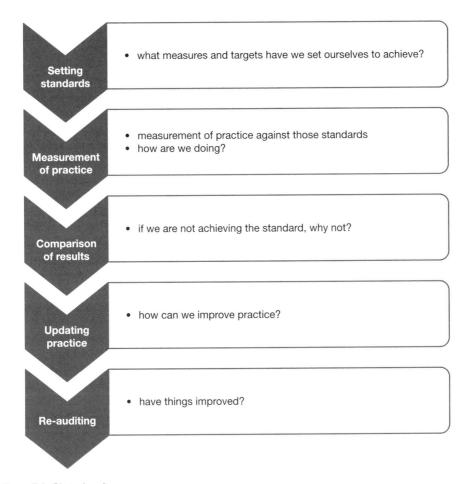

Setting standards
- what measures and targets have we set ourselves to achieve?

Measurement of practice
- measurement of practice against those standards
- how are we doing?

Comparison of results
- if we are not achieving the standard, why not?

Updating practice
- how can we improve practice?

Re-auditing
- have things improved?

Figure 7.6 Clinical audit stages.

ACTIVITY

When selecting a topic for clinical audit, it should be an area or topic that is relevant to improving patient outcomes, not merely for curiosity's sake. A review of adverse incidents or high-risk activities might be a good starting point.

Have a look to see what recent audits have been undertaken in your own area and then make a list of four appropriate topics for audit within your work area.

- What organisational factors should be considered prior to commencing?
- How will your audit contribute to improved patient outcomes/experience?
- How will record keeping contribute to your audit process?

Successful clinical audit requires structure, leadership and effective team working. It may be a profession-specific audit or it may be multidisciplinary, but the key issue is to involve all who will be affected at the planning stage to ensure buy-in and engagement. Any proposed changes in practice following an audit will be difficult to implement without the commitment of all concerned and it is important to note that audits require both funding and protected time and may result in increasing costs as well as increasing quality (NICE 2002).

Patient safety

In an interview with a national newspaper during 2014, Robert Francis QC said that if the NHS was an airline, it is so unsafe that 'planes would fall out of the sky all the time' (Donnelly 2014). Over recent years, scrutiny of safety incidents in healthcare has led to a recognised specialism of patient safety. The approaches and experiences of high-risk industries such as aviation have informed approaches now adopted in healthcare environments. A report from the World Alliance for Patient Safety (2008) outlined three main categories:

- Outcomes of unsafe medical care.
- Structural factors that contribute to unsafe care.
- Processes that contribute to unsafe care.

Patient safety can also be considered from three perspectives:

- The patient
- The professional
- The system.

Ambrose (2011) summarises the definitions of terms used when talking about patient safety:

- **Patient safety** – maintaining a safe environment and avoiding accidental harm to people receiving healthcare.
- **Patient safety incident (PSI)** – an event where something goes wrong which may be harmful to patients (either potential or actual).
- **Patient safety solution** – systems designed to prevent or mitigate risks of patient harm arising from healthcare.
- **Organisational resilience** – the system's intrinsic resistance to its organisational risks (Ambrose 2011).

ACTIVITY

Thinking back to the section on clinical audit, can you identify areas of patient safety (perhaps high-risk activities) that can be measured or monitored?

Consider the case in the earlier case study – how could this accident have been avoided?

Incident reporting

Incident reporting mechanisms are organised locally and nationally. The National Reporting and Learning System (NRLS) (2014), as part of the National Patient Safety Agency (NPSA), was set up in 2003. The NPSA was transferred into the NHS Commissioning Board Special Health Authority in 2012 to place patient safety at the heart of the NHS. The NRLS enables healthcare staff, patients and members of the public to report safety incidents, which allows collation of data and pictures to be built of safety incidents, and actions to then be taken where needed. An example of this is with childhood immunisations:

CASE STUDY

The introduction of a new immunisation schedule in 2005 using vaccines called Repivax and Revaxis resulted in a significant number of near misses in general practice and schools where health professionals administered the wrong product due to similar names and packaging. In one school 93 children received Repivax instead of Revaxis. As a result the manufacturer changed the packaging to make the vaccines more distinct and NHS Trusts were advised to:

- Ensure robust procedures existed to check correct selection of vaccines on every occasion.
- Raise awareness of packaging changes amongst immunisation staff.
- Review the risk management procedures for introduction of new vaccines and strengthen where needed.
- Continue to report patient safety incidents (www.nrls.npsa.nhs.uk/resources/?EntryId45 =59795).

Another example of a change in practice resulting from an NRLS study was of establishing a common 'crash call' in secondary care. In 2004 the NPSA carried out a feasibility study that revealed that services were not using standardised numbers for 'crash calls' and that this presented a risk of potential delays in summoning crash teams where agency staff moved from hospital to hospital and therefore a potential threat to patient safety. A patient safety alert was issued for trusts to standardise their numbers to 2222.

In 2009 the World Health Organization introduced the Surgical Safety Checklist as part of its 'Safe Surgery Saves Lives' global challenge. Use of the checklist in 8,000 procedures had demonstrated a reduction in deaths and complications (Haynes *et al.* 2009). During 2007, 129,419 incidents relating to surgery were reported to the NRLS. Of these, 271 resulted in the death of the patient and 1,105 reported as severe harm (National Patient Safety Agency 2009a). The checklist was adapted for England and Wales by the NPSA and requires surgical teams to complete checklists (*read out loud*) prior to the induction of anaesthesia (*sign in*), prior to the start of the surgical intervention (*time out*) and prior to any of the team leaving theatre (*sign out*). You can view a copy of this at www.nrls.npsa.nhs.uk/resources/?entryid45=59860.

ACTIVITY

Watch the video on YouTube entitled *Just a Routine Operation* (Bromiley 2011). This film has been made by an airline pilot whose wife died following induction of an anaesthetic for a routine procedure, leaving him to bring up their young children. Despite being surrounded by experienced staff, a lack of clear leadership, planning and decision making resulted in the tragic outcome. He investigated the actions using the principles used in the aviation industry (www.youtube.com/watch?v=JzlvgtPIof4).

REFLECTION POINT

Reflect on how the Surgical Safety Checklist might have influenced the potential outcome for the patient in the film.

Think about your work environment – how do teams work together to ensure that human factors are not the causative agent for poor outcomes?

Do you feel able to speak up when part of a team to voice your concerns?

What can healthcare learn from the aviation industry?

In commercial aviation, pilots and crew operate in an open, no-blame environment. Recording equipment operates throughout a flight, flying teams are frequently changed to minimise the development of bad habits and fit-to-fly licences and health checks are a regular feature. These principles can be applied to healthcare practice to increase patient safety and avoid complacency in teams used to working together.

Seven Steps to Patient Safety

Step 1   Build a safety culture.
Create a culture that is open and fair.

Step 2   Lead and support your staff.
Establish a clear and strong focus on patient safety throughout your organisation.

Step 3   Integrate your risk management activity.
Develop systems and processes to manage your risks and identify and assess things that could go wrong.

Step 4   Promote reporting.
Ensure your staff can easily report incidents locally and nationally.

Step 5   Involve and communicate with patients and the public.
Develop ways to communicate openly with and listen to patients.

Step 6   Learn and share safety lessons.
Encourage staff to use root cause analysis to learn how and why incidents happen.

Step 7   Implement solutions to prevent harm.
Embed lessons through changes to practice, processes or systems (National Patient Safety Agency 2004).

Whilst the Seven Steps to Patient Safety have been produced primarily for risk management and clinical governance teams, it also functions well as a safety manual for staff caring directly for patients.

REFLECTION POINT

Review the 'Seven Steps' and consider how they are embedded in your working environment.

- Are you aware of a 'safety culture'?
- Is there a strong focus on patient safety?
- Do you understand why certain activities have a clear procedure to promote safety?
- Do you know how to report an incident?
- How does your service communicate with the public?
- When something does go wrong, how do you learn from it?
- Can you think of any changes implemented as a result of a safety incident?

Medication errors

Medication errors may be defined as:

> any preventable event that may cause or lead to an inappropriate medication use or patient harm while in the control of the healthcare professional, patient or consumer.
>
> (National Co-ordinating Council for Medication
> Error Reporting and Prevention 2014)

Sometimes adverse drug events cannot be predicted. These are where the patient suffers a reaction, but this comes from the side effect profile of the drug or a bizarre reaction and not from an error in prescribing, dispensing or administration (Clinical Knowledge Summaries 2012). Errors occur when a mistake is made, for example prescribing or administering a drug to a patient with a known allergy to the product, or prescribing, dispensing or administering an overdose or administering a correctly prescribed drug via an incorrect route.

The *Safety in Doses* reports (National Patient Safety Agency 2007b, 2009b) demonstrated a year-on-year increase in the number of safety incidents being reported in relation to medications. Three types of incident emerged as being responsible for 71 per cent of fatal and serious harm from medication errors:

- Unclear/wrong dose or frequency.
- Wrong medicine.
- Omitted/delayed medicines.

Safety events can be related to prescribing, communication, labelling, packaging, dispensing, education, monitoring and use. Dispensing errors, calculation errors, monitoring errors and administration errors all play a part. Other factors such as distraction and interruption, fatigue, complicated prescriptions, insufficient training, unfamiliarity with the medication and new staff can all have an influence of the rate of errors.

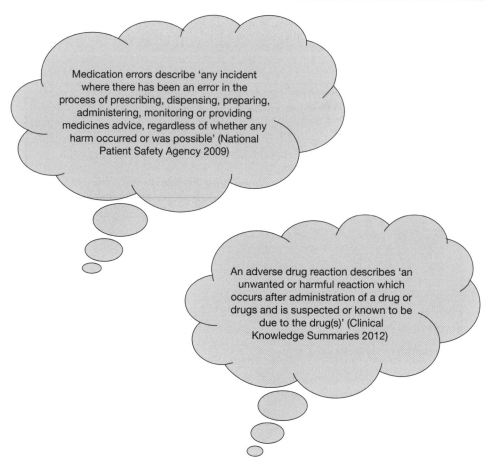

Figure 7.7 Medication errors.

ACTIVITY

Think about your working environment and how medications are administered.

- What actions can be taken to avoid interrupting staff administering medications?
- What actions would you take if you discovered a medication error?

Yellow Card System

The Yellow Card System enables anybody to report a suspected side effect from a drug. It is administered by the Medicines and Healthcare Products Regulatory Agency (MHRA) and the Commission on Human Medicines (CHM). The system collects information from both health professionals and the general public and enables the MHRA and CHM to monitor the safety profile of licensed drugs and to update advice where necessary. It is important to remember that all drugs have side effects. Patient safety incidents can be reported via the NRLS at www.nrls.npsa.nhs.uk/report-a-patient-safety-incident/.

Patient Safety First

The 'Patient Safety First' campaign ran between 2007 and 2010, aiming to focus on a safety culture and engaging staff to actively provide safer and improved care. The aim was to create a mindset of 'no avoidable death and no avoidable harm'. The approach was from both a leadership perspective and a clinical perspective.

One theme focused upon the deteriorating patient (National Patient Safety Agency 2007a). Research indicated that failure to recognise a deteriorating patient or to provide rescue treatment was a significant area in which unintended harm was happening. The NPSA analysed 576 deaths reported over a one-year period and found that 11 per cent of the deaths were due to deterioration that was not recognised or acted upon. This may have been where observations were not taken accurately, not communicated or not responded to appropriately. Other factors included communication breakdown in teams, delays in referrals and in the delivery of essential care. A NICE Guideline was released in 2007 in relation to the deteriorating patient and this can be accessed at: www.nice.org.uk/nicemedia/pdf/CG50FullGuidance.pdf (NICE 2007).

The 'Deteriorating Patient' intervention raises six areas as key to identifying and managing patients safely in secondary care:

* Physiological observations must be recorded for all adult patients in hospital care.
* Physiological observations should be undertaken and acted upon by staff trained to take them correctly and understand how to interpret them (clinical relevance).
* Track and trigger systems should be used.
* A graded response strategy should be used.
* An escalation protocol must be in place.
* A communication tool must be used.

The actions that a healthcare worker must take in response to changes in the patient's observations and conditions must be very clear and the escalation policy unambiguous. Some areas have used colour coding on charts or print the instructions on the charts. There should be an area for the healthcare worker to record changing status and actions taken, and for that member of staff to feel they can call for help if they have concerns about a patient irrespective of the observations.

ACTIVITY

In your clinical area:

* What are the guidelines for reacting to a change in the patient's observations (for example rapid pulse and hypotension)?
* Does your hospital have a rapid response or critical care outreach team?
* Does the system follow the NICE Guidelines?

Another project under the 'Patient Safety First' initiative is the prevention of venous thromboembolism (VTE) (Patient Safety First 2014). The National VTE Prevention Programme (2014) has been shown to save lives. The complication of VTE following hospitalisation is significant and can cause thousands of deaths each year. This programme is designed to ensure that all adult patients admitted to hospital are assessed for risk and provided with appropriate evidence-based preventative care according to national guidelines. Research at Kings College Foundation Trust has indicated a 40 per cent reduction in VTE events related to inadequate prophylaxis (Roberts *et al.* 2013).

REFLECTION POINT

In your service or workplace, how is VTE risk-assessed and are the appropriate interventions provided for patients?

Health and safety

A further consideration for all staff is their responsibilities under the Health and Safety at Work etc. Act 1974. This is the primary piece of legislation with regards to occupational health and safety in Great Britain. All workers have a right to working environments in which risks to their health and safety are controlled, but the employees also have a responsibility to help ensure this safe working environment is upheld.

What employers must do for you:

1 Decide what could harm you in your job and the precautions to stop it. This is part of risk assessment.
2 In a way you can understand, explain how risks will be controlled and tell you who is responsible for this.
3 Consult and work with you and your health and safety representatives in protecting everyone from harm in the workplace.
4 Free of charge, give you the health and safety training you need to do your job.
5 Free of charge, provide you with any equipment and protective clothing you need, and ensure it is properly looked after.
6 Provide toilets, washing facilities and drinking water.
7 Provide adequate first-aid facilities.
8 Report major injuries and fatalities at work to the Incident Contact Centre: 0845 300 9923. Report other injuries, diseases and dangerous incidents online at www.hse.gov.uk (Health and Safety Executive (HSE) 2014).
9 Have insurance that covers you in case you get hurt at work or are ill through work. Display a hard copy or electronic copy of the current insurance certificate where you can easily read it.
10 Work with any other employers or contractors sharing the workplace or providing employees (such as agency workers), so that everyone's health and safety is protected.

What you must do:

1 Follow the training you have received when using any work items your employer has given you.
2 Take reasonable care of your own and other people's health and safety.
3 Cooperate with your employer on health and safety.
4 Tell someone (your employer, supervisor, or health and safety representative) if you think the work or inadequate precautions are putting anyone's health and safety at serious risk (Health and Safety Executive 2009).

If there's a problem:

1 If you are worried about health and safety in your workplace, talk to your employer, supervisor, or health and safety representative.
2 You can also look at the HSE website for general information about health and safety at work.
3 If, after talking with your employer, you are still worried, you can find the address of your local enforcing authority for health and safety and the Employment Medical Advisory Service via HSE's website: www.hse.gov.uk (Health and Safety Executive 2014).

Fire safety: You can get advice on fire safety from the Fire and Rescue Services or your workplace fire officer.

Chapter summary

This chapter has explored definitions of quality and then considered different elements of quality, with a focus on patient safety:

• Healthcare settings provide highly complex interventions which inevitably introduce risk into the daily lives of patients and staff.
• These need to be managed effectively within systems that minimise and manage risk.
• Incidents that result in harm can have far-reaching consequences for patients and their families, but are also distressing for the staff involved and can have a significant financial impact on the NHS through the need for additional treatment and litigation.
• High-quality care and patient safety are everyone's business, and as such lead to good outcomes for patients and staff.

Further resources

Royal College of Nursing. 2014. *How Patient Safety Incidents Evolve*. Available at: www.rcn.org.uk/development/practice/cpd_online_learning/making_sense_of_patient_safety/how_patient_safety_incidents_evolve_-_two_scenarios.
Royal College of Nursing. 2012. Available at: *Patient Safety Human Factors* www.rcn.org.uk/development/practice/patient_safety/human_factors_-_what_are_they.
Royal College of Nursing. 2014. First Steps for Healthcare Assistants. Available at: http://rcnhca.org.uk/.
Patient Safety First. Available at: www.patientsafetyfirst.nhs.uk.
NICE. Available at: www.nice.org.uk/.
The NHS Constitution. Available at: www.gov.uk/government/publications/the-nhs-constitution-for-england.

References

Ambrose, L. 2011. 'Patient Safety', *InnovAiT* 4(8): 472–7.

Bromiley, M. 2011. *Just a Routine Operation* [YouTube] 6 July. Available at: www.youtube.com/watch?v=JzlvgtPIof4 [Accessed 16 July 2014].

Clinical Knowledge Summaries. 2012. *Adverse Drug Reactions* [online]. Available at: http://cks.nice.org.uk/adverse-drug-reactions#!topicsummary [Accessed 15 July 2014].

Donnelly, L. 2014. 'If NHS Were an Airline, Planes Would Always Be Crashing, Warns Mid Staffs Inquiry Chief' [online]. *Daily Telegraph*, *Health News*. Available at: www.telegraph.co.uk/health/healthnews/10853099/If-NHS-were-an-airline-planes-would-always-be-crashing-warns-Mid-Staffs-inquiry-chief.html [Accessed 27 May 2014].

Department of Health. 1989. *Working for Patients*. Cm 555. London: HMSO.

Department of Health. 1998. *A First Class Service* [online]. Available at: www.dh.gov.uk/en/Publicationsandstatistics/Publications/PublicationsPolicyAndGuidance/DH_4006902 [Accessed 29 May 2014].

Department of Health. 2002. *Learning from Bristol: The Department of Health's Response to the Report of the Public Inquiry into Children's Heart Surgery at the Bristol Royal Infirmary 1984–1995* [online]. Available at www.dh.gov.uk [Accessed 30 May 2014].

Erasmus, D. n.d. BrainyQuote.com [online]. Available at: www.brainyquote.com/quotes/authors/d/desiderius_erasmus.html [Accessed 30 December 2014].

Francis, R. QC. 2013. *Report of the Mid Staffordshire NHS Foundation Trust.* Public Inquiry [online]. Available at: www.midstaffspublicinquiry.com/report [Accessed 27 May 2014].

Jacks-Fowler, R. M. 2011. 'Clinical Governance', *InnovAiT* 4(10): 592–5 [online]. Available at: http://ino.sagepub.com/content/4/10/592 [Accessed 29 May 2014].

Haynes, A. B., Weiser, T. G., Berry, W. R., Lipsitz, S. R., Breiza, A. S., Patchen Dellinger, E., Herbosa, T., Joseph, S., Kibatala, P. L., Lapitan, M. C. M., Merry, A. F., Moorthy, K., Reznick, R. K., Taylor, B., Atul, A. and Gawande, A. A. 2009. 'A Surgical Safety Checklist to Reduce Morbidity and Mortality in a Global Population for the Safe Surgery Saves Lives Study Group', *New England Journal of Medicine* 360: 491–9 [online]. Available at: www.nejm.org/doi/full/10.1056/NEJMsa0810119 [Accessed 15 June 2014].

Health and Safety at Work etc. Act. 1974. London: HMSO.

Health and Safety Executive. 2009. *Health and Safety Law: What You Need to Know*. Available at: www.hse.gov.uk/pUbns/law.pdf [Accessed 15 July 2014].

Health and Safety Executive. 2014. *Guidance* [online]. Available at: www.hse.gov.uk/guidance/index.htm [Accessed 25 July 2014].

Keogh, B. 2013. *Review into the Quality of Care and Treatment Provided by 14 Hospital Trusts in England: Overview Report* [online]. Available at: www.nhs.uk/NHSEngland/bruce-keogh-review/Documents/outcomes/keogh-review-final-report.pdf [Accessed 27 May 2014].

Lee, H., Vlaev, I., King, D., Mayer, E., Darzi, A. and Dolan, P. 2013. 'Subjective Well-being and the Measurement of Quality in Healthcare, Centre for Health Policy, Institute for Global Health Innovation, Imperial College London, UK', *Social Science & Medicine* 99: 27e34.

Leigh Day. 2010. 'Basildon Hospital Admits to Safety Failings' [online]. Available at: www.leighday.co.uk/News/2010/March-2010/Basildon-Hospital-admits-to-safety-failings [Accessed 15 July 2014].

National Co-ordinating Council for Medication Error Reporting and Prevention. 2014. 'About Medication Errors' [online]. Available at: www.nccmerp.org/aboutMedErrors.html [Accessed 24 July 2014].

National Patient Safety Agency. 2004. *Seven Steps to Patient Safety* [online]. Available at: www.npsa.nhs.uk/sevensteps [Accessed 29 July 2014].

National Patient Safety Agency. 2007a. *Recognising and Responding Appropriately to Early Signs of Deterioration in Hospitalised Patients* [online]. Available at: www.npsa.nhs.uk [Accessed 27 July 2014].

National Patient Safety Agency. 2007b. *Safety in Doses: Improving the Use of Medicines in the NHS* [online]. Available at: www.nrls.npsa.nhs.uk/resources/?entryid45=61625 [Accessed 20 July 2014].

National Patient Safety Agency. 2009a. *WHO Surgical Safety Checklist* [online]. Available at: www. nrls.npsa.nhs.uk [Accessed 15 July 2014].

National Patient Safety Agency. 2009b. *Safety in Doses*: *Improving the Use of Medicines in the NHS* [online]. Available at: www.nrls.npsa.nhs.uk/resources/?entryid45=61625 [Accessed 22 July 2014].

National Reporting and Learning System. 2014. *Patient Safety* [online]. Available at: www.nrls.npsa. nhs.uk/home/ [Accessed 26 July 2014].

NICE. 2002. *Principles for Best Practice in Clinical Audit*. Oxford: Radcliffe Medical [online]. Available at: www.nice.org.uk [Accessed 22 July 2014].

NICE. 2007. *Acutely Ill Patients in Hospital: Recognition of and Response to Acute Illness in Adults in Hospital*. NICE Clinical Guideline 50. July 2007 [online]. Available at: www.nice.org.uk/nicemedia/ pdf/CG50FullGuidance.pdf [Accessed 15 June 2014].

Patient Safety First. 2014. *VTE Prevention* [online]. Available at: www.patientsafetyfirst.nhs.uk/ Content.aspx?path=/interventions/VTE-prevention/ [Accessed 15 July 2014].

Roberts, L. N., Porter, G., Barker, R. D., Yorke, R., Bonner, L., Patel, R. and Arya, R. 2013. 'Comprehensive VTE Prevention Program Incorporating Mandatory Risk Assessment Reduces the Incidence of Hospital-Associated Thrombosis', *Chest* 144(4): 1276–81.

Royal College of Nursing. 2014. *How Patient Safety Incidents Evolve* [online]. Available at: www.rcn. org.uk/development/practice/cpd_online_learning/making_sense_of_patient_safety/how_patient_ safety_incidents_evolve_-_two_scenarios [Accessed 15 July 2014].

Scally, G. and Donaldson, L. J. 1998. 'Clinical Governance and the Drive for Quality Improvement in the New NHS in England', *British Medical Journal* 317(7150): 61–5.

UBHT United Bristol Healthcare Trust Clinical Audit Central Office. 2005. *What Is Clinical Audit?* [online]. Available at: www.ubht.nhs.uk/clinicalaudit [Accessed 24 July 2014].

Weerakkody, A. 2012. 'Quality in Healthcare – Part 1 How Did It All Start? – A Historical Perspective', *Sri Lanka Journal of Obstetrics and Gynaecology* 34: 27–8.

World Alliance for Patient Safety. 2008. *Summary of the Evidence on Patient Safety: Implications for Research*. World Health Organization [online]. Available at: whqlibdoc.who.int/publications/ 2008/9789241596541_eng.pdf [Accessed 7 April 2014].

WHO. 2006. *Quality of Care: A Process for Making Strategic Choices in Health Systems* [online]. Available at: www.who.int/management/quality/assurance/QualityCare_B.Def.pdf [Accessed 24 July 2014].

WHO. 2009. *Surgical Safety Checklist* [online]. Available at: www.nrls.npsa.nhs.uk/resources/ ?entryid45=59860 [Accessed 4 July 2014].

www.nrls.npsa.nhs.uk/resources/?EntryId45=59795 [Accessed 4 July 2014].

Chapter 8

Legal aspects of healthcare delivery

Patricia Macnamara

LEARNING OUTCOMES

By the end of this chapter you will be able to:

1 Understand the ethical theory which has shaped the development of how our society is organised.
2 Relate the legal principles which reflect this.
3 Discuss how these uphold the dignity and worth of individuals.
4 Have an understanding of the Human Rights Act 1998 and Mental Capacity Act 2005 and how these affect healthcare practice.

Introduction

This chapter looks at how the law upholds and protects the rights of people undergoing medical care and treatment. The desire to care for the ill and the vulnerable is considered to be one of humanity's finest qualities and in our society this has led to the founding of the National Health Service (NHS) so that everyone can receive treatment that is free at the point of delivery. Our society also considers that its individual members should be free to make their own decisions about their lives, i.e. they should be able to exercise self-determination. This includes decisions about their own healthcare even if that decision will lead to avoidable death or disability and the professionals involved in their care should respect the decision. However, when such a decision is made there will always be questions about whether the person making it is capable of doing so. The law helps to provide the balance between protecting the individual from the unwanted interventions of others and protecting him or her from themselves. The law also helps to uphold the rights and dignity of those who cannot make their own decisions. The opening sections of this chapter develop some of the ethical theory from Chapter 5 before describing how this is reflected in the law.

Utilitarianism

One of the most influential theories about how society should be organised in order to bring about the greatest benefit for all its members is utilitarianism. Jeremy Bentham (1748–1832) is the name most closely associated with utilitarianism. He believed that:

Nature has placed mankind under the governance of two sovereign masters, pain and pleasure. It is for them alone to point out what we ought to do, as well as to determine what we shall do.

(Bentham 2005: 11)

Utilitarianism is called a consequentialist moral theory because the moral worth of an action is judged by the outcomes, or consequences, that it produces. A utilitarian, according to Bentham, should aim to bring about the 'greatest good for the greatest number'. Bentham believed that all human beings were of equal worth and value and as such each person's happiness was of equal importance. The founding of the NHS in 1947 can be seen as a part of the culmination of this view that the state should view all citizens as equal members of society with equal access to services on the basis of need.

The founding of NICE in 1999 continued this ethical tradition. NICE was originally set up in 1999 as the National Institute for Clinical Excellence, a special health authority, to reduce variation in the availability and quality of NHS treatments and care. Its name changed to the National Institute for Health and Clinical Excellence in 2005 (NICE 2013) and changed again in 2013 to the National Institute for Health and Care Excellence. The aim of NICE is to try to achieve the best use of resources available to the health service in order to ensure the best treatment for as many patients as possible across the entire country. As the NICE charter states:

NICE guidance helps health, public health and social care professionals deliver the best possible care based on the best available evidence.

(NICE 2013: 1)

One of the most effective ways of improving public health has been through immunisation. Smallpox has been eliminated throughout the world and it is hoped that the same can be achieved for polio in the near future (World Health Organization 2014b). While it is clear that immunisation against various diseases has produced great benefits for the population both at home and abroad there have been some instances of vaccines causing harm to the recipients. An example of this came to light in 1974 when Jack Ashley (1922–2012), then the Labour MP for Stoke-on-Trent, asked parliament what was to be done for children left damaged as a result of the whooping cough vaccination. Until this point the general public had not been aware that there were any potentially serious risks associated with this vaccine. Jack Ashley continued to campaign on behalf of children damaged by the vaccine because, as he said in 1977 in the House of Commons:

. . . the main beneficiary of the immunisation programme is society. It is not only the individual who benefits but the community at large, through a high level of population immunity, yet the risk is all to the individual . . .

(Hansard 1977)

This statement identifies one of the main objections to Bentham's formulation of producing the greatest good for the greatest number: what happens to the individual if they are not part of the greatest number? Is it acceptable to sacrifice individuals for the sake of the common good?

ACTIVITY

Smoking, drinking alcohol in excess and overeating are all regarded as harmful. There is often a feeling that the individual has made a choice and is responsible for their own misfortune when illness strikes.

Should they be held responsible for their misfortunes?

When do the rest of us have a moral duty to help others?

Does it make a difference if they are thought to be the 'architects of their own misfortunes'?

A solution to this problem was provided by John Stuart Mill (1806–73) and a fellow utilitarian. Mill declared:

> The only purpose for which power can be rightfully exercised over any member of a civilized community, against his will, is to prevent harm to others.

(Mill 1859: 1)

In this statement Mill is saying that the individual should be free to make his own decisions and the only acceptable constraint on that freedom is the harm that may befall others. The ability to make and execute one's own decisions is what is meant by autonomy. The abuse of alcohol was considered a major problem because of the social consequences that arose from the practice. This remains the case to the present day. Smoking was originally considered a harmless activity. However, by the 1930s German scientists had evidence that smoking was the cause of serious ill health (Proctor 1989). By the 1950s articles were appearing in British and American medical journals linking smoking and lung cancer. At this point the harm only seemed to be to the individual smoker and thus by Mill's definition there would be no grounds for curbing the behaviour of smokers or tobacco companies. However, by the end of the twentieth century the harm arising from passive or second-hand smoking had been established and this has led to legislation to restrict the activities of both smokers and tobacco companies. Ireland was the first country to institute a comprehensive national smoke-free law on smoking in all indoor workplaces in 2004. Non-smoking legislation was introduced in Scotland in 2006 and in the rest of the UK in 2007. This and similar legislation is justified by Mill's definition because of the harm caused to non-smokers by smokers.

Duty-based ethical thought

Intervening in the apparently autonomous choices of an individual is justified by a utilitarian by the prevention of foreseen harm to others. However, the outcomes of actions cannot always be accurately predicted either for individuals or for society and thus it has been argued that making decisions based on their outcomes is not a satisfactory foundation for ethical thinking. It is argued that it is better to have rules which will be implemented rather than trying to work out the consequences of an action.

The name most usually associated with this approach is that of a German philosopher, Immanuel Kant (1724–1804). Kant believed that the basis of moral action was duty and hence this school of ethical thought is described as duty based. This then gives rise to the question of how it is to be decided that something is a duty and must therefore be carried out?

Kant (2007) argued that there are three criteria to be considered when trying to determine a rule that must be obeyed. The first of these is that all humans are members of what he called a kingdom of ends. This means that everyone has their own ends or goals in life and these must be respected by everyone else. A human being can never be just a means to an end. At the end of the Second World War it was discovered that German scientists and doctors had carried out medical experiments on prisoners and concentration camp inmates with no regard for the welfare of these individuals, many of whom had died or were left with serious disabilities. The information gained from these studies was often scientifically sound but the way in which it was obtained was considered to be morally unacceptable because the people experimented upon were simply a means to the end of finding the results of the study. As a result of this the World Medical Association (2013) drew up the Declaration of Helsinki in 1964. This is a set of ethical principles established to regulate research involving human subjects. A key principle is that a human participant in research must never be regarded only as a means of obtaining data. The individual must as far as possible be a knowing and willing participant in the research and be able to leave the study at any time. Research also needs to be carried out involving those who cannot give consent, e.g. babies or people with dementia. Researchers need to respect these individuals as ends in themselves and never only a means to an end.

The second principle is that of impartiality. This means that all humans have the same standing and that no individual or group of people should be favoured or disadvantaged in relation to another.

ACTIVITY

NICE guidance states that couples experiencing infertility where the woman is under 35 years of age should be offered three cycles of IVF on the NHS. Some areas offer fewer cycles and some do not offer any. Is this an example of discrimination based on where someone lives and thus a failure to offer treatment impartially? The reason the age limit is set at 35 is that after this age IVF success rates are much lower and thus the treatment is felt to be too expensive in relation to the possible benefits. Should other treatments, e.g. kidney transplants, have an age-based cut-off point?

The NHS Constitution (2013) says:

> The NHS provides a comprehensive service, available to all irrespective of gender, race, disability, age, sexual orientation, religion, belief, gender reassignment, pregnancy and maternity or marital or civil partnership status.
>
> (NHS Constitution 2013: 3)

This binds the NHS to treating all patients impartially.

The third principle is that a moral duty must be universally binding, i.e. it applies in all places at all times without exception.

If all three principles are met then the rule would be a categorical imperative, meaning it must be obeyed by all, no matter the circumstances. This is why a categorical imperative has never been established, because there will always be an exception to the rule. It also fails to consider cultural differences. Most people accept that taking another human life is wrong but can think of exceptions to that rule, e.g. in defence of self or others. There is also a problem if there is a conflict between two or more principles, e.g. telling the truth would mean breaking a confidence. A duty-based ethic does not tell us how to resolve this conflict.

The Four Principles approach

The application of principles is a useful way of making us focus on the patient and can be helpful in avoiding self-interest. The Four Principles approach of Tom Beauchamp and James Childress was first introduced in 1985 as a tool to help healthcare professionals to make decisions (Beauchamp and Childress 2013). The principles to be taken into account are: autonomy, beneficence, non-maleficence and justice.

Autonomy

As already mentioned, this means that people who have the ability to make decisions should have these decisions respected. The NHS Constitution says:

> You have the right to accept or refuse treatment that is offered to you, and not to be given any physical examination or treatment unless you have given valid consent. If you do not have the capacity to do so, consent must be obtained from a person legally able to act on your behalf, or the treatment must be in your best interests.
>
> (NHS Constitution 2013: 8)

This acknowledges the autonomy of adults (someone over the age of 18) and thus their right to accept or to refuse treatment that is offered even when the refusal will lead to death or disability.

Beneficence

As healthcare professionals we are committed to doing good, and this is what beneficence, the second principle, means. So although a patient has the right to refuse treatment our legal, ethical and professional duty is to ensure that the decision is freely made by someone who understands the possible or actual consequences of the decision. Similarly, if someone cannot make his/her own decision then others must do so for him/her. The requirement that the professionals act in peoples' best interests if they cannot make their own decisions, e.g. because of dementia, recognises the principle of beneficence.

ACTIVITY

In Re E [1993] 1 FLR 386 a 15-year-old boy who was a Jehovah's Witness wanted to refuse blood products for the treatment of his leukaemia. His parents also wished to refuse the blood products on his behalf as they too were Jehovah's Witnesses. The judge overruled the refusal of consent on behalf of both the boy and his parents. He explained:

> Parents may be free to become martyrs themselves, but it does not follow that they are free in identical circumstances to make martyrs of their children.
>
> The decision was made in what the court felt were the boy's best interests, as it is obliged to.
>
> In this situation should the court be the final arbiter of best interests over the whole family?
>
> Do you agree with the judge's statement? Why?

Non-maleficence

This means that if we cannot actively do good then we should avoid making things worse. It also means that professionals have to know and acknowledge the limits of their own competence in order to avoid inflicting harm. In some instances, e.g. the outbreak of the Ebola virus in West Africa in 2014, there is no tested treatment available. Under these circumstances the World Health Organization (2014a) said that as the mortality rate was over 50 per cent it was acceptable to use untested forms of treatment as things could not be made worse than they already were. Where possible the consent of the patient should be sought before administering the drugs.

Justice

This means that patients should be treated fairly and equally when considering the distribution of resources and about who gets what when decisions about treatment are made. As already noted, NICE was established to try to ensure fairness for patients in England and Wales in the provision of treatment.

Human rights

So far we have looked at some of the tools developed to help us as healthcare professionals to make decisions. One common theme that has emerged is that all human beings are of equal worth and standing. This arises from an individual's status as a human being and does not rely on anything else. This is the basis of human rights. Human rights are inherent in the nature of human beings and it is essential that they be upheld to protect both humanity as a whole and the welfare of the individual. This means that institutions, including the NHS, must recognise and respect those rights.

A significant milestone on the journey of human rights came on 10 December 1948 when the General Assembly of the United Nations accepted the Universal Declaration of Human Rights (1948). This was the first global expression of rights to which all human beings are entitled.

The path to the Human Rights Act 1998

The Universal Declaration arose from the atrocities associated with the Second World War (1939–45). In Europe this led to the formulation of the Convention for the Protection of

Human Rights and Fundamental Freedoms, now the European Convention of Human Rights, in 1950. The Convention was an attempt to share common ideals among the nations of Europe and to establish a court to enforce them. It was hoped that this would prevent the terrible wrongs of the Nazi era from happening again. One of the leading members of the committee which drafted the Convention was the British lawyer Sir David Maxwell-Fyfe and Britain signed in 1951. Despite this the Convention was not incorporated into law in the UK as the Human Rights Act 1998 until 2 October 2000. The gap between 1998 and 2000 was to enable any necessary adjustments to be made to enable the Act to be enforced. One of the main changes that the Human Rights Act 1998 has brought about is that a British citizen who feels that their rights under the Act have been violated can have their case heard in a British court rather than having to go the European Court of Human rights in Strasbourg (Dimond 2015).

How does the Act work?

Section 2 of the Human Rights Act 1998 states that a court considering a question connected with a Convention right must take into account any relevant judgments, decisions, declarations or opinions of the European Court of Human Rights, together with other official decisions and opinions concerning the Convention. Section 3(1) states: 'So far as it is possible to do so, primary legislation (i.e. Acts of Parliament) and subordinate legislation (i.e. regulations and rules) must be read and given effect in a way which is compatible with the Convention rights.' This means that parliament and judges must ensure that both statute and case law are compatible with the Act as it has developed over the years since it was first signed in Europe. It also means that UK judgments can be cited in European cases.

The Human Rights Act applies to public authorities, including bodies which carry out public functions. Section 145 of The Health and Social Care Act 2008 states that a private nursing home providing publicly funded care is carrying out a public function and thus comes under the remit of the Act.

Key Articles of the Human Rights Act

Article 2 – the Right to Life

The Act consists of 18 Articles which must be considered. Article 2 concerns the right to life. 'Everyone's right to life shall be protected by law.' There are some exemptions, for example if death occurs while defending oneself against unlawful violence, or arresting someone, or putting down a riot. It should be noted that: the state must positively promote the right to life and so cannot ignore life-threatening situations, such as someone in prison threatening to commit suicide. It will also apply where a hospital's negligent treatment causes death.

CASE STUDY – SAVAGE V SOUTH ESSEX PARTNERSHIP NHS FOUNDATION TRUST (2010) EWHC 865 (QB)

Carol Savage committed suicide while a patient of the trust and her daughter Anna argued that the trust had breached her mother's right to life under Article 2 of the Human Rights Act. The courts agreed, saying that the trust had breached Article 2 as (a) it had the requisite knowledge, actual or constructive, of a real and immediate risk to the patient's life from self-harm, and (b) failed to do all that could reasonably have been expected of it to avoid or prevent that risk. Thus the patient's daughter was eligible to bring the claim as a victim under s7HRA1998 and compensation of £10,000 was awarded.

Article 3 – Protection against Torture

Article 3 concerns protection against torture: no one shall be subjected to torture or to inhuman or degrading treatment or punishment. There are no exceptions to this Article; however, there is room for argument about what is meant by 'inhuman' or 'degrading' treatment. The Court in Strasbourg has ruled that prescribed medication does not breach Article 3, even if it causes unpleasant side effects. The judgment stated that 'as a general rule, a measure which is a therapeutic necessity cannot be regarded as inhuman or degrading' Herczegfalvy v Austria [1992] 15 EHRR 437. This means that if a patient cannot give consent then the professionals do not breach Article 3 if they give treatment which can be shown to be in the patient's best interests. It is important that good records are made of these decisions and how they are reached so that if care is questioned in the future there is evidence of the clinical basis for how the treatment decisions were made and implemented.

Article 5 – Deprivation of Liberty

Article 5 is concerned with deprivation of liberty. *'Everyone has the right to liberty and security of person.'* The Article details the circumstances under which liberty can be taken away, including *'the lawful detention of persons of unsound mind'*. In England and Wales the Mental Health Act 1983 sets out the conditions under which a person with mental health problems can be forced to accept treatment for their mental health condition and the safeguards that are in place to protect the rights of such individuals from abuse of power. However, the Act does not apply to informal patients in mental hospitals or in care homes. In HL v UK 45508/99 (2004) European Court of Human Rights 471 it was decided that although a patient, HL a man with profound autism, had not objected to being admitted to hospital without the right to leave, he had been deprived of his liberty and as such this infringed his rights under Article 5. As a result of this, Deprivation of Liberty safeguards (DoLs) have been developed since 2009 to try to ensure that vulnerable adults can be protected and have their rights as human beings protected. There will be more discussion of this later in the chapter.

Article 8 – Private and Family Life

Article 8 concerns the right to private and family life. *'Everyone has the right to respect for his private and family life, his home and his correspondence.'* A public body may only interfere with this to the extent that is lawful and 'necessary in a democratic society' for specified reasons, including national security, public safety, the prevention of disorder or 'the protection of health and morals'.

ACTIVITY

Fred Maynard is 79 and lives alone in his own house. The District Nurse has been visiting in order to dress a venous ulcer. Fred tells her that he no longer wants the ulcer dressed as its 'too painful' but he would like her to continue her visits as she is the only person he sees each week. He would also like her to find out how much a single ticket to the Dignitas clinic would cost so that when the pain becomes too much he can arrange to go there.

What issues does this situation raise?

Fred and the District Nurse are both moral agents, what is the potential for a clash of autonomies? Under Article 8 what are the responsibilities of the District Nurse?

Article 8 has been cited in a series of cases concerning assisted suicide. Diane Pretty (1958–2002) suffered from motor neurone disease. She wanted the Crown Prosecution Service to guarantee her husband immunity from prosecution if he helped her to commit suicide. Assisting someone to commit suicide is a crime under the Suicide Act 1961. The Crown Prosecution Service refused to do this and so Mrs Pretty went to court to establish that the Suicide Act was incompatible with the Human Rights Act 1998 in a number of aspects. In particular it was claimed that Article 8 included the right to decide when and how to die. The courts rejected this argument and Mrs Pretty lost her case. She died of her condition in 2002.

A few years later in 2009 Debbie Purdy (1963–2014) also challenged the compatibility of the Suicide Act 1961 with the Human Rights Act 1998 arguing that it was a breach of her human rights not to know whether her husband, Omar Puente, would be prosecuted if he were to accompany her to the Dignitas clinic in Switzerland when she travelled there to end her own life. The House of Lords ruled that the lack of a clear policy was a breach of Section 8 of the Human Rights Act and ordered the Director of the Crown Prosecution Service to issue a policy stating when people in Mr Puente's situation could expect to be prosecuted. The policy was introduced on 25 February 2010 and can be found on the website of the Crown Prosecution Service (2014). Both the judges involved in the above cases and the Crown Prosecution Service have stated that it is not their role to change the law concerning assisted suicide or euthanasia. This can only be done by parliament. In 2012 the matter returned to court when Tony Nicklinson sought a ruling that a doctor in this country should be able to end his life as he was not able to travel abroad (R (Nicklinson) v Ministry of Justice 2012). He was unsuccessful and then refused nutrition and hydration and died shortly afterwards. In 2013 Lord Falconer introduced a private member's bill, The Assisted Dying Bill, which would, 'enable competent adults who are terminally ill to be provided at their request with specified assistance to end their own life; . . .'. As of early 2015 the bill is still working through parliamentary procedure but it is thought that it is unlikely to become law as it is a private member's bill and not part of the government's legislative programme.

The NHS Constitution (2013)

The Human Rights Act also provides the basis for the NHS Constitution (2013). The Constitution sets out rights for patients, public and staff. It outlines NHS commitments to patients and staff, and the responsibilities that the public, patients and staff owe to one another to ensure that the NHS works fairly and effectively. Patients are told in Section 3a that: '**You have the right** to be treated with dignity and respect, in accordance with your human rights' (NHS Constitution 2013: 8).

The Constitution goes on to say:

> **You have the right** to accept or refuse treatment that is offered to you, and not to be given any physical examination or treatment unless you have given valid consent. If you do not have the capacity to do so, consent must be obtained from a person legally able to act on your behalf, or the treatment must be in your best interests.
>
> (NHS Constitution 2013: 8)

The right of patients to accept or refuse treatment has long been recognised in English law, e.g. Bolam 1957 and The Mental Capacity Act 2005, and thus the Constitution echoes well-established legal principles. These legal principles in their turn rest on the recognition of the ethical principle that says an adult with capacity should be able to determine what happens to their body, in other words their autonomy should be respected.

The Mental Capacity Act 2005

The Mental Capacity Act 2005 now governs the law of consent for adults in England and Wales. There is a different act in Scotland and there is no Mental Capacity Act in Northern Ireland. It is based on five principles:

MENTAL CAPACITY ACT 2005: FIVE PRINCIPLES

1 Every adult has the right to make his or her own decisions and must be assumed to have capacity to make them unless it is proved otherwise.
2 A person must be given all practicable help before anyone treats them as not being able to make their own decisions.
3 Just because an individual makes what might be seen as an unwise decision, they should not be treated as lacking capacity to make that decision.
4 Anything done or any decision made on behalf of a person who lacks capacity must be done in their best interests.
5 Anything done for or on behalf of a person who lacks capacity should be the least restrictive of their basic rights and freedoms.

ACTIVITY

Maisie Parry is 85 years old. She has recently been admitted to hospital after a fall which resulted in a fractured hip. The ward staff and her son feel she cannot cope at home any more. Mrs Parry feels she can cope and says she would 'rather be shot' than leave her home.

What factors should be taken into account when deciding Mrs Parry's future?

In English law an adult is anyone over the age of 18. The law says that anyone over that age must be assumed to have capacity to make decisions about themselves. If there is any doubt about an adult's mental capacity then the following questions need to be resolved:

1   Is there an impairment of or disturbance in the functioning of a person's mind or brain?
      Examples of impairment could be a learning disability, dementia or permanent brain injury. Disturbances in the functioning of the mind or brain can arise from low oxygen levels, low blood sugar levels in a diabetic, being under the influence of certain drugs, e.g. diamorphine, both prescribed and recreational, and being drunk. A disturbance can usually be corrected but an impairment cannot. If it is decided that there is an impairment or disturbance then the professionals need to consider the following:
2   Is the impairment or disturbance sufficient that the person lacks the capacity to make a particular decision?
      This means that a person has to have the capacity to make a particular decision and the level of capacity needed will depend upon the seriousness of the decision that needs to be made. Someone may therefore be able to make decisions about what they would like to eat but not about whether or not to have an operation. This also means that because some individuals lack full capacity their rights to make choices and decisions about their lives cannot be ignored or overridden. The implications of this will be discussed shortly.

Capacity is important because we are asking someone to make a decision about their care or treatment. In order to make a decision, information is needed and the person must:

• Understand the information given to them.
• Retain that information long enough to be able to make the decision.
• Weigh up the information available to make the decision.

The question of what information and how much should be given is not easily answered. The Bolam case (Bolam v Friern Hospital Management Committee 1957) established the principle that patients had a right to know, *'the general nature and purpose of what is intended'*. Patients also have a right to know about 'grave or substantial risk'. The case of Mrs Sidaway in 1985 defined this as a risk greater than 1 per cent but it is not always straightforward for the professional to determine the level of risk as the information may not be available for newer procedures. The Sidaway case (Sidaway v Board of Governors of the Bethlem Royal Hospital 1985) also introduced the concept of the reasonable patient and gave the professionals the responsibility of determining what mattered to the patient when giving information – in other words a one-size-fits-all explanation will not do. Recognition of this principle is reflected in the GMC's guidelines on consent (General Medical Council 2008). These state that no single approach to treatment or care will suit every patient, nor apply in all circumstances. Individual patients may want more or less information. The guidance goes on to state that the amount of information shared with patients will depend on the individual patient and what they want or need to know. Some patients want to know as much as possible while others find that the more they learn the less able they feel to make a decision and therefore prefer to leave matters to the professional's judgement. Assumptions should not be made about a patient's understanding of risk or the importance they attach to different outcomes. An example of this would be to assume that a woman who is post-menopausal will be happy to have a hysterectomy. She may feel that her womb is an essential part of her identity as a woman and thus be unwilling to undergo such a procedure even though it may bring other benefits.

Having made a decision they must then be able to communicate what this is. This could be by talking, using sign language or even simple muscle movements such as blinking an eye or squeezing a hand. From this it can be seen that gaining consent from a patient is very important. The principles supplied by parliament do not mention consent forms. This is because the emphasis is on consent rather than the means by which it is recorded. A consent form is a means to an end, i.e. it should show that consent has been obtained. In ordinary situations, e.g. providing a wash or giving medication, the above have always been considered adequate means of agreeing to what is proposed. Consent forms for operations and other invasive procedures can help to remind all parties of what needs to be discussed and provide evidence of what has been agreed and by whom, e.g. the patient and the professional. They are not, however, usually a legal requirement. If a patient cannot sign a consent form but can give valid consent then the procedure can go ahead. It would be advisable for everyone involved to make detailed records of the discussions held and the decisions reached. The quality of the information provided and the patient's un-coerced agreement are what make consent valid, not a signature on a form. Patients also have the right to change their minds at any point before a procedure.

This tells us that respect for patients' autonomy is paramount if a patient has capacity. This includes the autonomy of patients who make decisions that others might consider to be unwise as we have seen from Section 1(3) of the Mental Capacity Act 2005. The assumption is that if treatment is suggested it must be because it is considered to be in the patient's best interests or it would not have been offered. However, patients may, and sometimes do, have a different understanding of their best interests to that of the professionals. An example of this arose in 1994 when a patient in Broadmoor with a diagnosis of paranoid schizophrenia refused an amputation which he was told was necessary to save his life. The patient accepted that this was the doctors' view but he disagreed and refused treatment. The judge held that he was competent, i.e. he had capacity. He understood the information he had been given and the possible consequences of his refusal but was able to reach his own decision in opposition to professional advice. A patient cannot be held to lack capacity because they do not agree with the professionals or because they make a decision that others consider to be irrational. The patient subsequently made a good recovery physically and was then deemed well enough mentally to be discharged into the community where he is said to be living happily (Re C 1994).

While the Mental Capacity Act 2005 stresses the importance of respecting and upholding the rights of patients with capacity to make their own decisions it also recognises in Sections 1(5) and (6) that not all adults have capacity and that decisions sometimes have to be made on their behalf. There are several mechanisms by which this can be done lawfully. The most important of these is an advance directive. To be lawful this has to be valid and applicable. Validity means that it was drawn up by a person over the age of 18 who had capacity at the time of making it. Applicability means that it applies to the treatment needed at the time it comes into use, Section 26(1) Mental Capacity Act 2005. An advance decision only comes into force when a patient has lost capacity. It can only be used to refuse treatment, e.g. to refuse ventilation but not to demand it. However, if decisions are being made about treatment it will be a factor to consider if a patient has said that they would want it. If the directive states that the patient refuses life-saving treatment then it must be in writing, signed and witnessed, Section 25 Mental Capacity Act 2005. It is not possible to ask for anything unlawful, e.g. a lethal injection. One of the most important issues to be considered when devising an advance directive is the difficulty of predicting the future. An individual may have seen members of the family suffering from cancer and draw up a directive accordingly but then suffer from a stroke. It is also difficult to predict what advances in the treatment of a disease will be made and thus what the prognosis will be. If a patient has an advance directive it will be useful if it is reviewed regularly in the light of any developments so that it is a true reflection of the patient's wishes.

If there is no advance directive then the next most important means of determining a patient's wishes is through someone who has a Lasting Power of Attorney (2014). This is set up by someone, known as the donor, who is over the age of 18 and while they have capacity. There are two types of Lasting Power of Attorney:

- health and welfare
- property and financial affairs.

An individual can make one or both. Those given the Lasting Power of Attorney are attorney(s). The donor chooses their attorney(s) who can be anyone they want and fills in the forms. These can be obtained from the Office of the Public Guardian online or through the post. They must be signed by the donor and witnessed and then registered with the Office of the Public Guardian. Unless the forms are registered the attorney(s) has no legal standing when decisions have to be made. Registration takes eight to ten weeks according to the government website (gov.uk). The sort of decisions that someone with a health and welfare Lasting Power of Attorney can make include:

- the donor's daily routine (e.g. washing, dressing, eating)
- medical care
- moving into a care home
- life-sustaining treatment.

It can only be used when the donor is unable to make their own decisions. The healthcare professional will therefore need to check that the attorney is registered with the Office of the Public Guardian as relatives may not understand the need for this. If there is more than one attorney then the forms will stipulate if each attorney can act individually or if they must make decisions jointly. A person with capacity may also end a Lasting Power of Attorney and this must be registered with the Office of the Public Guardian and the attorney(s) informed.

If a patient who lacks capacity has no advance directive or someone with a Lasting Power of Attorney, a Deputy of the Court of Protection may make decisions on the patient's behalf. This will be someone, usually family or a close friend, who has applied to the court to be made a deputy in order to act as a health and social welfare deputy on behalf of an individual who does not have capacity and where there is no other provision made.

If none of the above is in place then it is the responsibility of the healthcare professionals to act in the patient's best interests when deciding on any care or treatment to be given. The Mental Capacity Act 2005 gives some guidance on the factors that should be considered when trying to work out what is in a patient's best interests.

MENTAL CAPACITY ACT SECTION 4(6)

In determining for the purposes of this Act what is in a person's best interests, the person making the determination must consider, so far as is reasonably ascertainable:

(a) the person's past and present wishes and feelings (and, in particular, any relevant written statement made by him when he had capacity),

(b) the beliefs and values that would be likely to influence his decision if he had capacity, and

(c) the other factors that he would be likely to consider if he were able to do so.

The wording of the Act means that while an individual's wishes etc. need to be considered this does not mean that they will necessarily determine what happens to the patient. The doctor will have the final say about what constitutes best interests unless the courts intervene.

The final principle of the Mental Capacity Act 2005 is that any decision taken on behalf of an individual who lacks capacity must be the least restrictive of their rights and freedoms. This was as a result of a decision of the European Court of Human Rights usually referred to as the Bournewood case, HL v UK [2004] EHRC 471, which has already been mentioned in the discussion of Article 5 of the Human Rights Act.

CASE STUDY – BOURNEWOOD CASE, HL V UK [2004] EHRC 471

Mr L, a 49-year-old man with autism who lacked capacity, had been detained in Bournewood hospital for a few months in 1997. He was detained in his 'best interests' under the common law doctrine of necessity. The European Court of Human Rights held that he had been detained and thus Article 5 of the European Court of Human Rights, the right to liberty, applied. Further, it held that detention under the common law was incompatible with Article 5 because it was too arbitrary and lacked sufficient safeguards (such as those available to patients detained under Mental Health Act 1983). Finally, the European Court of Human Rights held that judicial review, which was the only way Mr L had been able to challenge his common law detention, did not provide the kind of rigorous challenge required by the European Court of Human Rights, Article 5(4). As a result of this judgment the Deprivation of Liberty procedures were incorporated into the Mental Capacity Act 2005.

In a recent judgment of the Supreme Court, Lady Hale stated:

> human rights are for everyone, including the most disabled members of our community, and that those rights include the same right to liberty as has everyone else.
>
> (P v Cheshire West & Chester Council; P & Q v Surrey County Council [2014] UKSC 19)

Deprivation of liberty is only permitted in three circumstances under the Mental Capacity Act 2005. These are when:

1   it is authorised by the Court of Protection by an order under Section 16(2)(a);
2   it is authorised under the procedures provided for in Schedule A1, which relates only to deprivations in hospitals and in care homes falling within the meaning of the Care Standards Act 2000 (see Schedule A1, para. 178);
3   it falls within Section 4B, which allows deprivation if it is necessary in order to give life-sustaining treatment or to prevent a serious deterioration in the person's condition while a case is pending before the court.

The Supreme Court found that there is a deprivation of liberty for the purposes of Article 5 of the European Convention on Human Rights in the following circumstances:

The person is under continuous supervision and control and is not free to leave, and the person lacks capacity to consent to these arrangements.

It was held that factors which are not relevant to determining whether there is a deprivation of liberty include:

• the person's compliance or lack of objection to their care arrangements,
• the purpose of the deprivation of liberty,
• the extent to which it enables them to live a relatively normal life.

The result of this decision is that anyone whose living arrangements fall under this definition will have been deprived of liberty and this can only be sanctioned via the courts in the three circumstances already mentioned. This will involve six assessments and aims to ensure that proper legal process is followed. Thus they will also gain the protection of regular independent reviews of their situation to ensure that the arrangements remain in their best interests.

The Mental Health Act 1983

The reason why deprivation of liberty safeguards have been developed under the Mental Capacity Act 2005 is because the law does not normally allow individuals to be detained unless they are convicted criminals. As we have seen, liberty is considered to be an essential part of human rights. However, people with a mental illness can be detained against their will. The Mental Health Act 1983 (which was substantially amended in 2007) is the law in England and Wales which allows people with a 'mental disorder' to be admitted to hospital, detained and treated without their consent – either for their own health and safety, or for the protection of other people (Scotland and Northern Ireland have their own laws about compulsory treatment for mental ill health).

People can be admitted, detained and treated under different sections of the Mental Health Act 1983, depending on the circumstances, which is why the term 'sectioned' is used to describe a compulsory admission to hospital. People who are compulsorily admitted to hospital are called 'formal' or 'involuntary' patients. In order to prevent abuse, carefully defined procedures must be followed and care must be reviewed. It is important to remember that a patient can only receive compulsory treatment for their mental illness. If they require treatment for physical illness then the Mental Capacity Act 2005 will need to be used. So if a patient with schizophrenia needs treatment for hypertension the principles of the Mental Capacity Act 2005 would be followed concerning their capacity to make a decision.

Parental responsibility

Anyone below the age of 18 is a child and children are not covered by the provisions of the Mental Capacity Act. When caring for children consent is essential and can be provided by:

- someone with parental responsibility for the child
- a 16- or 17-year-old
- a Gillick-competent child
- an order of the court.

So who has parental responsibility? The gestational mother has automatic parental responsibility from birth. This means that it does not matter if a donor egg has been used or if it is a surrogacy arrangement. The gestational mother retains responsibility until the child turns 18, is adopted or dies. The situation with fathers is slightly more complicated. In England and Wales, if the parents of a child are married to each other at the time of the birth, or if they have jointly adopted a child, then they both have parental responsibility. Parents do not lose parental responsibility if they divorce, and this applies to both the resident and the non-resident parent.

A father, however, has this responsibility only if he is married to the mother when the child is born or has acquired legal responsibility for his child through one of these routes:

- (from 1 December 2003) by jointly registering the birth of the child with the mother,
- by a parental responsibility agreement with the mother,
- by a parental responsibility order, made by a court,
- by marrying the mother of the child.

If the birth of a child was registered before 1 December 2003 then the father will need a parental responsibility agreement or order or to have married the mother in order to have parental responsibility, even if his name is on the child's birth certificate. Living with the mother, even for a long time, does not give a father parental responsibility. If the parents are not married, parental responsibility does not automatically pass to the natural father if the mother dies – unless he already has parental responsibility. If a father applies to the courts for parental responsibility the court will take the following into account:

- the degree of commitment shown by the father to his child
- the degree of attachment between father and child
- the father's reasons for applying for the order.

The court will then decide to accept or reject the application based on what it believes is in the child's best interest.

Since 6 April 2009 same-sex parents can register both parties to a civil partnership or same-sex marriage as the parents of a child with full parental responsibility for both adults if the child has been born as a result of fertility treatment in a centre licensed by the Human Fertilisation and Embryology Authority. Same-sex parents who do not fill these criteria will need a parental order from the court for both to have parental responsibility.

As children grow older they may wish to make decisions about their healthcare without involving their parents. The Family Law Reform Act 1969 Section 8 allows anyone of 16 or 17 years to give consent to medical or dental treatment without gaining consent from their parent or guardian. Young people below the age of 16 may give valid consent if they are said to be Gillick competent. In 1985 the House of Lords (Gillick v West Norfolk & Wisbech Area Health Authority 1985) ruled that:

> . . . whether or not a child is capable of giving the necessary consent will depend on the child's maturity and understanding and the nature of the consent required. The child must be capable of making a reasonable assessment of the advantages and disadvantages of the treatment proposed, so the consent, if given, can be properly and fairly described as true consent.

The court then went on to describe the basis on which the adults involved in the care of the child could decide if the child had the necessary maturity. Lord Scarman, one of the judges, said that the test was whether or not the child has 'sufficient understanding and intelligence to enable him or her to understand fully what is proposed'.

He went on to say:

> Parental right yields to the child's right to make his own decisions when he reaches a sufficient understanding and intelligence to be capable of making up his own mind on the matter requiring decision.

There will often be disagreements among the adults involved, both the professionals and those with parental responsibility, as to the level of maturity the young person has. If no agreement can be reached among all the parties involved including the patient then the courts will make the final decision (Glass v UK 2004). When the courts make a decision on behalf of a child they must act in the child's best interests (Children Act 1989). Since the Gillick case and the Children Act 1989 the courts have ruled that when a young person gives consent then their decision should be upheld. If, however, the young person wishes to refuse consent then that decision will be overruled as not being in the best interests of the individual. It has been argued that if someone has the maturity to give consent then their refusal of treatment should also be respected but this is not how the law has developed.

Confidentiality

Respect for confidentiality is also recognised as an important way of upholding the dignity and worth of the individual and respecting their autonomy. Patients and service users tell professionals things they may not want to share with anyone else. It is important that they feel that this information will not be shared indiscriminately as this would lead them to withhold potentially crucial information and this in turn could lead to ineffective care.

The importance of confidentiality in healthcare was recognised as long ago as the fifth century BCE in the Hippocratic Oath which obliged those who took it to swear not to reveal what they learnt about their patients. In more recent times, the right to confidentiality is seen to come from Article 8 of the Human Rights Act 1998. However, the duty of confidentiality is not absolute – there are times when it may be breached, when it should be breached and when it must be breached. The obvious occasion on which information about a patient or client may be passed on to someone else is with the patient or client's permission.

Trying to decide when confidentiality should be broken is more difficult. The law accepts that there is a concept of public interest.

CASE OF W V EGDELL [1990] 2 WLR 471

W was a patient in Broadmoor whose lawyers commissioned a report from Dr Egdell to assess W's mental health and his danger to the public. Dr Edgell found that W was still very dangerous and his report was not used by W's lawyers when bringing his case to the mental health tribunal. W's request for release was nevertheless refused. Dr Edgell was concerned that W might be successful on a future occasion and therefore disclosed his report to the authorities. W tried to sue him for breach of confidence. He failed in this as the judge held that Dr Edgell's action was in the public interest. It should be noted that the disclosure had not been to the general public, e.g. via a newspaper.

If a healthcare or social care professional is ordered to breach confidence via a court order then this must be obeyed. Failure to do so is contempt of court and can result in a prison sentence.

The last 25 years have seen considerable developments in technology and thus the ability for information to be widely disseminated. There were concerns that health and social care data could be accessed by those without a legitimate right to know this information. As a result the government commissioned Dame Fiona Caldicott to chair a committee with the task of investigating how all confidential information was handled by the NHS. As a result of the Caldicott committee's findings and recommendations, the role of Caldicott Guardians (2014) was introduced into healthcare in 1999 and social care in 2002. Every organisation that has access to patient or service user records is obliged to have a Caldicott Guardian. This is a senior person who is responsible for protecting the confidentiality of the information about patients and service users and enabling appropriate information sharing. More information about this role and its responsibilities can be found on the website of the Health and Social Care Information Centre (www.hscic.gov.uk/).

Chapter summary

- The law takes seriously the right of adults with capacity to make decisions about their own treatment.
- The obligation of the healthcare worker to ask for permission before treating someone shows recognition and respect for the patient's humanity. That recognition and respect continues to exist when individuals do not have capacity and is based on the fact that they are members of the human family and all humans are of worth and value.
- Healthcare workers must act in the best interests of the service user. This is further reinforced by maintaining, where appropriate, a person's right to decide who should have access to confidential information about them.

• The law underpins the delivery of healthcare and incorporates ethical principles to protect individuals within our care.

Further reading

Brazier, M. and Cave, E. 2011. *Medicine, Patients and the Law*, 5th edn. London: Penguin.
Dimond, B. 2009. *Legal Aspects of Consent*, 2nd edn. London/Salisbury: Quay Books.
Dimond, B. 2010. *Legal Aspects of Patient Confidentiality*. London/Salisbury: Quay Books.
Foster, C. 2013. *Medical Law: A Very Short Introduction*. Oxford: Oxford University Press.

References

Bentham, J. 2005. *An Introduction to the Principles of Morals and Legislation*. Whitefish, MT: Kessinger Publishing Co.
Beauchamp, T. and Childress, J. 2013. *Principles of Biomedical Ethics*, 7th edn. Oxford: Oxford University Press.
Caldicott Guardians. 2014. *Health and Social Care Information Centre* [online]. Available at: www.hscic.gov.uk/ [Accessed 10 November 2014].
Children Act. 1989. London: HMSO.
Crown Prosecution Service. 2014. *Policy for Prosecutors in Respect of Cases of Encouraging or Assisting Suicide* [online]. Available at: www.cps.gov.uk/publications/prosecution/assisted_suicide. html [Accessed 12 November 2014].
Dimond, B. 2015. *Legal Aspects of Nursing*, 7th edn. London: Pearson Education.
General Medical Council. 2008. *Consent: Patients and Doctors Making Decisions Together* [online]. Available at: www.gmc-uk.org/static/documents/content/Consent_-_English_0914.pdf [Accessed 15 October 2014].
Family Law Reform Act. 1969. London: HMSO.
Hansard. 1977. HC Deb 17 February 1977. Vol. 926: cc 879–90.
Health and Social Care Act. 2008. London: HMSO.
Human Rights Act. 1998. London: HMSO.
Kant, I. 2007. *Critique of Pure Reason*. London: Penguin Classics.
Lasting Power of Attorney. 2014. *Gov.uk* [online]. Available at: www.gov.uk/power-of-attorney/overview [Accessed 10 October 2014].
Mental Capacity Act. 2005. London: HMSO.
Mental Health Act. 1983. London: HMSO.
Mill, J. S. 2003. *On Liberty*. New York: Dover Publications.
NHS Constitution. 2013. *NHS Choices* [online]. Available at: www.nhs.uk/choiceintheNHS/ Rightsandpledges/NHSConstitution/Pages/Overview.aspx [Accessed 10 October 2014].
NICE. 2013. *NICE Charter London* [online]. Available at: www.nice.org.uk/Media/Default/About/ Who-we-are/NICE_Charter.pdf [Accessed 10 October 2014].
Proctor, R. N. 1989. *Racial Hygiene: Medicine under the Nazis*. Cambridge, MA: Harvard University Press.
United Nations. 1948. *Universal Declaration of Human Rights* [online]. Available at: www.un.org/en/ documents/udhr/ [Accessed 8 October 2014].
World Health Organization. 2014a. *WHO Statement on the 1st Meeting of the IHR Emergency Committee on the 2014 Ebola Outbreak in West Africa* 08/08/2014 [online]. Available at: www.who.int/media-centre/news/statements/2014/ebola-20140808/en/ [Accessed 12 October 2014].
World Health Organization. 2014b. *Poliomyelitis* [online]. Available at: www.who.int/mediacentre/ factsheets/fs114/en/ [Accessed 14 October 2014].
World Medical Association. 2013. *Declaration of Helsinki – Ethical Principles for Medical Research Involving Human Subjects 1964 and amended by 64th WMA General Assembly, Fortaleza, Brazil,*

October 2013 [online]. Available at: www.wma.net/en/30publications/10policies/b3/index.html [Accessed 10 September 2014].

Table of statutes

Children Act 1989.
Family Law Reform Act 1969.
Health and Social Care Act 2008.
Human Rights Act 1998.
Mental Capacity Act 2005.
Mental Health Act 1983.

Table of cases

Bolam v Friern Hospital Management Committee [1957] 1 WLR 582.
Gillick v West Norfolk & Wisbech Area Health Authority [1985] AC 112 House of Lords.
Glass v UK [2004] 1 FCR 553 (ECtHR).
Herczegfalvy v Austria [1992] 15 EHRR 437.
HL v UK 45508/99 [2004] ECHR 471.
P v Cheshire West & Chester Council; P & Q v Surrey County Council [2014] UKSC 19.
Re C (Adult, refusal of treatment) [1994] 1 All ER 819.
Re E [1993] 1 FLR 386.
R v Director of Public Prosecutions (Respondent), ex parte Diane Pretty (Appellant) & Secretary of State for the Home Department (Interested Party) [2001] UKHL 61.
R (on the application of Debbie Purdy) (Appellant) v DPP (Respondent) & Omar Puente (Interested Party) & Society for the Protection of Unborn Children [HL] [2009] UKHL 45.
R (Nicklinson) v Ministry of Justice (2012) EWHC 2381 (Admin), (2012) MHLO 77.
Savage v South Essex Partnership NHS Foundation Trust (2010) EWHC 865 (QB).
Sidaway v Board of Governors of the Bethlem Royal Hospital [1985] AC 871.
W v Egdell [1990] 2 WLR 471.

Chapter 9

Research and evidence-based practice

Shirley Jones

LEARNING OUTCOMES

By the end of this chapter you will be able to:

1   Explain the role of evidence-based practice in caring for patients.
2   Describe the stages of the research process.
3   Explain the difference between quantitative and qualitative research.
4   Effectively read a research paper to inform practice.

Introduction

When you visit a health professional you would like to be confident that the treatment or advice they offer is right and that it is based on some form of reliable evidence. You would not like them to 'guess' which treatment to give you. Fortunately there is the requirement and expectation of health professionals that all care is delivered using the best available evidence. This is termed 'evidence-based practice'.

But what do we mean by evidence-based practice (EBP)? If you read the literature you will come across a range of definitions and terminology, e.g. evidence-based medicine, evidence-based care, research-based practice and evidence-based nursing. Fortunately most of them say the same thing.

One of the earliest and most well-known definitions was provided by David Sackett and colleagues:

> Evidence based medicine is the integration of best research evidence with clinical expertise and patient values.

> (Sackett *et al.* 2000: 1)

From this definition we can see that the aim of EBP is to bring together three key elements to ensure we provide high-quality care which meets the needs, values and choices of the clients who access our services. These are:

- the expertise/experience of the healthcare professional
- the findings of externally provided good-quality research
- the preferences of the carer/patient/service user.

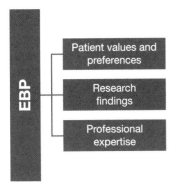

Figure 9.1 Components of evidence-based practice.

ACTIVITY

Make a list of reasons why you, and all healthcare practitioners, should be providing evidence-based care?

Here are some of the reasons you might have thought of:

1   To demonstrate that care given is of benefit and provides good outcomes for patients.
2   To provide consistency of care at all times.
3   We need to spend public money wisely and ensure best value for money.
4   To ensure that we are able to account for our actions. This is part of clinical governance.
5   To help practitioners develop professionally. It improves staff confidence when we understand the basis of the care that we give and can justify our decisions.
6   It is unethical to deliver poor or unsafe care.
7   To prevent complications occurring which are costly in terms of money, human suffering and the distress caused.

Despite agreement that EBP is a good thing, there is a lot less agreement about what counts as evidence and who should provide it. You may be aware of some highly publicised disputes within professional groups, and amongst politicians and consumer groups, about decisions relating to care which are not universally accepted. For example, some patient groups have protested about the withdrawal of certain drugs from NHS prescriptions, based on the recommendations of the National Institute for Health and Care Excellence (NICE). NICE was established to provide independent advice on the most effective way to prevent, diagnose and manage illness, and reduce inequality and variations in healthcare. However, the guidance they give is not always accepted by everyone. Many people do not agree with what NICE decides is good evidence. NICE considers cost, which is criticised, particularly by patient groups, as being driven more by political and financial needs rather than focusing on effective outcomes and what is best for service users.

Despite this, we all have a duty to strive to provide evidence-based care. Many of you may have experience of delivering care based on evidence provided as clinical protocols/

guidelines and for a practitioner this can reassure you that you are delivering good-quality care.

ACTIVITY

Find a set of guidelines for treatment or a treatment policy that relates to any of the care you give? Identify what is the aim of using this in practice?

What key elements does it contain?

You may have noted some of the following features:

1   It is based on a summary of best practice.
2   It gives you clear direction about how care should be delivered, what should be done, where, when and by whom.
3   It may provide a description of support systems to help you make decisions about appropriate care.
4   It aims to make sure everyone is providing the same care to patients and to improve patient outcomes.

Developing knowledge using research

Much of our everyday information is based on common sense and knowledge that we have acquired from a variety of sources, such as:

- By trial and error and practical personal experience.
- Acquired from people considered to be experts.

In health and social care settings, although we may think we know the answer to a problem or question, sometimes there are conflicting ideas about what may work best and until we have subjected the problem to rigorous scientific testing our knowledge may be merely guesswork. Common sense approaches are not good enough and may overlook factors which have not yet emerged. What may work in one situation may be dangerous in another. It is very evident that there are still gaps in knowledge and understanding about what works best. As practitioners we cannot afford to take risks when providing care. We need to be as certain as possible that doing something is better than doing nothing. Some of what we do can cause harm so we need to try and spot where that is happening and this requires knowledge. We need a solid base of structured, rigorously acquired knowledge to base practice on. Undertaking research is a way of achieving this.

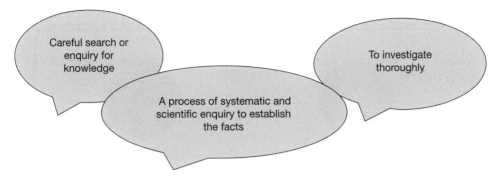

Figure 9.2 Common phrases to describe research.

What is research?

Various definitions of research can be found in the literature.

Underpinning all these definitions is an emphasis on several key steps:

1   Research is a structured, planned, logical and rigorous approach to finding out information.
2   Research tries to find answers to specific questions or to resolve specific problems which arise in health and social care.
3   It aims to extend and develop our current understanding of a topic or develop and establish new knowledge, new truths.

This development of new knowledge, new ways of understanding problems and how best to solve them by undertaking research is often termed **Empirical Research** (Ellis 2013). This approach implies that it is more than just looking up information which is new to us; this is about establishing new knowledge and new ways of understanding the world we live in, which will benefit everybody.

> ## STUDENT TIP
>
> When discussing research there are many specialised terms which might be unfamiliar to you. A useful tip is to make a glossary or list of common research terms. You could start this now with the term Empirical Research.

Understanding the research process

Identifying a research question and then undertaking research is a structured and planned process which usually follows a series of stages or a research cycle (Ellis 2013).

An understanding of research enables practitioners to effectively read published research and make judgements about the quality of the research to inform practice. In the following sections of this chapter we will consider how research is reported and how to read research articles and understand them. The format of published research usually mirrors the research process.

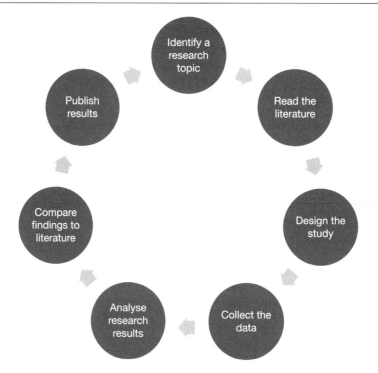

Figure 9.3 The research cycle, adapted from Ellis (2013).

STUDENT TIP

Remember that not all published research is good quality. You need to be able to read and evaluate research articles and then decide if the research is helpful to your practice.

How to read a research article

Most research studies follow a similar format although variations will reflect the research approach being used or the requirements of the publishing journal. Becoming familiar with the format can help you improve your reading and make sense of the reports. The following steps will help guide you through reading a published research article.

ACTIVITY

Find a research study published in a journal using your searching skills as outlined in Chapter 1.

Read the article alongside the rest of this chapter and see if you can identify the key components which are described below.

Step 1 – identify the title of the research article

This should be a concise and clear statement that indicates the research topic, the method used to collect the information, and who were the participants in the study. For example:

- A qualitative study of a nurse's experiences of supporting patients living with dementia in community settings.
- Effectiveness of shoulder supports in the management of stroke patients with shoulder pain. A randomised controlled trial.

This is followed by the author's name and information about their qualifications. This can be helpful to enable you to establish their experience as researchers or practitioners in the field. Contact details may also be provided.

Step 2 – read the abstract

The abstract is usually presented in a different way, in order to catch your attention. It is usually a paragraph and you should always read this because the abstract gives you a summary of the main research report. It will usually include information about the aim or objectives of the research, how information was collected and who from, and what the results are. Reading the abstract will give you enough information to know if the report is relevant to your needs and whether or not you wish to read the full article. It may be accompanied by keywords, which are helpful for searching related articles.

> **STUDENT TIP**
>
> Read the abstract several times to make sure you are clear what the report is actually about. Look up any words you do not understand.

Step 3 – read the introduction

The introduction provides some background information about the topic being researched and why it is being undertaken. It may contain references to other related research and work on the topic – although sometimes this material will be in a separate section headed Literature Review.

Usually a review of the literature on the subject is undertaken to ensure that the project is of potential benefit and there is a need for research (Punch 2006). This helps in several ways.

- To refine the research question for the current study.
- To find out what is already known – perhaps the answer to the question is already known.
- To identify any gaps in the literature; even when research has been carried out on a topic there may still be questions about its use in particular situations or with different groups of patients.
- To learn from the experiences of other researchers, in particular what methods they have used, what worked well, what problems they faced and what future recommendations they have suggested (Coughlan *et al.* 2013).

Step 4 – identify the research questions

The research question is the specific problem for which the author is trying to find an answer, e.g. what is the impact on the quality of life of stroke patients following rehabilitation in the community?

In many published papers the actual question may not be stated, this is often meant to be inferred from the title of the paper. Instead, the specific information the researcher wants to find out is often stated in the form of an aim, e.g. the aim of the study is to examine the quality of life of stroke patients following rehabilitation in the community.

Sometimes knowledge of the literature can also be applied to the formulation of a *Hypothesis*. This is a specialised research question, used only in quantitative research when the research seeks to explore links (such as cause and effect) between *variables* (Ellis 2010). A variable is simply a characteristic, an attribute or a factor that may vary, e.g. height, blood sugar levels, heart rate, exercise levels, medical condition, pain levels etc. A hypothesis will contain the following features:

- Indicate the relationship between variables.
- Predict the nature of the relationship.
- Indicate the population to be studied.

For example, in the study mentioned above the research is looking at:

- Quality of life (variable).
- Rehabilitation in the community (variable).
- Stroke patients (population to be studied).

A hypothesis could then predict the link between these variables. In this case a positive relationship is predicted.

- The quality of life of stroke patients improves following community rehabilitation.

We will be explaining more about variables and hypotheses later in the chapter.

STUDENT TIP

It is helpful to establish early on when reading that you are clear about what the research question is. Identify if this is in the form of a question or a research hypothesis.

Remember that not all research studies have a hypothesis.

ACTIVITY

Remember to add the specialised research terms to your glossary. The rest of this chapter will provide many more for the glossary, some of which are highlighted in bold print to help you.

Step 5 – understanding the methodology

The **methodology** describes the overall approach to research that provides a framework for the study and gives details about the way in which the researcher went about answering the question. This includes information about the **research design**, **sample**, **data collection tools** used to collect the information to answer the research question, and how that information (**data**) is analysed (Ellis 2013)

Quantitative and qualitative research

Broadly, research can be grouped into two main approaches or **methodologies**, **quantitative** and **qualitative** research. Using these terms is a useful way of distinguishing between different methodologies but in many projects both approaches may be combined.

Quantitative research

Quantitative research methodology is used to answer research questions that require a numerical element to them by collecting information (**data**) in a way that it can be measured and counted, i.e. quantified. The **data** collected is **numerical**; the focus is on numbers and frequencies. This is analysed using **statistics** (Parahoo 2014).

A key term used in quantitative research is *variable* (Ellis 2013). Remember, a **variable is simply a characteristic, an attribute or a factor that may vary and can be measured**, e.g. respiratory rate, age, eye colour. Understanding variables can sometimes seem very confusing, but this is simply terminology which is used to help explain the rules used in quantitative research designs and they are labelled using the following terms, **independent variable, dependent variable, extraneous (confounding) variable**. We will look at these terms in more detail later.

Quantitative researchers are interested in exploring relationships between variables:

- Are there any **associations** between variables such as possible links between causes and effect? For example, does eating red meat (variable) increase the risk of heart disease (variable)?
- What are the **frequency and occurrence** of variables? For example, how many women (variable) suffer from postnatal depression (variable)? How long (variable) does it last?

Quantitative research designs can be grouped as either those that are **Interventional (experimental)** or those that are **Observational (non-interventional)**.

Interventional (experimental/quasi-experimental) design

Interventional (experimental) research designs are used when researchers are trying to **detect a relationship between cause and effect** and are often used when testing a **hypothesis** (Ellis 2013). When conducting an experiment researchers often manipulate variables to determine the effect on other variables (cause and effect). For example, a researcher might want to compare the effectiveness of two types of pain medication to see which is best. The variable of interest is the type of pain medication. When a variable is manipulated by the researcher, it is called an **independent variable**. The experiment seeks to determine the effect of the independent variable on a measurable outcome, in this case the relief of pain. In this example, relief from pain is called a **dependent variable**.

In health and social care, this method is chosen when trying to determine if a treatment intervention is effective by manipulating participants exposure to the intervention (the **independent variable**) in order to measure what effect it has on the outcome (the **dependent variable**). These types of experiments are not happening in a laboratory but take place in clinical settings.

Consider the following hypothesis:

Low-fat diets result in weight loss for clinically obese patients.

The researcher is keen to see if their prediction of a link (cause and effect) between eating a low-fat diet and losing weight in people who are clinically obese is correct. The researcher is looking to see if there is a relationship between these two variables; **the independent variable** (the intervention of a low-fat diet) and the **dependent variable** (outcome measure of weight loss). In a study of this nature the researcher would need to exclude any other factors (known as **extraneous or confounding variables**) which might affect the outcome but are not part of the planned experiment and may confuse the interpretation of the results. Researchers address this in the study design by means of introducing some form of control. In this case the researcher would need to exclude other variables such as use of other types of dietary control, weight loss surgery or weight loss medication. Exclusion of these extraneous variables is essential to ensure the outcomes (weight loss) are due to the independent variable (low-fat diet) and not something else.

Controlling extraneous variables

This is usually managed in several ways. First, researchers identify **inclusion and exclusion criteria** which guide the selection of participants into the study (Ellis 2013). For example, researchers will only include participants who are clinically obese in the study and exclude any potential participant who is clinically obese but is either following a different diet or using weight control medication. This helps the researcher control the extraneous variables they can identify.

Another strategy researchers use to guard against extraneous variables influencing the outcome of a study is to randomly allocate the participants who have been recruited to the study into an **experimental group** who receive the intervention (hence why this is an **interventional design**) and a **control group** who do not (Ellis 2013).

The make-up of participants in both groups should be the same: equal number of men and women in each group, similar levels of obesity in groups, similar ethnic diversity, similar ages etc. This means that those variables which can be identified, but more importantly those that cannot (for example, motivation to stick to the diet), are likely to be equally present in both groups. It is crucial that at the start of the research the two groups do not differ significantly from each other. This is so that any change in the dependent variable being measured (weight loss) that occurs in the experimental group but not the control group during the research can be put down to the introduced independent variable (the low-fat diet). If the two groups differed, for example in terms of how much exercise they did, then the weight loss in the experimental group may not be due to the low-fat diet. A summary of the research design is described in Figure 9.4 below.

Participants in the study would have their weight measured at the start of the research and then at the end of the research. This is commonly referred to as a **pre-test/post-test design** and differences in weight loss for the groups would be compared.

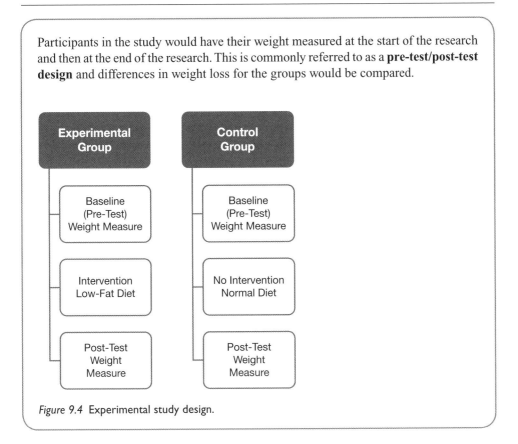

Figure 9.4 Experimental study design.

Randomised control trials and placebo

When experimental designs are used in clinical settings they are often called **randomised controlled trials (RCTs)** and are very commonly used to test the effectiveness of interventions. In some trials, such as drug trials, the control group may receive a **placebo** – which is an inactive form of the treatment. Participants are unaware that the intervention they are receiving is not the real one, this is known as **blinding**. In some studies the staff giving the drug or the placebo to the patient are also unaware which they are giving, this is known as a **double blinded RCT**. Placebos are used because there is much evidence that people report improvements when they participate in clinical trials mainly because they benefit psychologically from receiving the added attention. Blinding of staff and participants is a strategy used to control extraneous variables and strengthens the research design.

Quasi-experimental design

Sometimes researchers are not able to introduce controls when testing the effectiveness of interventions. This may be for many reasons including ethical issues such as being unable to deny participants treatment or that they are not able to randomly allocate participants. This design is known as **a quasi-experimental study** (Moule and Hek 2011). Researchers cannot be absolutely sure that the results they find are due to the intervention and not some unrelated factor (extraneous variable) they have been unable to control. This gives rise to weaker levels of evidence for use in clinical practice.

ACTIVITY

Write a definition for each of the following terms.

- Variable
- Independent variable
- Dependent variable
- Extraneous or confounding variable
- Hypothesis
- Experimental group
- Control group.

Check your understanding against the descriptions in the text above. These are useful terms to add to your glossary.

Observational (non-interventional) design

This type of quantitative research design is used when there is no intention to manipulate any variables (Ellis 2013). Researchers may seek to explore and describe variables in terms of their **frequency or prevalence** or may wish to see if there are any links, termed **associations/ correlations** between variables occurring naturally. For example, *is there an association between a sedentary lifestyle and the risk of developing heart disease?* Exploring associations using non-interventional approaches makes it difficult to be certain about cause and effect, because other causes may contribute to an effect. For example, a high salt intake may also cause heart disease.

When using this approach researchers may identify links after they have occurred, by looking back in time to see if there are possible reasons, i.e. **retrospectively**. This was the case in identifying the link between smoking and lung cancer. They may also study variables exploring links as they occur in the future, i.e. **prospectively**, such as monitoring people's age and the onset of Alzheimer's disease. Where multiple points of data are collected over a period of time, for example when participants in a study are tested every three years to check for the onset of Alzheimer's, this is known as a **longitudinal** study.

A common non-interventional quantitative research design is a **survey**. You will have seen political opinion polls reported in newspapers and magazines. Possibly you have been stopped in the street by a market researcher and asked to participate in a survey about your shopping preferences. Many of you will have completed the compulsory household census which happens every 10 years. These are all surveys.

A survey is a largely **descriptive type of research design** where large amounts of information can be collected quickly from a large number of participants. For example, a random sample of patients being discharged from hospital could be surveyed using a postal questionnaire in which they are asked to rate their levels of satisfaction with the quality of the care they have received. This can quickly produce data on patients' opinions and preferences.

This information can be counted and summarised. A survey describes things as they are. In some cases it is possible to see if there are any **associations** between data on the variables collected. For example, information about a patient's age, gender or their clinical condition could be compared to how they rate their levels of satisfaction; you may find older patients are happier with the care they received than younger patients. As surveys collect information often at one point in time, they are often called **cross-sectional**.

Qualitative research

Qualitative research is mainly **descriptive** and is used when the aim of the research is to understand human experience, perceptions, motivations, intentions and behaviour (Parahoo 2014). Researchers usually focus on understanding peoples interpretations of their situation, exploring the meanings, beliefs, attitudes and experiences of participants. Qualitative research can help us to determine why people do the things they do and what affects behaviour and relationships over time. It can also help us to make a link between what people say they do and what they actually do. Further it enables interpretation of people's behaviours, opinions and interactions within the context of their natural environment. It also helps us to capture the way in which people interpret events and experiences and relationships.

These types of questions are very important in answering many questions about living with illness, disability and also about the quality of care patients experience. For example: *What is it like to suffer with depression? Why do patients feel they are not being treated with dignity?* Qualitative researchers do not seek to explain cause and effect and are not trying to control the situation; instead, qualitative researchers view the context in which the study is taking place as an inherent part of the research. Qualitative research designs are therefore aimed at describing these perceptions, enabling participants to talk in depth about their experiences, usually by interviewing and listening to people's stories. The information generated is in the form of the participants' own words and is known as **narrative data.** The data is analysed by looking at common **themes** which arise.

The term qualitative research is a broad term used to describe a range of research approaches such as **ethnography**, **grounded theory and phenomenology** (Parahoo 2014). The different types of qualitative research look at different forms of human activity and behaviour and are outlined in Table 9.1.

Table 9.1 Summary of qualitative research approaches

Qualitative research design	Main use
Ethnography	Studies groups of people and cultures. For example, psychiatric in-patient setting, ward culture.
Grounded Theory	Seeks to develop a theory of process, action or interaction. For example, how do family support mechanisms help people develop coping skills when they have a diagnosis of a terminal illness?
Phenomenology	Investigates the meaning of an experience from the view of individuals who have experienced the same phenomena. For example, what is it like to be a parent of a child who is severely disabled?
Qualitative	Does not use a specific named method but follows rules of qualitative research.

ACTIVITY

Read the two examples below and then list the ways in which the research approaches taken by Sunitha and Mark differ.

Mark is a community nurse whose client group includes a small number of people who are suffering from cancer. Mark is concerned that he does not know enough about how these clients feel about having cancer and therefore cannot help them as well as he would like to. He decides that the way to improve his knowledge is to undertake a small research study in which he interviews a few of his patients about how they feel about having cancer.

Sunitha is a family support worker who has been assigned to work in a large inner-city housing estate. She is keen to develop a project to support families with young children. She wants to map out the potential size of her client group, so she can develop an appropriate service.

She wants to find out a number of things about her clients. She wants to find out the number of families living on the estate, how many have children, what are the age ranges of the children, how many children are at school, how many parents work, and how many are single parents. She plans to collect this data by posting out a questionnaire to all residents on the estate.

The ways in which the two studies differ can be summarised as follows:

1   Sunitha wants to collect a lot of information about a large number of people so she can determine the numbers in each group. Mark wants to collect information about how a small number of people feel about their condition. He does not intend or need to collect a lot of data in number form, but wants to know what it means to people to have cancer.
2   Sunitha knows exactly what information she wants to collect. The kind of information Mark collects may be quite varied – he does not know what patients will say about their condition.
3   Sunitha can collect the data she wants fairly quickly by sending out a postal questionnaire to a large number of households which contains specific questions and tick box answers for families to complete. She does not need to meet with the families. Mark might take quite a long time collecting the information he needs through interviewing his patients. He will be directly involved in collecting the data from the patients he meets in his work.

We can see that there is a difference between the type of data that is collected and the volume of data that is collected. The two cases above illustrate the main differences between qualitative and quantitative research. Table 9.2 summarises this.

Table 9.2 Main differences between quantitative and qualitative research

Qualitative research	Quantitative research
Focuses on unknown	Focuses on known issues
Data in words	Data in numbers
Searches for meaning	Searches for trends or cause and effect
Small number of participants	Large number of participants
Researcher interacts with people being studied	Researcher is distant from people being studied

---

ACTIVITY

Look at the research questions below and decide which would lend themselves to:

(a) quantitative methodology
(b) qualitative methodology.

1   How many children under five have attended A&E departments in the last month?
2   Why do some people become drug addicts?
3   What is the relationship between income and type of housing?
4   What is the incidence of postnatal depression in one GP surgery?
5   What is the overall success rate in exams in a college of health studies?
6   What does it feel like to be a client of a social worker?
7   What are cancer patients' perceptions of the value of complementary therapies?

Your answers should look like the list below. The highlighted words identify key aspects underlying the choice of the most suitable research methodology.

1   **How many** children under five have attended A&E departments in the last month? **Quantitative**
2   **Why** do some people **become** drug addicts? **Qualitative**
3   What is the **relationship** between income and type of housing? **Quantitative**
4   What is the **incidence** of postnatal depression in one GP surgery? **Quantitative**
5   What is the overall **success rate** in exams in a college of health studies? **Quantitative**
6   What does it **feel like** to be a client of a social worker? **Qualitative**
7   What are cancer patients' **perceptions** of the value of complementary therapies? **Qualitative**

ACTIVITY

In the article you are reading, did the researchers use a quantitative or qualitative research methodology or a combination of both?

If the study is quantitative research – can you identify:

- If the design of the study is interventional or observational?
- The variables the researchers are interested in studying?
- The type of variable, i.e. independent, dependent, extraneous?
- Are the variables being manipulated by the researchers or are they being observed as they naturally occur?
- Is the data being collected numerical?

If the study is qualitative research – can you identify:

- The type of qualitative research approach?
- Is it clear why they have chosen this approach?
- Is the data being collected in the participants' own words, i.e. narrative data?
- Is the researcher interacting with the participants to collect data?

Do you think the researcher has chosen the best methodological approach to answer their research question? Why?

STUDENT TIP

There are other types of research methodologies, such as Action Research, Mixed Methods Research, and it is worth undertaking some further reading on this topic.

Step 6 – identifying the participants in the study – the sample

After the researcher has decided which methodology and research design best suit the needs of the research question, the next decision they need to make is about who (or what) should participate in the research. Two key terms you need to understand are **population** and **sample**.

Population, sometimes called the **target population** is the entire set of subjects who are of interest to the researcher, for example all people who are obese. The population the researcher is interested in might not be made up of people but could be a community, an event such as feeding patients, hospital records or laboratory samples. However, whatever the basic unit is, i.e. people or hospital records, the population comprises all of the units the researcher is interested in (Boswell and Canon 2014). Usually in most studies you will read to support your practice the sample will be made up of people.

The term **sample** describes a smaller group, a subset of people or units, chosen to represent the population in a research study (Boswell and Canon 2014). Researchers use samples rather than populations for reasons of cost and time. It would be almost impossible to conduct research on an entire population. The example in Figure 9.5 illustrates this.

Imagine the government launched a campaign in England to encourage children in primary school to participate in more sport to reduce the risk of obesity developing in later life. The population in this case would be all the children in primary schools in England. In order to test if the campaign had been a success, researchers would have to question all the children in this group. This is clearly impracticable. Therefore, a smaller number of children, i.e. **a sample**, would be selected, and based on the results of that sample a conclusion would be drawn about the total population of children in primary school.

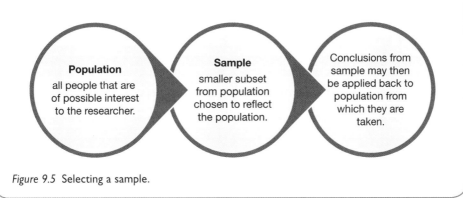

Figure 9.5 Selecting a sample.

Whilst sampling is widely used in research it does have limitations. Samples may not always fully reflect the population they are meant to represent. Approaches to sampling vary in quantitative and qualitative research.

Quantitative sampling

In quantitative research the sample is selected at random from the identified population and is often called **probability sampling** (Boswell and Canon 2014). This means that every member of the population has an equal chance of being included in the sample. The people included in this sample are **representative** of the whole population.

Imagine you are interested in studying people with high blood pressure. You would need to include people in your sample who reflect all characteristics of the population who suffer from high blood pressure. This would have to include participants who suffer with high blood pressure including both male and female, different age ranges, different ethnic groups, people underweight, of normal weight or obese.

The ways in which samples are collected in research is a crucial feature of the research design. Some of the common procedures are:

- simple random sampling
- stratified random sampling
- cluster sampling.

Achieving a representative sample is often very difficult but it is the best sample to have. However, in practical terms, cost and time, researchers often access a sample that is easily available. This is called **convenience** sampling. This is not ideal as it is not completely random; you only include participants you can get. This limits the extent to which we can be confident that the results would reflect the views of the whole population, therefore we cannot make valid inferences about the larger group from which the sample is drawn. This is called **generalisability**. When a sample is not truly random, then the sample may not be truly representative of the population. This introduces an element of **sampling error/bias**.

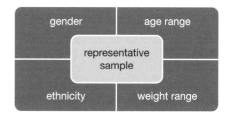

Figure 9.6 Representative sample.

EXAMPLE OF CONVENIENCE SAMPLING

In the example of children's activity levels, it would be best if a random sample of children from all primary schools in England were included. To do this a list of names of all the children – known as the **sampling frame** – could be uploaded into a computer and a smaller list could be randomly generated.

However, due to time constraints researchers might use just several primary schools from across England from which to draw the sample. This would be a convenience sample and not truly representative.

Sample size in quantitative research

How many people you need to include in a sample is a major issue for quantitative researchers and there is no simple answer to this. Generally, quantitative researchers try to use the largest sample possible. The larger the sample, the more representative it is likely to be (Boswell and Canon 2014).

When researchers are testing a hypothesis using RCT, they estimate the sample size mathematically using a technique called a **power analysis**, to ensure they include enough subjects to gather sufficient data.

ACTIVITY

Look at the two research studies described below. If you were looking at the findings from the two surveys which do you think would provide the most reliable information?

1   A researcher administered questionnaire to a random sample of 1,000 people.
2   A researcher administered questionnaire to a convenience sample of 30 people.

You would probably find the information from research study 1 to be the most reliable because the researcher has collected information from a random sample, which is a sample that represents the population as a whole. The researcher can say with more confidence that the results are generalisable. In example 2, this is a convenience sample and not representative. The results would be useful but would not be generalisable to a wider population.

Qualitative sampling

Sampling is approached differently in qualitative research because the aim is to understand the meaning of individuals in given situations. Sampling needs to be more *purposeful*, it is not random and is classified as a **non-probability** sample (Parahoo 2014). In qualitative studies researchers need to pick participants who are very knowledgeable and have experience of the topic of the study. For example, if a researcher *is interested in understanding what it is like to be a mother caring for a child with autism,* only mothers of children with autism would be included in the study. This is often referred to as a **purposive sample** or a **theoretical sample**. Participants are recruited based on the judgements of the researcher as to their suitability to provide information which answers the research question. Such samples are selected for a specific purpose and are non-representative samples. Therefore there is no intention to use the sample to make inferences about a wider population.

Sample size in qualitative research

In qualitative studies the researcher is looking for meaning in the data and is not concerned with trying to generalise findings to a wider situation (Parahoo 2014). Consequently the sample size is generally much smaller than that used in quantitative studies, but will vary depending on which type of qualitative approach is used. Phenomenological studies which focus on the unique experiences of individuals may only have small numbers such as 6–10. However, in ethnographic studies which look at people in cultural groups and settings, or in grounded theory which seeks to develop understandings and theory of basic social processes such as awareness of dying or coping with cancer, the sample numbers may be bigger.

When you read qualitative studies you may see the researcher refer to '**saturation**' of data. What this means is that when deciding how many people to involve in the study, the researcher will collect data until the ideas that are developing are saturated, i.e. no new information is being collected. For example, when exploring with patients what it is like to live with cancer, researchers will approach new cancer patients to include in the study until the same information keeps recurring.

ACTIVITY

In the research paper you are reading can you identify what type of sample is used for the study?

How many participants are included in the sample?

Are the researchers trying to make generalisations or not?

Is the sample appropriate?

There are many other types of sample and it is worth undertaking some further reading around this topic. Add sample definitions to your glossary.

Step 7 – what method is used to gather information – data collection tools

Generally in quantitative research, because the aim of the data collection is to quantify information, researchers need to use a structured approach which will enable them to collect information in a consistent way from all participants and which will enable them to count the responses. In qualitative research, a more open and flexible approach is required which allows the participants to respond in their own words (Punch 2006). Here the researcher is more concerned with being able to record in words what the participants have said.

Whichever approach is used the common tools or techniques used in data collection are:

- Questionnaires
- Observation
- Interviews.

However, the layout and structure of the data collection tools will vary depending on whether the researcher is wishing to collect quantitative numerical data or qualitative narrative data. We will now consider these tools in more detail.

ACTIVITY

Some of the advantages and disadvantages of research tools are considered in the following sections. Think about whether or not these are relevant to the study you are reading.

Questionnaires

These are very popular means of gathering data and most people have some experience of completing questionnaires. Highly structured questionnaires are used in quantitative research. The questionnaires make use of a range of **rating scales** and **closed-ended questions** sometimes called **fixed response** questions which are easy and quick to complete. They may also include some open-ended questions which allow participants to answer in their own words (Ellis 2013). They can be sent out by post, email or more recently there has been the development of online questionnaires. This reduces the need for direct contact between researcher and participants.

In some studies researchers develop their own questionnaire specifically for the study. However, for many topics there may well be already established questionnaires and scales which can be used, for example depression questionnaire scales, quality of life questionnaire scales.

EXAMPLE OF COMMON SCALES AND QUESTIONS USED IN QUESTIONNAIRES

A Rating scale

This allows evaluation of a topic.

On a scale of 0–10, where 0 means extremely dissatisfied and 10 means extremely satisfied, how satisfied are you with the care you have received from the community nursing team?

Extremely dissatisfied ---------------------------------------Extremely satisfied

0   1   2   3   4   5   6   7   8   9   10

B Likert scale

This allows measurement of attitudes towards a topic, by asking participants to rate their level of agreement with a statement; from strongly agree to strongly disagree.

Strongly agree	Agree	Undecided	Disagree	Strongly disagree
I feel confident that I can read a research report effectively				

C Closed-ended question

Are you satisfied with the care you have received?   Yes   No

D Open-ended question

What is your opinion of the quality of care you have received?

Some of the common advantages and disadvantages of using questionnaires to collect data are listed in Table 9.3.

Table 9.3 Advantages and disadvantages of questionnaires

Advantages	Disadvantages
Relatively inexpensive	Difficult to design a good questionnaire
Can be used with large numbers of participants	Respondents often have a fixed choice of answers, which may not truly represent their views
Provide large quantities of information which is easy and quick to handle.	Participants might not fully understand the questions or may misinterpret them

Table 9.3 continued

Advantages	Disadvantages
Provides replies which are anonymous and therefore likely to be more honest	Incorrectly completed
No contact with researcher, limits potential researcher influence on participants responses	Return rate of questionnaires is generally low

Interviews

Interviews require the researcher and the participant to meet face to face, in order to have a conversation. The researcher is seen as the primary instrument for data collection (Punch 2006).

There are three main types of interview (Moule and Hek 2011):

- **Structured** – this is where the researcher uses a set list of questions, '**interview schedule**', like a verbal questionnaire to ensure a consistent approach is used with all participants. This is a suitable tool for the collection of **quantitative data**.
- **Semi-structured** – this is where a researcher has a list of topics, which need to be discussed in the interview but no set format is used. The interviewer uses a topic guide to ensure all topics are covered but is flexible in its approach. Participants are encouraged to respond freely about all topics. This is a suitable tool for the collection of **qualitative data**.
- **Unstructured** – this is where the researcher sets a topic but encourages the respondent to talk freely about the subject and does not guide or direct the flow of the discussion. This is a suitable tool for the collection of **qualitative data**.

Interviews are usually conducted on an individual basis but can sometimes be conducted with a group, known as a **focus group**. These are becoming very popular as they can be used to gather information quickly about collective views in relation to a wide range of topics, such as provision of health and social care services.

The advantages and disadvantages of using face-to-face interviews are summarised in Table 9.4.

Table 9.4 Advantages and disadvantages of interviews

Advantages	Disadvantages
Interaction enables researcher and participant to clarify questions and answers	Interaction with researcher may influence the responses given by the participant. The researcher may be influenced also by the participant
	Not anonymous
In structured interview likely to get a higher response rate than using a questionnaire	Time consuming
In semi-structured and unstructured interviews researcher can pursue interesting issues raised by the respondent. The process allows for flexibility	Difficult to capture data accurately especially if the interview is not recorded. Note taking disrupts flow of interview

Advantages	Disadvantages
Non-verbal cues can be observed, e.g. body language, facial expression	Difficult to anticipate any problems which may arise
Often easier for participants to express their ideas verbally rather than in writing	May be more difficult to analyse information

Observation

This enables a researcher to see first-hand what is happening in a situation and to see how people behave and respond. Research observation can be approached from two different angles (Moule and Hek 2011):

- **Non-participant observation** – here the researcher is outside the situation and acts only as an outsider looking in. For example, you may be interested in seeing how elderly patients are supported during mealtimes on a ward. To do this, you may observe mealtimes on the ward and record what you see. You are not involved in helping with the task.
- **Participant observation** – here the researcher joins in the group and is part of the situation being observed. In the above example you would work alongside the staff at mealtimes and gain first-hand experience of the situation.

The same principles of high or low structure used in other tools can also be applied in observations. For example, if you wanted to undertake a study designed to measure the workload of healthcare assistants in residential homes you could begin by listing every task care assistants carry out in their work. You could then observe care assistants at work and record the frequency of each task and the time taken for each task. Table 9.5 shows an example of how this might look.

Alternatively, if we were using a low structure in the same observations you might start the study with a much more open approach and simply divide the categories of care into those involving direct care with residents and those that do not involve direct care. The researcher in this instance would write down in some detail the nature of the task and any observations relating to it.

Table 9.5 Example of a highly structured observation schedule

Area of work	Time	Time	Time	Time
Walks with resident to toilet				
Helps resident with dressing				
Serves meals to residents				

EXAMPLE OF A LOW-STRUCTURED OBSERVATION SCHEDULE

Working directly with resident

TASK:

Comment:

Not working directly with resident

TASK:

Comment:

The advantages and disadvantages of participant and non-participant observation are summarised in Table 9.6.

Table 9.6 Advantages and disadvantages of participant and non-participant observation

Advantages of participant observation	Disadvantages of participant observation
Being in the setting and a member of the group may give access to a wide range of information	May become too involved and lose objectivity
Gain a better understanding of what is relevant and what is not relevant in a situation	Participants may be influenced by the presence of the researcher which affects their behaviour
Large amounts of information may be generated	Difficult to record information when part of the situation
Researcher may gain the respect of the group	Researcher could be seen as a threat
Advantages of non-participant observation	*Disadvantages of non-participant observation*
Researcher may be more objective if not involved in the situation	Difficult to fully understand a situation from looking in
Researcher can be more focused and plan observations	Access to useful and relevant observations may be limited
Easier to record	May not record the most relevant information

STUDENT TIP

You can read about different data collection tools in much more detail in any basic textbook on research.

Step 8 – confirming the validity and reliability of data collection tools

When using tools such as questionnaires to collect data it is important to consider two key aspects about the tool.

1 Does the tool measure what it is intended to measure?
2 Does the tool provide the same results when repeated over and over again?

These two concepts are validity and reliability (Parahoo 2014):

* **Validity** – a ruler may be a valid measuring device for length, but isn't very valid for measuring volume. A ruler is intended to and does effectively measure length and for this purpose is a valid tool.
* **Reliability** – let us imagine that you have a piece of wood that is 70 cm long. You measure it once with the ruler – you get a measurement of 70 cm. Measure it again and you get 70 cm. Measure it repeatedly and you consistently get a measurement of 70 cm. The ruler is a measure which produces reliable results when used repeatedly. This could be either when measured by the same person (single rater – **intra-rater reliability**) or by different people using the tool (multiple raters – **inter-rater reliability**).

These two concepts are used when discussing data collection tools in quantitative research, because the tools are generally highly structured and designed to be independent and not influenced by the researcher when used in collecting data, thus reducing **bias**.

However, in qualitative research, it is not usually the case that rigid data collection tools are used. Therefore different criteria are needed to assess the accuracy of the tools used. Because the researcher interacts with participants, it is much harder to ensure that the researcher does not unduly influence or **bias** the information collected. **Trustworthiness** is a term used to cover this and is addressed by strategies outlined in Table 9.7.

Table 9.7 Criteria for trustworthiness

Term used	What does it mean?	How is it achieved?
Credibility	Is there a good fit between how the researcher presents the findings and what the participants said?	Researcher should ask the participants to check the initial information recorded is accurate
Transferability	Can the findings be useful in other settings?	Researcher needs to clearly describe the research setting and the participants
Dependability	Is the research process logical and easy to follow?	Researcher needs to have kept good records of what was done and why
Confirmability	When the data has been interpreted, it is clear that this is based on the information collected	Do the participants agree with the interpretation of the researcher?

ACTIVITY

It might be that when you are reading a research paper it is difficult to assess if the researcher has considered the validity and reliability of the tool or the trustworthiness of the study. Look to see if these are mentioned or if they have demonstrated some of the processes in the research paper you are reading.

Step 9 – consider the protection of participants in the study – research ethics

All research involving human participants should be reviewed by a research ethics committee to ensure that the study is appropriate and does not pose any serious risks to the participants (Moule and Hek 2011). Key areas they consider are:

1   Does the study pose any risk of harm to participants?
2   Is participation in the study entirely voluntary?
3   Are participants asked to give informed consent?
4   Is the privacy and confidentiality of the participants protected?
5   Can participants withdraw from the study at any time?
6   Are participants treated fairly?
7   Are participants fully informed about the study?
8   Are participants told the truth about the study?
9   Is the study design suitable?
10 Will the study results be made available to the participants and published for others to read?

ACTIVITY

Look to see if Ethical Approval is discussed in the research paper you are reading.

Have the rights of participants been protected?

Step 10 – reading and understanding the results

This is the section in which the findings of the study are reported. You may feel that reading the results of research can be quite daunting, but try not to panic. There are some simple tips which you might find helpful:

1   Go back and read the abstract again. This will have included a summary of the results and conclusions.
2   Remind yourself what question the researcher set out to answer.
3   If the results section contains tables, figures and charts, then make sure you read the captions that accompany them carefully. Do not get overwhelmed by the figures.
4   Take your time, make sure you read carefully.
5   If you need help, ask a more experienced colleague.

When you are reading the results it is important to realise that you do not see the individual data produced by each participant but rather an interpretation and summary of the data. The researcher should have clearly stated how the results of the study were analysed and if they used any software tools to support them. They should also tell you if other researchers were involved in this process to help check the accuracy of the results.

Presentation of quantitative results

For quantitative studies which have collected numerical data, the results are presented statistically using either **descriptive** or **inferential statistics** (Moule and Hek 2011). Let us consider these concepts.

First, why use statistics? Imagine that the researcher has collected information from 200 patients using a questionnaire about waiting time for clinic appointments. They could simply give you a spreadsheet of each of the individual responses and say 'Here, this is what we found. However, it is much easier if the researcher summarises the data for you and presents it in a way that is quick and easy to understand. This is exactly what descriptive statistics are all about.

Descriptive statistics summarise the data in a study and give us information about the frequency, distribution and range of some of the variables in the study. For example, we might see summaries of information about participants, their gender, age range and ethnicity. The exact nature of the results will of course depend on the individual research project.

The results may be presented in terms of a series of visual presentations such as graphs, bar charts, pie charts. Tables may also be used. In each case the table or graph should be clearly labelled and presented so you can identify the results. When reading tables and graphs you may notice the researchers often use the term **N**, followed by a number, N = 126. This refers to the number of participants included in a study sample. Other key terms used when describing quantitative data are terms such as **mean**, **median and mode**. These are terms which refer to average values for the data, for example the average age of participants included in the study, average waiting time for clinic appointment. **Range** refers to the spread of data from the lowest to the highest value, for example the youngest to the oldest participant included in the study, shortest to the longest waiting time for a clinic appointment. Associated with the range of the data you may see references to the term **standard deviation**. This gives information about the spread of the data from the average (mean) score. Some data can be spread widely from the mean score while other data sets are grouped more closely to the mean. Let us look at a couple of examples.

Table 9.8 shows some demographic data which has been collected, analysed and summarised so it is easy to read. It is always useful when reading a research paper to be able to identify who are the participants included in the study and what we know about them.

Let us consider presentation in the form of a bar chart. In this example a researcher has undertaken a survey to identify how women rated their levels of satisfaction with care they received in the local maternity unit over a period of three months. The following information was collected:

Level of satisfaction with care	N = 940
Very satisfied	658
Satisfied	235
Dissatisfied	47

Table 9.8 Example of a frequency distribution table

Frequency distribution of demographic characteristics of participants in a study

Characteristics	N = 107	Percentage (%)
Gender	Male 92	86.0
	Female 15	14.0
Marital status	Married 76	71.0
	Single 31	29.0
Age	Mean 71.2 years	
	Range 52–85 years	
Ethnicity	White 65	60.7
	Black 28	26.2
	Asian 14	13.1
Religion	Christian 46	42.9
	Jewish 12	11.2
	Muslim 15	14.2
	Atheist 3	2.8
	No religion 31	28.9

The researcher calculates the percentage frequency for each of the group responses and decides to present it graphically using a bar chart. From this we can quickly and easily see that 70 per cent of all women were very satisfied, 25 per cent were satisfied and 5 per cent were dissatisfied with the care they received.

It is important to remember that descriptive statistics do not draw conclusions about the data. They are used simply to describe the main features of the data in quantitative terms.

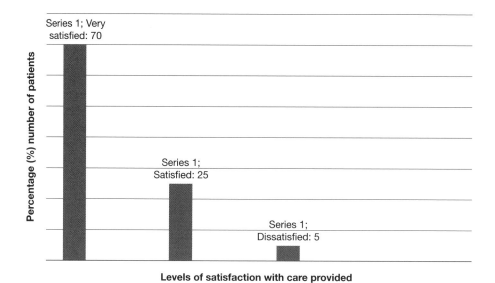

Figure 9.7 Example of a bar chart indicating patient satisfaction with care provided in a maternity hospital.

This includes summarising, tabulating, organising and displaying data for the purpose of describing the sample of individuals, or events that have been measured or observed. They are usually found in all quantitative research reports.

Inferential statistics

Often in quantitative studies the researcher may wish to find out if the results they have found from the sample can be generalised to the wider population from which the sample was selected. This requires the researcher to go beyond describing the data and start to draw conclusions about the data. The researcher tries to draw intelligent guesses about the population based on the sample. They do this mathematically using inferential statistics. In studies where researchers identify hypotheses as the main research question, then this will be tested using inferential statistics.

Statistical significance refers to whether or not any differences observed between groups of people in a study are real or not, that is, they are just due to chance. Linked to statistical significance is the term **Probability**. This is a measure of how likely an event is to occur. It is reported in studies by the term **P**, where a score of 1 indicates it will definitely happen and a score of 0 indicates it definitely will not happen. We see this written in research using values expressed for example as $P < 0.001$ or $P > 0.05$ (< means less than; > means greater than). Usually in health research, the lower the number the better, as it is indicating that it is unlikely that the differences observed in the results occurred by chance.

Inferential statistics are quite challenging and there are many different tests which can be used depending on the data. It is not possible to consider this in this chapter. However, when reading results it is the responsibility of the researcher to make clear which tests they have used and indicate if results are significant or not.

ACTIVITY

If the research paper you are reading is a quantitative study:

- Can you identify if the results are reported using descriptive statistics in the form of tables, graphs, bar charts, etc.?
- What information do these provide, e.g. demographic data, frequency of variables under study?
- Have the researchers aimed to draw conclusions about the data to generalise findings to a wider population by using inferential statistical tests?
- Have the results been tested to see if the findings are statistically significant?
- Which are the variables of interest they are testing?
- Are the results reported using a $P < >$ value?

Presentation of qualitative data

Qualitative research studies are likely to produce large amounts of data in the form of words. If a researcher has undertaken in-depth interviews with ten participants and each interview has lasted an hour, this will have generated individual interview transcripts and collectively produced a huge number of words. This initial data will need to be reduced and reported in such a way that is meaningful to the reader. The most common method of reporting the analysed qualitative data is to identify themes in it. Qualitative data analysis requires the researcher to make judgements about the significance of recurring ideas, the strength or frequency of ideas, and to consider the emphasis participants have placed on ideas in order to finally determine what the key themes are. To ensure a rigorous approach is followed many researchers will ask another researcher to check their interpretation (peer review) or return the findings to participants to get their feedback. They also keep detailed notes about the decisions they make and why, which provides an audit trail.

The findings are often presented under the theme headings to provide structure. These themes usually contain some element of description together with the analysed meaning and interpretation. Themes are often illustrated by inclusion of **anonymised direct quotes** taken from the original raw data, to demonstrate the validity of the theme. Sometimes the results may be supported by a visual summary of how themes were derived, or how they all interrelate.

The focus of qualitative research is on the exploration of human experience in a specific context and it is not the intention to generalise findings to a wider population. However, when reading qualitative findings you may feel that the research study context is similar to your own work environment and that the description of participants in the study shows similarity to your own clients. You may decide then that the findings of the study are useful to inform your practice, a concept known as **transferability** (Parahoo 2014).

ACTIVITY

If the research paper you are reading is a qualitative paper, can you identify the steps the researcher took to ensure the data analysis was rigorously conducted?

- Did they seek help from another researcher to check the data analysis process, or did they go back to the participants?
- How did they report the findings?
- Did the findings include quotes taken from participants?
- Did they include a visual summary of the findings?

Step 11 – focus on the discussion and conclusion

In these sections the results of the study are discussed in more general terms. These may be identified under separate headings or integrated. Aspects of the discussion may focus on:

1   An explanation of what has been found and how this relates back to the original research question.
2   How the findings of the study support or contrast the findings of other researchers. This will link back to the literature review.
3   Strengths and weaknesses of the current study.
4   Links to practice.
5   Summary of the research study.
6   Recommendations for future research.

Sometimes if the study has been funded by an organisation this is stated at the end of the report. This is important to note as you may feel funding is influential in shaping the work. For example, if it was a study about sugar in processed foods and had been funded by the companies that produce sugar, this may have influenced the way the study was conducted and hence the results.

ACTIVITY

Look at the study you are reading. The discussion can help you decide if the findings of the study can be used in practice.

• Does the weakness in the research limit the use of the findings?
• Are you convinced the findings are meaningful and could be used as evidence to support practice?

Step 12 – finally, the references

The final information provided in the research article should be the references supporting all sources cited in the main text. These can be very useful if you wish to follow up on any of them. You should be able to link references cited in the text with the full reference at the end of the paper (see Chapter 1).

Conclusions

Reading and understanding research papers takes practice. The steps outlined in this chapter have tried to provide you with a structure to follow and a series of questions to ask each time you review a study. It is useful to develop a systematic approach to reading so as to develop a more critical approach and to help you make a judgement about the quality of the study and its relevance to your practice.

STUDENT TIP

To help develop a systematic approach to reading a research article it is useful to use a tool in the form of a proforma. These usually consist of a series of questions covering all the aspects of the study. Many are available in the textbooks on research. An easy one to use is Moule and Hek's Critical Appraisal Framework (2011).

Systematic reviews

Many research articles are available and it would be impossible for practitioners to read all that is published on a specific topic. **Systematic review** is a research methodology that seeks to address this problem by locating all the published research studies on the topic, evaluating the quality of the studies and producing a summary outcome of the integrated study results. There are specialised electronic sites which contain systematic reviews that you can access. The Cochrane database is one such site.

ACTIVITY

Try using Google to access the Cochrane Library.

Explore the site to learn more about systematic reviews.

Search the site using keywords to see if you can locate a systematic review on a topic relevant to your practice.

Chapter summary

- All care that is provided to patients needs to be supported by the best available evidence.
- Good quality research is a key feature of EBP. Research is a systematic approach to discovering new knowledge.
- The two major approaches of qualitative and quantitative research are used in health and social care research.
- As consumers of research it is important to read research effectively and focus on the key areas of a research report, namely, title, abstract, research question, literature review, methodology, sample, data collection tools, ethical considerations, results and conclusions for practice. A critical appraisal framework will help you do this.
- Understanding research terminology is important and worthwhile – persevere in reading research and keep a glossary to help you.
- Reading research enables practitioners to keep up to date.

Further resources

The National Institute for Health and Care Excellence (NICE) – provides national guidance and advice to improve health and social care. Available at: www.nice.org.uk

Evidence Based Nursing Practice – the site gives an insight into why EBP is important by outlining some of the fundamental principles. A resource page acts as a gateway to other websites. These sites are useful in gaining a deeper understanding of EBP and provide further information to assist with the process. Available at: www.ebnp.co.uk/index.htm

NHS – this website overviews the different types of research undertaken to find better ways of looking after people. Available at: www.nhs.uk/Conditions/Clinical-trials/Pages/Introduction.aspx

The Institute of Work and Health – this website provides useful explanations of many of the key terms used in the chapter. It is also helpful for understanding statistics. Available at: www.iwh.on.ca/what-researchers-mean-by

SCIE's Research Mindedness learning resource – produced to help students and practitioners of social care and social work make more effective and extensive use of research in their studies and in practice. Available at: www.scie.org.uk/publications/researchmindedness

Flying Start NHS 2015 – this site provides useful resources to support your understanding of research Available at: www.flyingstart.scot.nhs.uk/learning-programmes/research-for-practice/

Further reading

Griffiths, F. 2010. *Research Methods for Healthcare Practice*. London: Sage.
Le May, A. and Holmes, S. 2012. *Introduction to Nursing Research*. London: New York: Routledge.

Jolley, J. 2013. *Introducing Research & Evidence Based Practice for Nursing & Healthcare Professionals*. London and New York: Routledge.

References

Boswell, C. and Cannon, S. 2014. *Introduction to Nursing Research: Incorporating Evidence-based Practice*, 3rd edn. Burlington MA: Jones & Bartlett Learning.

Coughlan, M., Cronin, P. and Ryan, F. 2013. *Doing a Literature Review in Nursing, Health and Social Care.* London: Sage.

Ellis, P. 2010. *Evidence-based Practice in Nursing*. Exeter: Learning Matters.

Ellis, P. 2013. *Understanding Research for Nursing Students*, 2nd edn. London: Sage/Learning Matters.

Moule, P. and Hek, G. 2011. *Making Sense of Research: An Introduction for Health & Social Care Practitioners*, 4th edn. London: Sage.

Parahoo, K. 2014. *Nursing Research: Principles, Processes and Issues*, 3rd edn. London: Palgrave Macmillan.

Punch, K. F. 2006. *Developing Effective Research Proposals*, 2nd edn. London: Sage.

Sackett, D. L., Straus, S. E., Richardson, W. S., Rosenberg, W. and Haynes, R. B. 2000. *Evidence-based Medicine: How to Practice and Teach EBM*, 2nd edn. Edinburgh: Churchill Livingstone.

Chapter 10

Improving public health

Dr Andy Stevens and Sarah Kraszewski

LEARNING OUTCOMES

By the end of this chapter you will be able to:

1 Understand the role and function of public health.
2 Consider how you can support the public to protect their own health.
3 Understand how the use of research and data informs public health policy.
4 Demonstrate awareness of common screening programmes and the criteria that informs them.

Introduction

Public health encompasses population-based approaches with collective responsibility for health, protection of health and disease prevention. The state undertakes a key role in public health. This is linked to socioeconomic factors and the wider determinants of health and partnership working amongst all the groups that support the health of the nation (Faculty of Public Health 2010).

The Health and Social Care Act 2012 made major changes to the delivery of public health services in England and reorganised national bodies related to care quality, and the professional regulation of care workers, and funded health-related organisations. Section 30 of the Act relates to the local appointment of directors of public health and other sections relate to transfer of responsibility for the provision or commissioning of many adult health services from health to local authorities. Despite representations to the contrary, there remains a split in the commissioning of children's services between the NHS (0–5 years) and older children and young people's services (5–18 years) that move to local government.

While transitional problems will naturally occur, these organisational changes should benefit the provision of public health services in England. The main reasons for this are historical. We are used to a national health service, but before the Second World War, local health and social care provision was in the hands of a variety of organisations, some charitable, but increasingly funded and managed by local or county councils and coordinated locally by the Medical Officer of Health. This was particularly effective at times of epidemics, but also for public health innovations in local communities. Joint planning (between the centrally managed NHS and local authority departments) and more particularly joint funding of projects has been difficult in the area of general health improvement, given that this was not central to the priorities of either body. The new legislation, with a focus on localism, shifts more emphasis towards the local authority again.

We should anticipate that new initiatives will result in a broader range of public health services work opportunities, with non-traditional employment areas. In this chapter, we will look at what we mean by public health, the way we consider health and well-being in communities and the types of activities undertaken by public health workers. The case studies in this chapter therefore take a different approach in that they are about projects or communities rather than about individuals or their families.

History

It would be impossible to do complete justice to the historical development of public health here (see Berridge *et al.* 2011). The earliest measures (provision for public baths, toilets and clean drinking water) can be found in the first cities in the Indus Valley (around 3300 BCE), and some medical interventions such as vaccinations can be found in China (around 1000 BCE). The first modern development of organisations for public health can be attributed to Edwin Chadwick (1800–90) who conducted surveys of living conditions of the urban poor in Victorian cities, reformed the poor law system and local councils to provide a range of regulation of public health hazards (such as slaughterhouses, burials and mains water supplies) and established the profession of 'sanitary inspectors', now known as environmental health officers. Technical developments in sewer building and the development of theory were important in establishing our understanding of the processes of infection.

European countries with world empires, during the late nineteenth century, were particularly interested in protection of the public from diseases found in the tropics such as malaria and dysentery, which resulted in the development of colonial medicine. It was from research into germ theory that we discovered that infection was spread through water and other agents (or vectors) rather than in the air (the name 'malaria' literally means 'bad air'). As a result of scientific developments, a biomedical phase of public health led to the dominance of public health medicine at the beginning of the twentieth century.

More recent phases of public health result from understanding of the influence of social inequality, and lifestyle in life expectancy and the distribution of disease and ill health. A widespread recognition of the limitations of medical interventions in the 1980s and acknowledgement of the importance of social determinants of health have resulted in a more broadly based approach to public health, including political solutions in public policy.

Definition

Let us start by considering what we mean by public health. It is what it says – the health of the public – but what does that mean in practice? First, it is an approach that considers populations, not individuals. The 'public' are communities that can be geographically defined (such as 'Londoners' or the Northeast), or sections of a population (such as premenopausal women or manual workers who smoke) and categories of a population that can be compared, for example on the grounds of age, sex, racial or cultural group. Health (or well-being, which largely means the same thing) is about not being ill. Given that most health service provision is about ill health perhaps local services should be renamed 'injury and illness services', rather than health centres. Each population is likely to have different needs and require particular services.

CASE STUDY

Homeless people have been identified as having high health and social care needs. The average life expectancy in England for a homeless person is 47 years, compared to an average of 77 years (Crisis 2011).

A recent report estimated that there are 2,000 people who sleep rough and a further 40,000 living in hostels in the UK. Both groups have significantly higher levels of drug dependence, physical and mental ill health than the average population and are more difficult to find and provide services for (such as medical treatment, welfare and employment services).

Most regular health and social care services do not see these clients even though they have significant needs. One specialist local service, the Cambridge Access Surgery (a GP surgery dedicated to homeless patients), found the following health problems in a random sample of patients:

- Drug dependence (62.5%)
- Mental ill health (53.7%)
- Alcohol dependence syndrome (49.1%)
- Dual (mental health and drug) diagnosis (42.6%)
- Injuries/assault (26.4%)
- Hepatitis C virus antibody positive (17.6%)
- Respiratory diseases (16.7%)
- Liver disorders/abnormalities (15.7%)
- Other infections (13.9%)
- Other health problems (31.5%).

It is estimated that the costs to government of addressing the health and social concerns of homeless people is between £24,000 and £30,000 per person each year (Department of Communities & Local Government 2012).

REFLECTION POINT

Think about your workplace and local area that your service supports.

What are the common health and social care problems that you encounter?

What barriers do your clients encounter when trying to access services?

Public health is mainly interested *in preventative health* measures and identifying the factors that make people ill. A good initial definition of public health is:

the science and art of promoting and protecting health and well-being, preventing ill-health and prolonging life through the organised efforts of society.

(Faculty of Public Health 2010)

It is worth reflecting on some of the important elements involved in this statement which correspond to the four domains set out in the Department of Health Public Health Outcomes Framework:

The **four domains** of the Department of Health Public Health Outcomes Framework:

- Improving wider determinants of health.
- Health improvement.
- Health protection.
- Healthcare, public health and preventing premature mortality (Department of Health 2012).

Let us first consider what might be meant by the 'organised efforts of society'. This is rather vague, but it does point out an important difference between public health and other healthcare services, which is that responsibility for public health provision is shared across a variety of agencies and across communities not just health services.

Theoretical approaches

Environmental

The health of any group of people is obviously affected by their age, genetic predispositions and their lifestyle choices, but it is also affected by the social, environmental and political circumstances in which they find themselves. Such environmental factors are significant in determining their exposure. These factors will influence the level of their exposure to infection and pollutants, diet and opportunities. Each of these factors is a determinant of people's health. Figure 10.1 is very commonly used to express how determinants of health affect populations.

Access and support from your local community networks will influence your lifestyle choices (e.g. to learn music, smoke, socialise with peers or to play sports) and also influence the quality of living and working conditions, which include access to services such as schools, fresh food, work and leisure activities. Some of these factors have significantly more influence on long-term well-being than others. Consider the following quote from the Marmot report:

> Inequalities in educational outcomes affect physical and mental health, as well as income, employment and quality of life. The graded relationship between socioeconomic position and educational outcome has significant implications for subsequent employment, income, living standards, behaviours, and mental and physical health.
>
> (Marmot 2010: 24)

No matter which country you are considering, access to education has a greater effect on the health of populations than all interventions from health and social care services.

> Higher educational attainment is associated with healthier behaviour. Those educated to degree level were shown not only to be more likely to be in full-time employment than

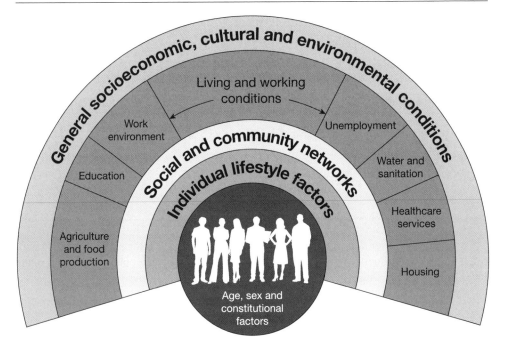

Figure 10.1 Dahlgren and Whitehead's Rainbow Model of Health, adapted from Dahlgren and Whitehead (1991).

those with lower educational attainment, but also less likely to smoke and be over-weight and more likely to exercise regularly and eat healthily.

(Marmot 2010: 66)

From an environmental perspective on public health, you can see that teachers, lecturers and other educational personnel make a significant contribution to the health of the public. Children who attend school are also often target populations for school health initiatives, such as those relating to diet, exercise and immunisation, as well as receiving education relating to safe sex and the dangers of drugs.

ACTIVITY

Consider one or more of the life and working areas of the Dahlgren and Whitehead Rainbow (agriculture and food, work and unemployment, water and sanitation, healthcare services, housing) and list all the professions that can make a contribution to public health.

You will find, as you do this, that the implications for public health range across a wide range of jobs that would not consider themselves public health professions, yet their work has significant implications on the health of communities.

Some of the professions in your list will be working in regulatory authorities and others in private businesses or not-for-profit organisations, but there are health and safety issues for staff and customers. If you had chosen housing, for example, your list should not only include town planners, architects, builders (painters, carpenters etc.), housing officers, power engineers, but also the police and fire services. If people do not feel safe in their streets, if they are poorly maintained or not well lit, they will be less likely to take exercise or participate in community social activities. This will affect their well-being and their physical and mental health, as they are vulnerable by becoming isolated. Buildings that are unsafe or poorly maintained (such as restaurants or some industries) are also visited by environmental health officers. Environmental health services have a broad range of duties all related to public health, so should appear in most lists.

Life course

Another approach to public health considers the long-term effect of different lifestyles and adverse or good environmental conditions. Taking no exercise for a week will not make you ill, but never taking exercise will have grave implications for your cardiovascular system, particularly if combined with a poor diet. Drinking alcohol every day even within recommended limits will also have implications on a population even if some individuals cope with this better than others. Life course analysis of populations provides useful insights into disease trends, genetic effects and ethnic, gender and regional inequalities in health. There are various models of approach based on accumulation of risk, birth cohorts and chains of risk (such as alcohol dependence leading to unemployment, then homelessness then respiratory illness). These approaches have context (like the environmental model) but also relate this to time which involves critical periods (such as adolescence) and can take into account a variety of susceptibility and resilience factors (Kuh *et al.* 2003). A study of nutritional effects on cancer prevention provides a clear life course approach illustrated in Figure 10.2.

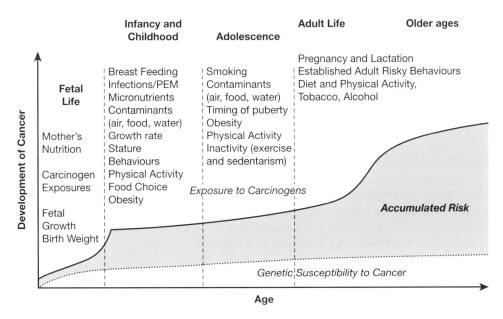

Figure 10.2 Model of accumulated risk of cancer, adapted from Uauy and Solomons (2005).

Life course approaches tend to justify the importance of early intervention which emphasises the importance of public health provision with preschool children or even *in vitro* within maternal health initiatives.

CASE STUDY

The EarlyBird research project monitors obesity in cohorts of children from 5 years to 16 years and has been producing research findings for over a decade. While this research has indicated that social inequalities between families and access to healthy open spaces are not influential factors, it does indicate that most excess weight gain occurs before school age and diet not exercise is the key determinant for weight management in children. While it is convenient for public health programmes on children's weight management to be set in school as it is easier to work in this setting, this research clearly indicates that such interventions are too late. Until puberty, obesity is confined to small groups of children whose behaviour patterns differ from the majority, so identification and concentrating dietary support on relevant children would be most effective. These and other findings have significant implications for public health practice and can be viewed on the EarlyBird website (www.earlybirddiabetes.org; EarlyBird Diabetes Trust 2014).

Environmental and life course approaches can be and are usefully used in combination to understand patterns of disease and the influence of determinant of health in populations.

Social capital

You may come across theories that relate to the concept of social capital in public health research and policies. Social capital has been defined as 'the ability to secure benefits through membership in networks and other social structures' (Portes in Lucas and Lloyd 2005: 66). This involves a sense of belonging (or isolation) or engagement, and a resource of human capital (which includes family, friendships, membership of social clubs, churches, societies etc.) in the local community. Such human capital can act as a buffer against stress resulting from life changes and is a powerful influence on well-being. The work of Robert Putnam has been very influential in identifying indicators of social connection within communities and their importance to well-being. Putnam distinguishes between 'bridging' capital – activities which draw people together from different backgrounds – and 'bonding' capital – which offers a sense of identity (Putnam and Feldstein 2003). This approach has political implications and has been criticised for ignoring stress caused by social conformity (Mutaner and Lynch 2002), for ignoring power inequalities (Navarro 2007) and for explaining the inevitability of poverty and encouraging 'top-down' approaches ignoring the views of ordinary people (Welshman 2006). Some groups can be high on bonding social capital, but disruptive to society (e.g. street gangs, Ku Klux Klan or the Mafia).

ACTIVITY

Assessment or measurement of social capital in a local community is often called 'community profiling' or 'asset management'. It is often necessary to undertake this when seeking funding for public health projects. Two main approaches to this have been to survey the community and ask people who they trust, or to count the number of social organisations within the area.

Consider how you might approach community profiling in a local area that you know. Bear in mind cost-effectiveness and the likelihood of having limited resources. You may want to look for ideas from the Internet – try searching for 'social capital measurement tools'.

Questionnaires would be a thorough way of assessing a community, but you may get a low response in an area with low social capital, or even a hostile one if you went door-to-door as you might be viewed with suspicion. Conversely, simply counting social groups and clubs will not indicate the quality of social networking within them and they may exclude most of the community. The World Bank (web.worldbank.org) is a useful international data source and also has useful information on surveying. They have a tool (SOCAT) which you may find useful to consider. Go to the website and in the search box type SOCAT or Social Capital for more general information.

There are other ways of assessing community needs, which do not require you to do your own surveying, through the use of public statistics. We will now look at how useful these are at assessing a locality.

Assessing determinants of health

Epidemiology and causes of ill health

In order to understand the health needs of a population, it is necessary to use epidemiology. Epidemiology is simply the study of patterns of disease and ill health in a population and identification of likely causes or risks of disease. While some of the statistical processes involved in epidemiology can be complex, if you can understand a bivariate graph (a graph that shows the relationship between two variables) or chart then you can use epidemiological data. Three simple concepts that will help you to understand statistics are prevalence (how many in a population – usually given as a percentage), frequency (the rate at which something occurs) and trend (changes in prevalence – commonness – or frequency over time).

Local statistics show the varying influence of different determinants on the health of a community. Poverty and unemployment is less damaging to the health of the poor in a community which is mutually supportive. People who live in an environment with a high crime rate are likely to become more isolated and take less exercise. Epidemiological statistics can indicate likely causes of illness, and also allow us to target interventions on people that need them most. Statistics allow us to assess a community to justify a public health intervention, to plan how to deliver services efficiently and to monitor how effective those interventions have been. This is why local and national government collect statistics on a regular basis and make them available for us to use.

ACTIVITY

Figure 10.3 shows two bivariate graphs from an annual Health & Social Care Information Centre (HSCIC) (2012) report.

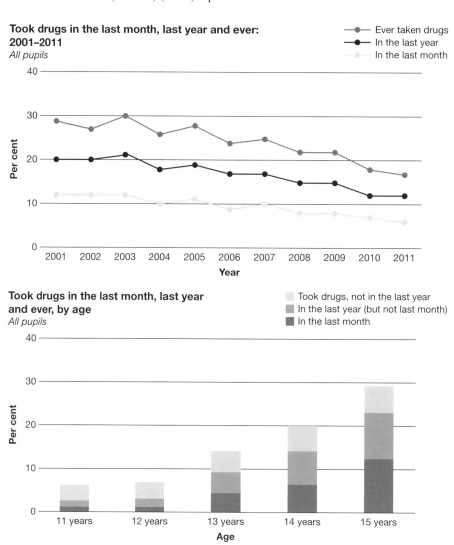

Figure 10.3 Two bivariate graphs, adapted from an annual HSCIC (2012) report.

Look at these charts and see what you can learn from them.

Which one do you think demonstrates prevalence and which demonstrates a trend?

In which age group for example do drug users proportionately experiment with drugs most and which age group has the most regular users?

Do these charts indicate that drug use is becoming an increasing problem?

The top chart indicates a similar decline in all drug activities over time – so it is a trend. The bottom chart indicates drug activities over difference ages. There are fewer younger children taking drugs, but those who do are mainly experimenting. By 15 years, they are mainly regular drug users. This chart indicates patterns of prevalence at different ages. It is to be expected with addictive drugs, that most of those who are likely to take drugs (less than 30 per cent) have probably tried them by this age. We could also have generated a similar chart comparing prevalence between males and females, across ethnic groups or geographical regions.

ACTIVITY – USING STATISTICS

Why not start by looking at your own neighbourhood (www.neighbourhood.statistics. gov.uk; Office for National Statistics 2014)? On this site you can look at different levels of detail from local authority to ward by typing in your postcode. On the left you will find links to all sorts of data for your locality, but type your postcode on the left and you get summary charts which are easier to interpret. You can find charts and tables on age distribution, housing, general health, employment and education.

Now compare your community with two different areas – more wealthy/poor, urban/ rural. If you can't find their postcodes compare your neighbourhood with one in Bath (BA1 2NA), Liverpool (L8 1XN) and West London (SW7 2NB).

Look at the differences in charts for type of house occupancy, employment and educational qualifications for example.

You will find that urban communities will have higher flat occupancy, wealthier communities have higher educational and employment levels and rural areas more family occupancy. Each of these variables are relevant to public health, so you can start comparing areas in which you live and work.

ACTIVITY – COMPARING PUBLIC HEALTH DATA

The UK Observatory Interactive Maps (www.apho.org.uk/default.aspx?QN=HP_ INTERACTIVE2012) operate at two levels (local district and county level). Open this webpage and click on the County Level Atlas. You can now put your cursor on the map or the graph and find that the public health needs and service performance appear on the large table on the left. Look up your own work or home area and see which priorities most need tackling in comparison with national performance. Then go to the District Level Atlas for a more detailed view of your locality. Play around with these two atlases and you will find that you can download data summaries and reports that will be useful to you.

Health protection and health improvement

Health protection is concerned with preventative actions to protect against any threat to the nation's health. This could be in relation to infections and outbreaks of disease, maintaining the quality of air, water supplies and other environmental concerns.

Health improvement encompasses areas such as screening for particular conditions such as cervical, breast and bowel cancer, lowering rates of teenage pregnancy and maintaining effective immunisation coverage.

Health screening

There are a number of different screening programmes operating in the UK, such as those for cervical cancer, bowel cancer and breast cancer. Before any screening programme is set up, clear criteria have to be applied to the proposed test, treatment and the screening programme to ensure that it is valid and worthwhile – i.e. that it will reduce mobility and mortality from the condition or disease in question (UK National Screening Committee 2014, www.screening. nhs.uk/criteria).

The condition

The condition that is the subject of screening should be an important health problem. Furthermore, the health problem should have robust epidemiology and have a reliably detectable marker or risk factor that can form the basis of the screening. For example, the bowel screening test looks for faecal occult blood; the cervical screening test looks for particular changes in a certain set of cells. Alongside a screening test, cost-effective primary prevention measures should be implemented as far as practicable, such as dissemination of lifestyle advice and symptom awareness for early diagnosis.

The test

There must be a clear and robust evidence base to support the proposed test, which needs to be simple, safe and accurate. It is also necessary to be able to clearly identify the target group with defined parameters and cut-off points. Furthermore, the test needs to be acceptable to both the health professionals and the target population from a clinical, social and ethical standpoint. Prior to any programme commencing, evidence-based care pathways must be agreed, to address investigations for positive results and further treatment. It is essential that the infrastructure for managing positive results and a call and recall system are in place. The test itself needs to be a cost-effective one and the risk–benefit profile addressed. There is little point launching a screening programme that may do more harm to the population than good.

The treatment

There should be an effective evidence-based treatment identified for cases diagnosed through screening, and policies that use the evidence base to determine who is treated and how to optimise patient outcomes.

The screening programme

Quality assurance standards must be in place. There have been a number of high-profile reports over the years of lapses in quality assurance, for example in cervical screening which has led to either women being given false positive results and hence receiving treatment not needed, or conversely not being recalled for treatment when they should have been called back, with distressing consequences. Participants in the process need to be provided with sufficient information to make an informed choice about whether they wish to be screened or not. At times there will be pressure from the public to widen access to a screening programme, but any decision to do so must be justified via the evidence base. The programme has to be cost-effective and evidence based, and steps must be taken to ensure there are sufficient staff to administer the scheme. Literature for patients must also be made available (UK National Screening Committee 2014, www.screening.nhs.uk/criteria).

WHO (Wilson and Jungner 1968) – 10 principles which should govern a national screening programme:

1   The condition is an important health problem.
2   Its natural history is well understood.
3   It is recognisable at an early stage.
4   Treatment is better at an early stage.
5   A suitable test exists.
6   An acceptable test exists.
7   Adequate facilities exist to cope with abnormalities detected.
8   Screening is done at repeated intervals when the onset is insidious.
9   The chance of harm is less than the chance of benefit.
10 The cost is balanced against benefit.

REFLECTION POINT

Think about a screening programme that you have had experience of, either personally or as a health professional.

How does it map to the 10 principles above?

A good example of a screening programme that is run in accordance with the principles above is the NHS Cancer Screening Programme, which is delivered by the NHS and coordinated as part of Public Health England. The programme currently consists of three screening strands: breast screening, bowel screening and cervical screening. Up-to-date information on the programmes can be accessed at www.cancerscreening.nhs.uk (NHS Cancer Screening 2014). Prostate cancer awareness is also addressed but there is no formalised screening programme as currently there is no reliable test that meets all the criteria.

Other examples include the antenatal and newborn screening programme which includes newborn hearing screening, blood spot screening, Down's syndrome screening and others. Other adult screening programmes include the abdominal aortic aneurysm screening and diabetic retinopathy screening (UK National Screening Committee 2014, www.screening.nhs.uk/programmes).

The chlamydia screening programme was launched as a means to address the rising prevalence of chlamydia infection in the under 25s, and the associated longer-term health impact of chlamydial infection. Using a simple self-swab or urine test, young people under 25 can access screening and treatment discreetly, hopefully avoiding any long-term health implications from the infection. Further information on this screening programme can be accessed at www.chlamydiascreening.nhs.uk (National Chlamydia Screening Programme 2014).

For all screening programmes, they are only going to be successful if the target group comes forward and attends screening. Promoting the uptake of national screening programmes is a core health promotion activity for healthcare practitioners, as is being able to answer questions regarding attendance results and, where appropriate, treatment. Some people may be reluctant to attend, especially if they perceive the test to be uncomfortable or embarrassing. It may also be that service provision is not easily accessible (clinic timing, location, male or female practitioner) or the individual may be part of a 'hard to reach' group such as those with a learning disability, travellers or homeless people. It is important that service provision takes account of the profile of the area.

CASE STUDY – SOCIAL MARKETING

The West Midlands utilised a fully integrated social marketing campaign to raise awareness and identify any behavioral changes in relation to cervical screening. They identify a range of reasons as to why women may not attend, such as embarrassment, anxiety, discomfort of test, lack of understanding of benefits, cultural reasons and inconvenient appointment times, and this research can help health practitioners consider ways to promote attendance for this and other screening services.

What's Pants but Could Save Your Life? Available from: http://thensmc.com/resources/showcase/whats-pants-could-save-your-life?v (West Midlands Cervical Screening Quality Assurance Reference Centre/NSMC 2011).

Media campaigns are sometimes used to disseminate positive messages about screening programmes or lifestyle changes and high-profile cases sometimes temporarily increase attendance – the 'Jade Goody effect' being one example. Jade Goody was a reality television star who tragically died from cervical cancer at a young age in 2009. Attendance for cervical cytology screening improved dramatically for a short period but the effect was not sustained. Television soap dramas often carry storylines about characters accessing screening and living with cancer which can sometimes communicate unrealistic messages to the public. Change4Life (2014) is an NHS-driven campaign designed to reach people across the lifespan via television advertisements, an Internet site, Twitter and Facebook. Further information can be found at www.nhs.uk/change4life.

REFLECTION POINT

The Internet is a wonderland of information which varies greatly in terms of quality and accuracy. Consider which sources you could reliably recommend to communities as appropriate resources to support them in protecting their health.

Immunisation

The two public health interventions which have had the greatest impact have been clean water and vaccination. Immunisation or vaccination can be described as the most effective preventative medical intervention in the world.

Vaccination has three broad aims:

- To protect the individual from infectious diseases, associated mortality, morbidity and long-term ill health.
- To prevent outbreaks of disease.
- Ultimately to eradicate infectious diseases.

From these aims you can see that immunisation has a population-based public health approach.

Vaccination history can be traced back to Ancient Greece, but the familiar names associated with the development of vaccination are Edward Jenner and Louis Pasteur. You can read more about the history of vaccinations at www.nhs.uk/Conditions/vaccinations/Pages/the-history-of-vaccination.aspx (NHS Choices 2014) and at www.historyofvaccines.org (The College of Physicians of Philadelphia 2014).

ACTIVITY

Review the history of vaccination at www.nhs.uk/Conditions/vaccinations/Pages/the-history-of-vaccination.aspx (NHS Choices 2014).

What impact has vaccination had on the health of the population – think in broad terms about this? What are the risks of not vaccinating the population? You may find it interesting to talk to elderly people about their childhood experiences before vaccination was introduced.

AIMS OF VACCINATION

To protect those at highest risk (selective immunisation strategy)

or

To eradicate, eliminate or contain disease (mass immunisation strategy)

Mass immunisation strategies aim to eradicate diseases (for example, smallpox has been eradicated worldwide) or to eliminate in regions (for example, the Americas have been polio-free for some years now). The point at which a disease no longer constitutes a significant public health problem is called 'containment'. Selective immunisation strategies target areas of the population at highest risk. Immunity conferred via vaccination is termed either 'active' (long term) or 'passive' (short term).

ACTIVITY

Can you think of examples of a mass immunisation strategy and of a selective immunisation strategy?

ACTIVE IMMUNITY

'Natural' active immunity may follow infection.

'Artificial' active immunity is induced by vaccination.

PASSIVE IMMUNITY

'Natural' – from mother to baby during breastfeeding.

'Artificial' – administered from injection of human immunoglobulin (from human blood products). The protection is immediate but only for a few weeks.

It is important to understand that, like the health screening programmes, vaccination programmes also require a robust evidence base, structure and quality assurance to ensure they are successful as a public health intervention. Surveillance and research establishes the disease incidence, age distribution, trends and complications/mortality and informs the need to establish a vaccination programme. Surveillance also monitors the impact of a vaccination programme, in terms of disease incidence, susceptibility, vaccine uptake, vaccine safety and adverse events (World Health Organization 2014).

The NHS operates a vaccination programme from birth all the way through to later life, based on surveillance data and the evidence base. The schedules are frequently updated to respond to changes in disease trends. For example, recent updates have been the introduction of rotavirus vaccination for babies, to offer pertussis (whooping cough vaccine) to pregnant women to offer protection to their newborns in the first two months of life and a new programme of HPV vaccination introduced several years ago aimed at decreasing the incidence of cervical cancer. The up-to-date UK vaccination schedules can be accessed at: www.nhs.uk/Conditions/vaccinations/Pages/vaccination-schedule-age-checklist.aspx (NHS Choices 2014).

The Green Book is the up-to-date guide to vaccinations, vaccination procedures and vaccine-preventable diseases in the UK, and can be accessed online at: www.gov.uk/government/collections/immunisation-against-infectious-disease-the-green-book (Department of Health 2014).

Legislation

Non-communicable diseases cause a significant burden in both health and economic terms (Galbraith-Emami 2013). Frequently these types of diseases are caused by the consumption of tobacco, alcohol or poor dietary choices or by lifestyle behaviours. One means of response is through the use of public health legislation to reduce the population's exposure to risk factors.

The World Health Organization has identified key areas where public health legislation might be an effective tool:

*   Protecting people from tobacco smoke and banning smoking in public places.
*   Warning about the dangers of tobacco use.
*   Enforcing bans on tobacco advertising, promotion and sponsorship.
*   Raising taxes on tobacco.
*   Restricting access to retailed alcohol.
*   Enforcing bans on alcohol advertising.
*   Raising taxes on alcohol.
*   Reducing salt intake and salt content of food.
*   Replacing trans fats in food with polyunsaturated fat.
*   Promoting public awareness about diet and physical activity, including through mass media (World Health Organization 2011).

REFLECTION POINT

Look at the list above and consider which of the actions have been implemented in the UK and think about how effective they might be.

English smoke-free legislation is an example of public health law and was introduced in July 2007, and was associated with a reduction in hospital admissions for severe childhood asthma in the first year of 12 per cent and a further 3 per cent in the following two years (Millett *et al.* 2013). A similar study showed a more than 3 per cent reduction in hospital admissions for myocardial infarction in men and women over 60 years and men under 60 years (Sims *et al.* 2010).

ACTIVITY – SEAT BELTS

Some public health interventions lead to unexpected results. Most developed countries make it compulsory to wear seat belts in cars. One of the most successful UK social marketing campaigns was by RoSPA (Royal Society for the Prevention of Accidents), starting in 1971, which promoted the wearing of seat belts in cars to reduce accident injury and fatalities. Data from the 17 countries that owned 80 per cent of the world's cars in the 1970s show that in 13 countries motor accident fatalities increased significantly, in comparison with the four countries where they did not. The UK introduced seat belt laws in 1983 on the promise that it would save 1,000 lives a year, but despite 95 per cent compliance, accident fatalities and injuries also increased.

Reflect on the reasons why road accident fatalities and injuries increase when you make people wear a seat belt in cars.

Why do you think the legislation is still in force in over 80 countries in the world?

All safety measures introduced into cars tend to make drivers feel safer. Research has suggested that seat belts provide reassurance which results in drivers driving faster and more recklessly. This increases the number of road accidents and consequently the number of deaths and injuries to other road users. In the 23 months following the UK seat belt legislation there was an increase in deaths of pedestrians (by 8 per cent), cyclists (by 13 per cent) and unbelted rear passengers (by 25 per cent). This is explained by the 'risk compensation hypothesis' in which, Adams (1999) suggests, risk-taking is balanced by perceived hazards. When a safety measure is introduced, hazards appear to be reduced which may lead to increases in risk-taking or 'risk compensation', or it may result in 'risk displacement', in this case from the car driver to other road users. This behavioural change adjustment has also been suggested in high-risk sexual practices following condom promotion campaigns and the availability of better HIV treatment (Richens *et al.* 2000).

Chapter summary

This chapter has provided an overview of the role of public health and the variety of approaches undertaken to improve health outcomes at a population level approach.

- We have considered epidemiology and its role in public health approaches.
- Health protection and health improvement are key components of public health programmes.
- The burden of poor health is significant both economically and in terms of human suffering.
- Public health approaches seek to prevent ill health and prolong life through population approaches.

Further resources

UK Faculty of Public Health. Available at: www.fph.org.uk.
Royal Society for Public Health. Available at: www.rsph.org.uk.
NHS Cancer Screening. Available at: www.cancerscreening.nhs.uk/.
The Green Book (Immunisation against Infectious Diseases). Available at: www.gov.uk/government/collections/immunisation-against-infectious-disease-the-green-book.
The World Health Organization. Available at: www.who.int/en/.

References

Adams, J. 1999. *Cars, Cholera and Cows*, Policy Analysis No: 335 (4 March 1999) [online]. Available at: www.cato.org/sites/cato.org/files/pubs/pdf/pa335.pdf [Accessed 15 July 2014].
Berridge, V., Gorsky, M. and Mold, A. 2011. *Public Health in History*. Maidenhead: Open University Press.
Change4Life. 2014. *Change4Life* [online]. Available at: www.nhs.uk/change4life/Pages/change-for-life.aspx [Accessed 17 July 2014].
Crisis. 2011. *Homelessness: A Silent Killer* [online]. Available at: www.crisis.org.uk [Accessed 11 July 2014].
Dahlgren, G. and Whitehead, M. 1992. *Policies and Strategies to Promote Social Equity in Health* (background document to WHO – Strategy paper for Europe.) Copenhagen: World Health Organization.
Department of Communities & Local Government. 2012. *Evidence Review of the Costs of Homelessness*.

Available at: www.gov.uk/government/uploads/system/uploads/attachment_data/file/7596/2200485. pdf [Accessed 17 July 2014].

Department of Health. 2012. *Healthy Lives, Healthy People: Improving Outcomes and Supporting Transparency.* London: HMSO.

Department of Health. 2014. *The Green Book* [online]. Available at: www.gov.uk/government/collections/immunisation-against-infectious-disease-the-green-book [Accessed 18 July 2014].

EarlyBird Diabetes Trust. 2014. *EarlyBird Diabetes* [online]. Available at: www.earlybirddiabetes.org [Accessed 19 July 2014].

Faculty of Public Health. 2010. *What Is Public Health* [online]. Available at: www.fph.org.uk/what_is_public_health [Accessed 15 July 2014].

Galbraith-Emami, S. 2013. 'Public Health Law and Non-communicable Diseases', *UK Health Forum* [online]. Available at: http://nhfshare.heartforum.org.uk/RMAssets/Reports/Public%20Health%20Law%20FINAL.pdf [Accessed 25 July 2014].

Health and Social Care Act. 2012. London: HMSO.

Health & Social Care Information Centre (HSCIC). 2012. *Smoking, Drinking and Drug Use Among Young People in England in 2011* [online]. Available at: www.natcen.ac.uk [Accessed 15 July 2014].

Kuh, D., Ben-Shlomo, Y., Lynch, J., Hallqvist, J. and Power, C. 2003. 'Life Course Epidemiology', *Journal of Epidemiology and Community Health* 57: 778–83.

Lucas, K. and Lloyd, B. 2005. *Health Promotion: Evidence & Experience.* London: Sage.

Marmot, M. 2010. *Fair Society, Healthy Lives: A Strategic Review of Health Inequalities in England Post-2010* [online]. Available at: http://www.instituteofhealthequity.org/projects/fair-society-healthy-lives-the-marmot-review [Accessed 13 July 2014].

Millett, C., Lee, J. T., Laverty, A. A., Glantz, A. A. and Majeed, A. 2013. 'Hospital Admissions for Childhood Asthma after Smoke-Free Legislation in England', *Pediatrics*. Available at: http://www.ncbi.nlm.nih.gov/pubmed/23339216 [Accessed 17 July 2014].

Mutaner, C. and Lynch, J. 2002. 'Social Capital, Class Gender and Race Conflict, and Population Health: An Essay Review of Bowling Alone's Implications for Social Epidemiology', *Journal of Epidemiology* 31(1): 261–7.

National Chlamydia Screening Programme. 2014. [online]. Available at: www.chlamydiascreening.nhs.uk [Accessed 17 July 2014].

NHS Cancer Screening. 2014. [online]. Available at: www.cancerscreening.nhs.uk/ [Accessed 19 July 2014].

NHS Choices. 2014. *The History of Vaccination* [online]. Available at: www.nhs.uk/Conditions/vaccinations/Pages/the-history-of-vaccination.aspx [Accessed 15 July 2014].

Putnam, R. D. and Feldstein, L. 2003. *Better Together: Restoring the American Community.* New York: Simon & Shuster.

Navarro, V. 2007. *Neoliberalism, Globalization, and Inequalities: Consequences for Health and Quality of Life.* New York: Baywood.

Office for National Statistics. 2014. Neighbourhood Statistics [online]. Available at: www.neighbourhood.statistics.gov.uk [Accessed 17 July 2014].

Richens, J., Imrie, J. J. and Copas, A. A. 2000. 'Condoms and Seat Belts: The Parallels and the Lessons', *The Lancet* 355(9201): 400–3.

Royal Society for the Prevention of Accidents. 2014. *ROSPA* [online]. Available at: www.rospa.com/ [Accessed 22 July 2014].

Sims, M., Maxwell, R., Bauld, L. and Gilmore, A. 2010. 'Short term Impact of Smoke-free Legislation in England: Retrospective Analysis of Hospital Admissions for Myocardial Infarction', *British Medical Journal* 340: c2161.

The College of Physicians of Philadelphia. 2014. *The History of Vaccines* [online]. Available at: www.historyofvaccines.org [Accessed 23 July 2014].

Uauy, R. and Solomons, N. 2005. 'Diet, Nutrition, and the Life-Course Approach to Cancer Prevention', *Journal of Nutrition* 135(12): 2934S–2945S.

UK Observatory Interactive Maps. 2014. 'Health Profiles Interactive' [online]. Available at: www.apho. org.uk/default.aspx?QN=HP_INTERACTIVE2012 [Accessed 5 July 2014].

UK National Screening Committee. 2014. [online]. Available at: www.screening.nhs.uk/ [Accessed 15 July 2014].

Welshman, J. 2006. 'Searching for Social Capital: Historical Perspectives on Health, Poverty and Culture', *Journal of the Royal Society for Promotion of Health* 126: 268–74.

West Midlands Cervical Screening Quality Assurance Reference Centre/NSMC. 2011. *What's Pants but Could Save Your Life?* [online]. Available from: http://thensmc.com/resources/showcase/whats-pants-could-save-your-life?v [Accessed 15 July 2014].

Wilson, J. M. G. and Jungner, G. 1968. *Principles and Practice of Screening for Disease*. Public Health Paper Number 34. Geneva: WHO.

World Health Organization. 2011. *Global Status Report on Noncommunicable Diseases 2010.* Geneva: WHO [online]. Available at: http://www.who.int/nmh/publications/ncd_report_full_en.pdf [Accessed 26 July 2014].

World Health Organization. 2014. *Immunization Surveillance, Assessment and Monitoring* [online]. Available at: www.who.int/immunization/monitoring_surveillance/en/ [Accessed 18 December 2014].

Chapter 11

Health promotion

Dr Fiona McMaster

LEARNING OUTCOMES

By the end of this chapter you will be able to:

1   Understand the psychological, social and environmental factors that can influence a person's lifestyle choices.
2   Describe models and theories around health promotion and behaviour change.
3   Start to work with individuals and groups on making positive lifestyle choices.
4   Understand key areas for health promotion in the UK.

Introduction

In this chapter, we consider how health promotion fits into health and social care. We will look at some of the reasons why we promote health, and think about our own health behaviours. We'll think about the aspects of life that health professionals want to encourage and change, and think about some approaches to health promotion, including some models and theories that you might find useful in creating health-promoting activities. We'll also discuss how we can do health promotion according to some of the World Health Organization (WHO) behaviours, and finally cover some of the main controversies that this interesting area of work might include.

Let's start with an activity to think about health behaviours.

Thinking about healthy living

ACTIVITY

What do you love to do?

Think about what you love doing most. If you weren't reading this book right now, what would you like to be doing?

If you are not feeling very inspired, here are some of the things my third-year BSc students said to me recently:

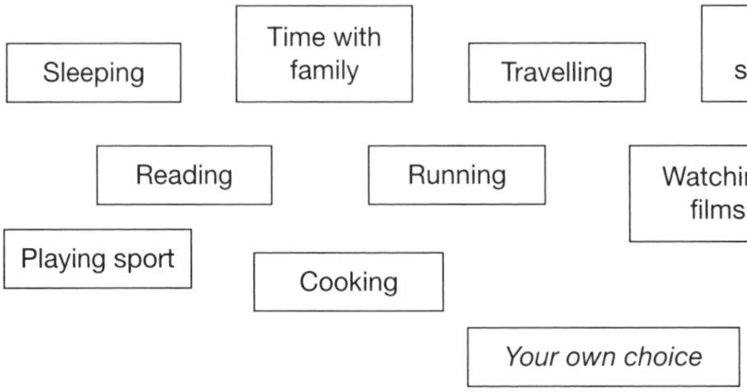

Figure 11.1 Example responses from Anglia Ruskin Public Health students.

Why do you love it?

Think about why you love your chosen activity. It might be that it:

- Relaxes you
- Makes you feel good
- Cheers you up
- Helps you forget about other worries.

Now, consider how you would feel if you woke up tomorrow to see the following headline about the leisure time activity that you love most:

READING KILLS

WATCHING FILMS SHORTENS LIFE

How would you feel?

- 'I don't believe it'
- 'I'll stop this immediately'
- 'I don't care – my grandfather read books every day and he lived to 100 years old'
- 'I want to see more evidence'
- 'I'll ask my doctor'
- 'I'll carry on anyway – the newspapers can't really be trusted'
- 'Everything is bad for you these days, I do far worse'.

So far, we don't think that reading or watching films actually kill people (although you could argue that they are contributing to sedentary lifestyles and decreasing physical activity, so be careful!), but these kinds of headlines about smoking, drinking and eating unhealthily are frequently on the covers of our newspapers.

Behaviour choice and health promotion

Before we think about how we can promote health, we should think about *why* we choose unhealthy behaviours and what might prevent us from being healthy. Many of us know what we *should* be doing, so why is it so hard to make the 'right' choice?

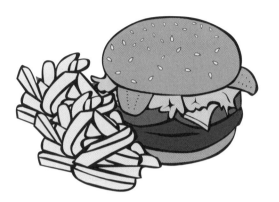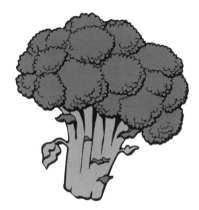

Figure 11.2 Do you always make the healthiest choice?

What did you eat last night? Could your meal have been any healthier? If it could, think about what stopped your meal being as healthy as it could be?

Barriers to healthy living

One element that health promoters often miss is consideration of the barriers that all of us encounter when we are trying to be as healthy as we would like. For cooking a healthy evening meal, these barriers can include how we feel, but could also include external factors like how much healthy food costs, or even who in the house is in charge of cooking the meals.

ACTIVITY

Now let's think about exercise. Current guidelines indicate that we are not getting enough physical activity on a daily basis. Even if you are a star sportsperson, there may be days when you just don't want to exercise, and for the rest of us it can be even harder to find the motivation to get up and go to the gym, or go outside for a walk.

What kinds of things stop you from exercising?

Look at the person in Figure 11.3 – there are lots of reasons why it is difficult to find time to exercise. Which, if any, of these are similar to your situation?

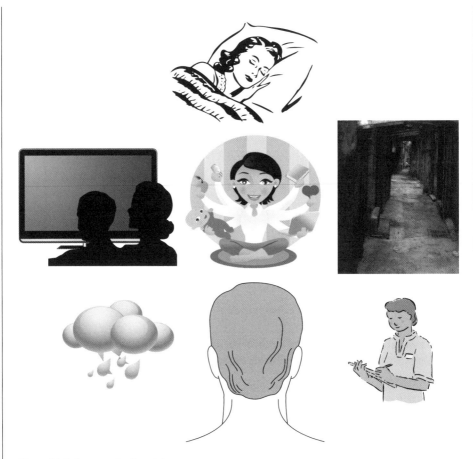

Figure 11.3 Reasons for inactivity.

What helps you to do some physical activity?

Can you make a list of ten things that could encourage you to do 30 minutes of physical activity each day:

1	6
2	7
3	8
4	9
5	10

Thinking about what kinds of things are barriers and what might encourage people to make healthy choices is a key part of promoting healthy living.

What is health promotion?

The WHO defines health promotion as 'The process of enabling people to exert control over and to improve their health' (World Health Organization 1996: 1).

Another definition of health promotion is:

> If you think health is X and if X is what you want, then you should do A, B C.
>
> (Seedhouse 2004: xiii)

You can see that we use 'health promotion' for a range of different activities that focus on improving and maintaining good health, and ultimately preventing disease. In health and social care contexts, it is becoming increasingly important to use all contacts with patients as a potential opportunity to work collaboratively with a patient to help them become healthier, if this is something that they would like. The areas in which we might work through health and social care roles may include weight management, addictions like smoking, alcohol and illicit drugs, and we might also help make it easier for patients to take their medications. All healthcare practitioners are involved in health promotion at some level, whether that is trying to avoid an outbreak of a food-borne disease by inspecting the hygiene of kitchens, performing smoking cessation counselling, or developing policy to make access to care easy for more marginalised groups. Unlike some other areas of healthcare, health promotion draws from academic disciplines like sociology, social policy, psychology and education to develop models to think about how we interact with our environments, and how something that might not seem to be connected to health can have a big impact on our health.

ACTIVITY – DISCUSSION POINT

Think about changes in all the ways in which our health has been improving over the past 100 years. Which do you think has had the greatest impact: the improvement of drugs and medical technology, or changes in working patterns and practices?

Changes in how we think about health

The way we think about health has changed over the last 100 years. You might have noticed that how you think about health – as a student of a health discipline – might be very different from some of your friends who are not involved in this kind of work.

Approaches to health promotion

Back in 1999, Ewles and Simnett used five categories to define health promotion approaches, shown in Table 11.1.

Table 11.1 Ewles and Simnett's Five Categories for health promotion approaches (1999)

Model	Aim	Example from obesity
Medical	Freedom from disease and disability.	Encouraging patients to seek early detection and treatment of heart disease.
Behaviour change	Individual behaviour that leads to freedom from disease.	Persuading patients to reduce their weight by eating less and choosing healthier options.
Educational	Patients and populations who know and understand enough about their health to make decisions about their health behaviours.	Giving patients information about the danger of being overweight, helping patients learn how to control portion size and perhaps cook differently.
Client centred	Working with the patient on their own terms.	Only working on obesity if it is something that is important to the client.
Societal change	Creating an environment that enables healthier living.	Making healthy options available, food labelling.

It is easy to be in favour or against any one of these approaches; however, Ewles and Simnett argue that they are all valid if the practitioner is acting with the underlying goal of improving health.

These models are helpful for thinking about the activities that might help to promote health, but we should think in more depth about some of the psychological theories around promoting health, and most specifically how these can help us understand why we and our patients can make choices that do not encourage health.

Theories and models can help

Theories for health promotion

There are many theories that help us understand health behaviour, help us design health promotion interventions and even think about how we might promote health with individuals in healthcare settings. There are so many theories that we could write a whole book just about theory. Here, we will introduce you to a few of our favourite theories, and give you some names of other approaches that you might like to look up by yourself. You will notice that some of these theories have been developed by psychologists, others by sociologists and anthropologists, and all have been used to develop interventions.

There are different ways we can look at health promotion, and theories try to explain change at either an individual, group, community or whole population level.

1. Rainbow Model of Health (Dahlgren and Whitehead 1991)

If we think about how these different factors or levels interact, the 'Rainbow' Model of Health is a good place to start. As Figure 11.4 shows, at the centre of this theory is the individual patient and factors about their life that cannot be changed, such as their age, and their genetic make-up. In the next ring of the rainbow, there are **individual lifestyle factors** that reflect

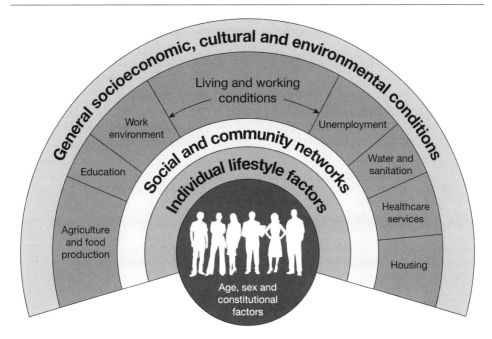

Figure 11.4   Dahlgren and Whitehead's Rainbow Model of Health, adapted from Dahlgren and Whitehead (1991).

the choices an individual makes about their eating, exercise, alcohol, tobacco use and sexual activities. After this is a layer which Dahlgren and Whitehead call **social and community networks** which includes significant others, social relationships and social support. **Living and working conditions** is the next rainbow layer and includes both access and opportunities for education and training, employments, welfare, housing, transport and other factors like running water, sanitation and food availability. The broadest layer is **general socioeconomic, cultural and environmental factors**, which include elements such as public policy, employment, availability of services, and other broad societal factors like taxes, food and fuel availability, and which could have an influence on behaviour.

2. Social Cognitive Theory (Bandura 1973)

In this theory, like the Rainbow Model above, we think about individuals' behaviour as tied into the environments in which we live (Figure 11.5). Social Cognitive Theory developed from Bandura's earlier *social learning theory* (Bandura 1973) and incorporates research from sociology, cognitive psychology and political science. This theory explains that we are influenced by our environment, but also that we have an influence on our environment. Bandura calls this **Reciprocal Determinism**, and it is a cornerstone concept of social cognitive theory – 'reciprocal' meaning 'two-way', and 'determinism' showing that we can both *actively change* our environments but also *be changed by* them. Other key concepts include **self-efficacy**, which describes a person's belief in their own ability to do something – in health promotion, this is usually used to think about whether someone feels capable of making a health behaviour change. One example could be the extent to which women feel like they could encourage their boyfriends, husbands and fathers to get screened for colorectal cancer.

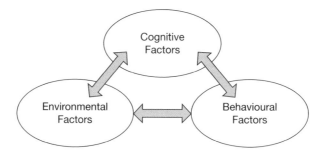

Figure 11.5 Social Cognitive Theory, adapted from Bandura (1973).

3. Health Belief Model (Hochbaum 1958)

The Health Belief Model was first described in the 1950s, and has been a widely used framework in research and in developing interventions (Janz 1984; Strecher and Rosenstock 1997; Glanz *et al*. 2008). There are several key constructs of this model:

Perceived susceptibility or how likely you think it is that you will get a disease, usually in the context of a health behaviour. For example, if a smoker considers how likely it is they will get lung cancer or emphysema.

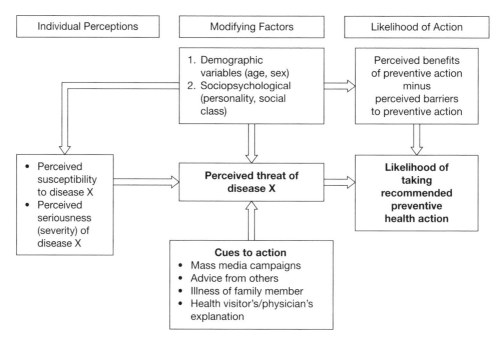

Figure 11.6 The Health Belief Model, adapted from Hochbaum (1958).

Perceived severity or how bad it would be if you got the disease. For a patient, this may include thinking about medical interventions like drugs and surgeries, the impact on the individual – such as the amount of pain or inconvenience it may cause, and also social implications such as the effect the condition might have on working, family and social life.

Perceived benefits or if you see any benefits in doing something healthier than the regular behaviour. This could include financial – smokers often think about the money they would save if they quit smoking, and what they would rather spend it on. Another benefit could be making friends and family happy with your decision.

Perceived barriers or something that would prevent you from making changes to improve health. Like the benefits, the barriers might not be directly related to health and could include things that impact on family and friends.

ACTIVITY

Think about these constructs from the Health Belief Model and how they might apply in two or three different health-promoting contexts. Use the example below as a guide for your answers:

Construct	Example: smoker	Example: cancer screening	Example: taking the contraceptive pill as advised (same time, every day)
Perceived susceptibility	Likelihood of getting lung cancer or emphysema, or being short of breath when climbing stairs or playing sport.		
Perceived severity	How bad it would be to have these conditions – 'everyone has to die from something' or 'how bad could it be'.		
Perceived benefits	If I gave up smoking, it might mean I could buy that coat I have wanted for ages, or go on holiday next year.		
Perceived barriers	I have a stressful job, my friends/family are all smokers. Even if I quit, I would still be breathing in their smoke.		

How would the consideration of these factors help you to decide how to promote health with an individual or a group?

4. Stages of Change Model (Prochaska and DiClemente 1983)

The models and theories we have looked at so far have involved elements of psychology and cognition. In this model, the Stages of Change Model, or the Transtheoretical Model (TTM), there is less focus on cognition and more on the practicalities of behaviour change (Prochaska *et al.* 2008). In this, there is a 'cycle' where patients move through a series of different 'stages' that eventually lead to a change in behaviour. For health promoters, if you agree with the TTM, you would deal with a patient in a different way according to their 'stage' of change. Let's have a look at the stages in this theory and apply them in Peter's journey from being a smoker – to stopping smoking:

Pre-contemplation is where Peter doesn't have any intention of changing his behaviour. He is happy to smoke, doesn't think it is a problem and certainly would not consider quitting smoking in the next six months.

Contemplation is where Peter starts noticing that smoking is affecting his life. He could be realising it is harder to play football without getting out of breath, or realise that he is coughing more than he has before. He has decided that he would like to quit smoking sometime soon, perhaps in the next six months or so.

Preparation By now, Peter has rehearsed his argument for stopping smoking. He knows that he will feel better (eventually), or he has read and heard enough about the benefits of stopping smoking, and he is tired of people nagging him to stop. Winter is coming, and he doesn't want to keep having to go outside for a cigarette break. He has stopped smoking as many cigarettes as he used to so it won't be quite so much of a shock to stop altogether. Peter has even decided when he is going to quit – 13 December, when it is a good friend's birthday.

Action is the stage when lifestyle change has occurred. For smoking, this means total abstinence rather than just cutting down, because of the serious health risks with any number of cigarettes smoked each day. For Peter, it is from 13 December, when he stops smoking. It is a daily struggle not to smoke and Peter has gone to his GP to ask for help with finding a local smoking cessation counsellor. He has also started to go to the gym a little because he is concerned about putting on weight now he isn't smoking.

Maintenance is the period when the temptation to lapse or relapse is still there, but less frequent than when the behaviour has recently been changed. For Peter, he is thinking about cigarettes less frequently and has strategies to distract himself when he does get tempted.

Termination is when the original behaviour does not tempt the individual at all. For Peter, it is five years since he stopped smoking – it is almost as if he never smoked at all. Even when he is under pressure at work, or in social situations (times when he used to smoke most), he never thinks of smoking.

You can see that the stages of change (Figure 11.7) can be applied to many different behaviours and settings; for some behaviours around health it is extremely difficult to get to the 'termination' stage. Most researchers consider that 'maintenance' is the realistic target for behaviours like weight control, exercise or consistent use of a condom.

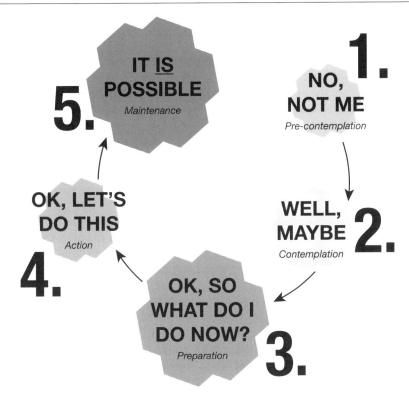

Figure 11.7 Stages of change.

ACTIVITY

Think about three issues where you would like to promote health.

How could you target your health promotion activity according to the 'stage' of change?

	Behaviour 1:	*Behaviour 2:*	*Behaviour 3:*
Pre-contemplation			
Contemplation			
Preparation			
Action			
Maintenance			

5. Theory of Reasoned Action, Theory of Planned Behaviour (Ajzen and Fishbein 1980)

The Theory of Reasoned Action, and the extended Theory of Planned Behaviour have the central position that *intention to change* a behaviour leads to *behaviour change*. However, in these theories there are two main factors which are thought to influence the intention to change, and these are the **attitude**, which is coloured by the beliefs around the behaviour, and an evaluation of the outcome of changing the behaviour, the **subjective norms**, in turn influenced by beliefs that are 'normal' in a particular group or community, and the individual's motivation to comply. In the Theory of Planned Behaviour, intention is also thought to be influenced by **perceived control** which derives from beliefs around control and perceived power.

6. Self-Determination Theory (Deci and Ryan 1985)

Self-Determination Theory (SDT) is a newer theory to explain the reasons *why* we do certain behaviours (Figure 11.8). Compared to some of the other theories, SDT reflects more about what motivates people to make changes, classifying them broadly as internal and external motivations. At the centre of their argument, Deci and Ryan suggest that the behaviours we are intrinsically motivated to do have one or more of three things: novelty, pleasure and challenge. You can see how this works for someone who likes running – there is the novelty of new trails and running routes, the challenge of getting faster and beating your previous race time, and the pleasure of seeing your results improve as well as the natural 'high' from the endorphins produced during exercise. Sadly for health promoters, it is difficult to think of novelty, pleasure and challenge around encouraging stopping behaviours that some people love, like smoking, drinking, eating unhealthy foods or avoiding sexual encounters that could be deemed 'risky'. Instead, we may be encouraging our patients and clients to change by talking about external sources. Some of these external sources could be positive, such as wanting to please a family member or prevent a disease. However, some external sources can be negative – like if you are shamed or made to feel guilty if you don't make the change. From research, it seems that blame, shame and financial reward do not lead to lasting change. Where health promoters may be able to make a difference, according to Deci and Ryan, is where we support individuals along three goals: autonomy, competence and relatedness. In this, they think that we might be more likely to change our behaviour if it is consistent with our core values and the change has congruent meaning.

CASE STUDY

Jo has been a smoker since she was 16. When she was 26, she gave up smoking because she was pregnant and she was very keen to protect her baby. Once the baby was born, she started smoking again, but was very careful never to smoke in front of him. Jo got into the habit of having a shower and changing her clothes as soon as she got in from work, before she started playing with her son, just as her doctor and health visitor told her. When the baby was small, this was easy to do, but as he has grown older, Jo has noticed that it is more difficult. 'Now he is 4 years old, he runs to me when I come home from work. But instead of cuddling him, I push him away because I need to shower and take off my smoky clothes.' Jo eventually decided that her smoking was indirectly causing her to push her son away, and she was worried about the impact this might have on her relationship with her son. 'I had a bad time with my mum when I was growing up – nothing is more important than my relationship with my child.'

ACTIVITY

Think about a change that you have made in the past in your own life.

What made you decide to make a change?

How hard was it to stick to this decision?

---

7. Tannahill's Model of Health Promotion

Finally, we have a model that is specifically designed to address the activities in which people promoting health regularly engage. For Tannahill (Downie *et al*. 1990), health promotion consists of three basic activities that may overlap (Figure 11.9).

This model is widely used, especially in the UK, and shows clearly that health promotion involves helping people to understand about their health behaviours and how they may impact on health and disease (**health education**), helping people get to screening and immunisation services (**prevention**), and setting laws and policies such as taxes around the health areas in question (**health protection**).

ACTIVITY

Here are a few theories that are commonly used in public health. See if you can find out more about each:

- Self-efficacy
- Social support and social networks
- Stress and coping
- Diffusion of interventions
- Locus of control

How theories can help

One of the common characteristics of successful health promotion interventions is that they are informed by theories (French 2004; Nutbeam 2004). Because of the results of many research studies, we think that behaviour change approaches can make a difference to the health of a nation.

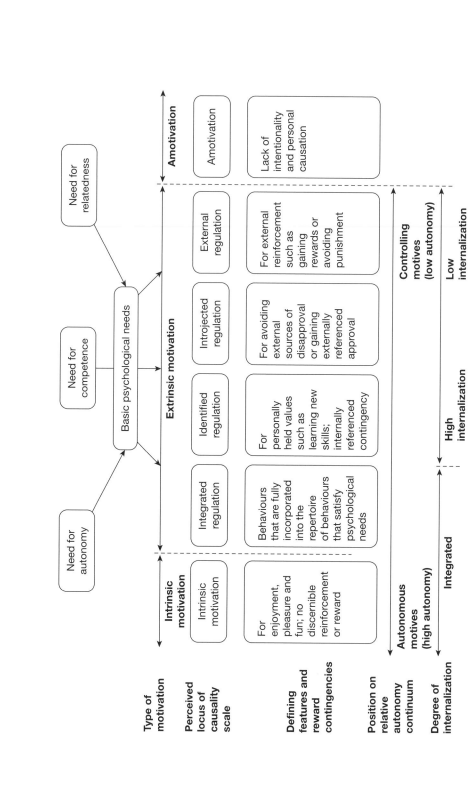

Figure 11.8 Self-Determination Theory, adapted from Deci and Ryan (1985).

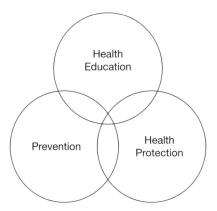

Figure 11.9 Tannahill's Model of Health Promotion, adapted from Downie *et al.* (1990).

Controversies of health promotion

When you start to promote health, you may find people who think it is not appropriate to try to change people's behaviour and who believe that this is an element of the 'nanny state', where the government takes away individual responsibility. In a democracy like the UK, a key societal value is freedom of choice; however, the government may choose to intervene when a choice could be harming more than just the individual who is making the choice.

ACTIVITY

Which of the following do you think would be reasonable policies?

Which are unreasonable?

Try to give a justification for each answer:

- Fining people if they don't wear a seat belt.
- Fining people if they don't wear a helmet when riding a motorbike.
- Making people smoke outside.
- Increasing the price of cigarettes to £100 per pack.
- When giving people on welfare/benefits money, giving it in the form of vouchers for fruit and vegetables.
- Prosecuting bar owners if they allow any customers to get drunk.
- Refusing to employ someone with a Body Mass Index (BMI) of over 24.

How to promote health with patients

As we have seen in the models and theories around health behaviour, there are many different factors that influence health. If we are involved in health promotion, we could help patients individually or within groups and communities.

Working with individuals

We all like to feel special and at the centre of our universe; so do our patients! Everyone wants to have care and respect, and an understanding of our own unique set of circumstances and how they may affect our ability and motivation to make healthy choices. With all the competing pressures of work and family, it can be a big challenge to work with patients around behaviours that they have been doing for years, are not interested in changing, or even don't see that there is any problem with how they are currently living.

Fortunately, there are several evidence-based ways that you can work with individuals. Many of these rely on good communication strategies, as covered in Chapter 3.

Motivational interviewing

Developed in the 1980s by two psychologists, motivational interviewing (MI) is widely used in healthcare settings. There are lots of pieces of research – a strong evidence base – that show us that this is a technique that can help to change behaviour. It is also in line with the NHS policies on *Values, Dignity and Respect* and the underlying model that NHS services should help individual patients feel empowered about their health.

In MI, practitioners have conversations about change with their patients (Miller and Rollnick 2013). Rather than **directing** the conversation (where a practitioner tells the patient what to do) or a wholly **following** style (where good listening strategies are used to hear more about a patient's experiences in the trust that they will solve their own problems eventually), MI uses a **guiding** style of communication where patients can express their own situation, values and views but also seek the expertise of the practitioner. To start with, you can use strategies such as agenda-mapping to discuss what areas of change a patient may like to work on during that particular session, to try to find reasons why a patient might like to change in line with their values rather than solely focused on the specific behaviour.

Another important component of MI is reflective listening, and this is a skill that also comes into other approaches to promoting health. In a reflection, you make a statement rather than a question. This statement should be based on something that the patient has already said, or that you can guess from their demeanour – not an excuse to slip in advice that comes from nowhere!

Forming a reflection is not difficult, but it does take a bit of practice. For example, if you met a patient who said 'I am sick and tired of everyone telling me how to run my life. I like smoking and it is just about the only bad thing I do', you would first think about how they are feeling:

- Angry
- Frustrated
- Annoyed.

And then you can form a sentence that shows this. For example, 'You are fed up with everyone giving you advice.'

If you keep your tone neutral, you will see that this kind of approach encourages people to open up about their feelings, particularly if they are frustrated about their health or angry about having to be in a hospital or care setting.

ACTIVITY

Try some reflections for yourself:

Statement	Your reflection 1	Your reflection 2
'There is nothing wrong with going out and drinking on a Friday night, I'm not harming anyone'		
'I HATE the idea of taking medication every day. I really don't want my life to be run by tablets'		
'My grandfather still smokes 20 cigarettes a day and he hasn't had a cough ever. Why should I listen to you?'		
'I don't know why I can't lose weight – I keep trying the latest diet. I think I have about 50 diet books at home'		
'We have so many people who have had heart attacks in my family, to be honest I am scared to talk to the doctor in case I find out bad news'		

Miller and Rollnick (2013) talk about four processes involved in motivational interviewing; these are **engage**, **focus**, **evoke** and **plan**. Before you can start really working with someone on promoting their health, you should be engaged with them and have some rapport – after all, you are talking to them about deeply personal habits that might have deep meaning. Only when you have a collaborative relationship will you be able to start thinking about a particular behaviour with your patient (**focus**) and then be able to move onto finding reasons for why they might consider making a change for themselves (**evoke**) and finally start thinking of an action **plan**.

You can probably see the links with some theories here – the way you have a conversation might be different according to the 'stage of change' that a person is at. Similarly, you might be trying to link to values and meaning – similar to elements of the Self-Determination Theory.

Motivational interviewing is used quite a lot by practitioners and fits with other approaches, such as behaviour modification, cognitive behavioural therapy and techniques from health literacy.

Promoting health with groups

There are many different groups that occur within the field of health promotion. You will encounter groups of colleagues and groups that form because of an intervention or health activity that you do.

From your experience so far, what groups do you think health promoters may work with? What do you think they may do?

We have started a table here with what Ewles and Simnett (2005) consider to be key purposes of groups in health promotion. There are gaps for you to fill in and make you think about the possible roles you may have in the future:

Purpose of group	Possible group	Possible health-promoting activities
Mutual support		
Group counselling		Smoking cessation
Mutual support		Walking group
Raising awareness	Existing groups such as teams	
Education	New parents Patients newly diagnosed with a chronic disease	

Working with groups is a major skill that we often neglect. As well as communication being very important, you may have to manage group dynamics and different personalities at one time. It can be really helpful for patients in some situations to be a part of a group so they can become more confident and perhaps increase their self-efficacy on a particular behaviour.

Working with a group also means considering where and when you will have meetings and what your ground rules are for participation.

If you like working as part of a group, you may like to think about different styles of leadership – are you more 'directive', preferring to give clear instructions and structure around your health-promoting activity? Or are you more 'collaborative'/'participative' where power may be with the members of the group and move between people at different points during your activity? There are times when each approach may work best – as a general guide, you should consider the needs of the group and be willing to be flexible.

Promoting health with communities

Working with communities can be similar to working with groups; however, when you are promoting health in a community there may be a broader range of activities such as community development, outreach work (where you try to access difficult-to-reach populations such as drug users), campaign work and health information.

Working with communities is one way in which health promoters try to address health inequalities. It is very important for health promoters to work in partnership with the community – we have seen from research studies that interventions that do not have input from the community are less likely to work effectively. The tools that health promoters have found useful in encouraging participation include:

- Being open, especially about plans and policies.
- Responding to the needs of the community – as the community perceives them.
- Plan from within the community rather than in a remote centre.
- Encourage networks – with the Internet and social media, this is easier than ever before.
- Involve the key stakeholders – and include a wide range of individuals and organisations.

Priority areas for health promotion

All disease areas and lifestyle factors are potential areas for health promotion. From giving information about services, to encouraging screening, to changing the fundamental lifestyle habits that can lead to disease and finally to self-management of a chronic condition, we could spend a lot of time with everyone in promoting these areas.

We have seen through models and theories that health promotion can really only occur when there are good economic, environmental, genetic, behavioural, social and access to healthcare factors. How countries and governments respond to the interplay of these factors can differ widely. At the moment, in the UK, there is a tradition of trying to address the social determinants of health, placing particular emphasis on groups or individuals who may be at risk due to an underlying condition such as poverty, poor housing, pollution or discrimination (Royal College of Nursing 2012). These risk conditions can be seen to affect at-risk groups (the unemployed, recent immigrants, black and minority ethnic groups, the homeless, travellers), and also affect risky behaviours (drug use, unsafe sex, diet, smoking and lack of exercise).

ACTIVITY

Choose one of the risk factors.

How could health promotion directly address one of these risk factors?

In addition to social determinants, the UK has key priorities around behaviours that increase risk of disease, namely:

- Smoking
- Diet and nutrition
- Physical activity.

In 2013–14 there has been increased attention on alcohol consumption (Public Health England 2014) and also targeted attempts to reduce overweight and obesity. In part, this is in response to the ageing population in the UK. With increased potential for more years of poor health, most health professionals are keen to encourage healthy ageing which includes the modification of these less healthy choices.

To accompany prevention activities in health promotion, you may also be involved in encouraging a new behaviour in your patients. Screening is an important tool in public health and is thought both to improve lives by early detection of disease, and also to save the government money in treating diseases when they are less advanced. Screening may happen in childhood, particularly for genetic conditions, but it happens throughout the life course. This includes targeted screening for breast and cervical cancers in particular groups of the population, or where there is a high risk, like screening for tuberculosis for people arriving from countries where tuberculosis is prevalent.

There are many possibilities in health promotion. In this chapter we have talked about some of the behavioural theories that can inform how we work with patients. We have shown some strategies for how you could work in a health-promoting way. For some of you, patient care is where you will want to work, but there are also other ways in which you can have a career in health promotion, designing and evaluating campaigns for particular audience 'segments' or groups, or thinking about policies that can affect healthy living at a community or even wider level.

Chapter summary

- Health promotion encompasses a range of strategies and models which can be used to inform how we work with patients.
- Emphasis is on empowering individuals and groups to make their own decisions concerning lifestyles and their management.
- There are a number of lifestyle behaviours identified as requiring input from healthcare workers.
- Health promotion includes individual, group and community approaches.
- Health promotion requires a range of skills including motivational interviewing.

Further resources

The Faculty of Public Health. Available at: www.fph.org.uk.
Public Health England. Available at: www.gov.uk/phe.
The Royal Society of Public Health. Available at: www.rsph.org.uk/en/health-promotion/.

Journals

Health Promotion International. Available at: http://heapro.oxfordjournals.org/.
Patient Education and Counselling. Available at: www.journals.elsevier.com/patient-education-and-counseling/.
Health Promotion Practice. Available at: http://hpp.sagepub.com/.
The American Journal of Health Promotion. Available at: www.healthpromotionjournal.com/.

Further reading

Evans, D., Coutsaftiki, D. and Fathers, C. P. 2014. *Health Promotion and Public Health for Nursing Students*, 2nd edn. Sage: London.
Ewles, L. 2005. *Key Topics in Promoting Health: Essential Briefings on Prevention and Health Promotion*. Edinburgh: Elsevier.
Ewles, L. and Simnett, I. 2003. *Promoting Health: A Practical Guide*, 5th edn. London: Bailliere Tindall.
Green, J. and Tones, K. 2010. *Health Promotion: Planning and Strategies*, 2nd edn. London: Sage.
Katz, J., Peberdy, A. and Douglas, J. 2002. *Promoting Health: Knowledge and Practice.* Basingstoke: Palgrave Macmillan.
Naidoo, J. and Wills, J. 2005. *Public Health and Health Promotion: Developing Practice*, 2nd edn. Edinburgh: Bailliere Tindall.

References

Ajzen, I. and Fishbein, M. 1980. *Understanding Attitudes and Predicting Social Behaviour.* Englewood Cliffs, NJ: Prentice Hall.
Bandura, A. 1973. *Social Learning Theory*. Englewood Cliffs, NJ: Prentice Hall.
Dahlgren, G. and Whitehead, M. 1991. *Policies and Strategies to Promote Social Equity in Health.* Stockholm: Institute for Futures Studies.
Deci, E. L. and Ryan, R. M. 1985. *Intrinsic Motivation and Self-determination in Human Behaviour.* New York: Plenum.
Downie, R. S., Fyfe, C. and Tannahill, A. 1990. *Health Promotion: Models and Values.* Oxford: Oxford University Press.
Ewles, L. and Simnett, I. 1999. *Promoting Health: A Practical Guide*, 4th edn. London: Bailliere Tindall.
French, J. 2004. 'Protecting and Promoting Health – Behavioural Approaches', in Pencheon, P., Guest, C., Melzer, D. and Muir Gray, J. A., eds, *Oxford Handbook of Public Health Practice*. Oxford: Oxford University Press.
Glanz, K., Rimer, B. K. and Viswanth, K., eds. 2008. *Health Behaviour and Health Education: Theory, Research and Practice*. San Francisco, CA: Jossey-Bass.
Hochbaum, G. M. 1958. *Public Participation in Medical Screening Programs: A Socio-Psychological Study* (Public Health Service Publication No. 572). Washington, DC: Government Printing Office.
Janz, N. K. and Becker, M. H. 1984. 'The Health Belief Model: A Decade Later', *Health Education Quarterly* 11(1): 1–47.
Miller, W. and Rollnick, S. 2013. *Motivational Interviewing: Helping People Change*. London: Guilford.
Nutbeam, D. 2004. 'Effective Health Promotion Programmes', in Pencheon, P., Guest, C., Melzer, D. and Muir Gray, J. A., eds, *Oxford Handbook of Public Health Practice*. Oxford: Oxford University Press.

Prochaska, J. O. and DiClemente, C. C. 1983. 'Stages and Processes of Self-Change of Smoking: Toward an Integrative Model of Change', *Journal of Consulting and Clinical Psychology* 51: 390–5.

Prochaska, J. O., Redding, C. A. and Evers, K. E. 2008. 'The Transtheoretical Model and Stages of Change', in Glanz, K., Rimer, B. K. and Viswanth, K., eds, *Health Behaviour and Health Education: Theory, Research and Practice*, 5th edn. San Francisco, CA: Jossey-Bass.

Public Health England. 2013. 'Our Priorities for 2013–14' [pdf]. *Public Health England* [online]. Available at: www.gov.uk/government/uploads/system/uploads/attachment_data/file/192676/Our_priorities_final.pdf [Accessed 5 January 2015].

Royal College of Nursing. 2012. *Health Inequalities and the Social Determinants of Health* [pdf]. Royal College of Nursing Policy Briefing #01/12 [online]. Available at: http://rcn.org.uk/_data/assets/pdf_file/0007/438838/01.12_Health_inequalities_and_the_social_determinants_of_health.pdf [Accessed 5 January 2015].

Seedhouse, D. 2004. *Health Promotion: Philosophy, Prejudice, and Practice*, 2nd edn. Hoboken, NJ: Wiley.

Strecher, V. and Rosenstock, I. M. 1997. 'The Health Belief Model', in Glanz, K., Lewis, F. M. and Rimer, B. K., eds, *Health Behaviour and Health Education: Theory Research and Practice*, 2nd edn. San Francisco, CA: Jossey-Bass.

World Health Organization. 1986. *Ottawa Charter for Health Promotion* [pdf]. World Health Organization [online]. Available at: www.euro.who.int/_data/assets/pdf_file/0004/129532/Ottowa_Charter.pdf [Accessed 5 January 2015].

Chapter 12

Safeguarding individuals and families

Dr Chris Thurston

LEARNING OUTCOMES

By the end of this chapter you will be able to:

1   Identify the signs, symptoms and effects of abuse.
2   Understand how the inter-professional team can use protocols and policies related to vulnerable individuals at risk.
3   Reflect upon issues of confidentiality with regard to safeguarding.
4   Understand how to escalate suspected cases of abuse.

Introduction

A significant number of individuals have experienced violence within their lives; this could be partner, sibling or parental abuse. Many people are vulnerable and 'vulnerable groups' include those who would be vulnerable under any circumstances, for example where the adults in a family are unable to provide an adequate livelihood for their household for reasons of disability, illness, age or some other characteristic. An indicative list of the kinds of individuals who make up vulnerable groups includes families that experience poverty; ethnic minorities; migrants; individuals who are disabled, either physically or linked to learning disabilities; individuals who are homeless; individuals who abuse substances; the older person and people who are isolated; individuals with low levels of education; individuals who are unemployed and underemployed; sex workers; people with mental health challenges; travellers; asylum seekers; individuals who are gay or bisexual; and people who are experiencing abuse (sexual, emotional, neglect, physical or financial). Abuse can be seen as:

> A violation of an individual's human and civil rights by any other person or persons. Abuse may consist of a single or repeated acts. It may be physical, verbal, or psychological, it may be an act of neglect or an omission to act, or it may occur when a vulnerable person is persuaded to enter into a financial or sexual transaction to which he or she has not consented, or cannot consent. Abuse can occur in any relationship and may result in significant harm to, or exploitation of, the person subjected to it.
>
> (Department of Health 2000: 9)

Abuse statistics

Domestic abuse statistics

- Domestic violence relates to 16 per cent of all recorded violent crime (Walby and Allen 2004).
- 45 per cent of women and 26 per cent of men have experienced at least one incident of interpersonal violence in their lifetimes (Walby and Allen 2004).
- In any one year, there are 13 million separate incidents of physical violence or threats of violence against women (Walby and Allen 2004).
- Two women a week are killed by a male partner or former partner.
- This constitutes around one-third of all female homicide victims (Department of Health 2005) (adapted from fact sheet *Statistics: Domestic Violence*, Women's Aid n.d.).

Child abuse statistics

- One child dies each week as a result of cruelty.
- About 5,000 minors are involved in prostitution in Britain.
- Nearly 23,000 children are looked after by local authorities.
- 25 per cent of all rape victims are children.
- Each year approximately 30,000 children are on child protection registers.
- Children with learning disabilities are at a greater risk of experiencing all forms of abuse and neglect (adapted from Thurston 2013).

Elder abuse statistics

- Both older men and women can be at risk of being abused.
- In 2004 the Prevalence Study (House of Commons Health Select Committee 2004) indicated that 4 per cent of older people experienced abuse.
- At least 342,000 people experienced abuse in their own homes (adapted from Action for Elder Abuse n.d.)

The following scenario introduces the challenges that a healthcare professional may be faced with. Professionals have to work jointly in a risky situation in which a family are finding it difficult to trust anyone.

CASE STUDY – THE JONES FAMILY

The family has experienced emotional trauma in recent years, and Granny Jones (Daisy) has moved into the family home following the death of her partner. Her son (Frank), who is unemployed, is suspected of abusing her and taking her pension. She is terrified she will be removed to an old people's home because she is unable to care for herself properly, especially as she is occasionally incontinent. Her daughter-in-law helps her with her personal needs. Daisy has to sleep downstairs and her bed is in the dining room. The family is hostile to social workers and health visitors who have expressed concerns about the welfare of the children in the past. Daisy feels frightened and embarrassed, and does not want any outside involvement and resents any interference in her life from outside the family.

Reasons for abuse

When discussing abuse and how to protect families it is valuable to explore why abuse occurs. There are three main groups of perspectives surrounding the theories of abuse (Kay 1999; Corby 2006; Walker and Thurston 2006; Wilson and James 2007).

Psychological themes emphasise the innate and emotional qualities of the perpetrator of abuse. This approach argues that some people have within themselves from birth an attribute which increases the risk of them harming others – the impetus comes from a physiological or involuntary aspect of human activity.

Social psychological themes emphasise the active relationship between the perpetrator of abuse, the individual receiving the abuse and their personal surroundings. This includes the power imbalances that may occur between a child and adult or between partners. This approach sits between the individual characteristics and the social environment. Therefore how the 'individual is able to relate to their immediate environment is seen as the cornerstone for these perspectives', consequently '*the political and wider social implication in the deterioration of neighbourhoods or social networks is often ignored*' (Walker and Thurston 2006: 45). This again places the responsibility or blame for the abuse on the individual perpetrator who is different from people who do not abuse.

Sociological themes emphasise the links between the social environment and the political climate as one of the major factors for the presence of violence and abuse. Exploring this theme of abuse is uncomfortable as the theme of safeguarding individuals is raised to the level of society rather than the individual, that in a given circumstance, such as poverty, unemployment, ill health or addiction, any person has the potential for becoming abusive. This means healthcare workers have to acknowledge that their daily intervention for individuals and families is frequently inadequate to support family stress, if there is no acknowledgement of the broader influence of the person's environment (Walker and Thurston 2006).

While all these approaches have merit, they should not be seen in isolation; rather, it is a combination or mix of all three which can be used to explore the general reason as to why abuse occurs. Other equally important elements relate to attachment, especially for a child and their carers. This chapter will not explore these further approaches; however, the healthcare practitioner needs to be aware of the risk of personal judgement about the reason behind the abuse, as exhaustion when caring for a relative, adult or child, or other health element may not be obvious but could be present.

Risk factors

It is difficult to describe what a typical abuser looks like and why that specific person may abuse. While it can be seen as statistically more likely to be men rather than women in some areas of abuse, when it comes to physical abuse this is more balanced: 50 per cent of each gender. There is no particular social class, culture or religion which could be seen as more at risk. Therefore it is useful to highlight some specific factors, which do not determine that abuse *will* occur, but may highlight the stress leading to increased risk when undertaking assessment of individuals and families.

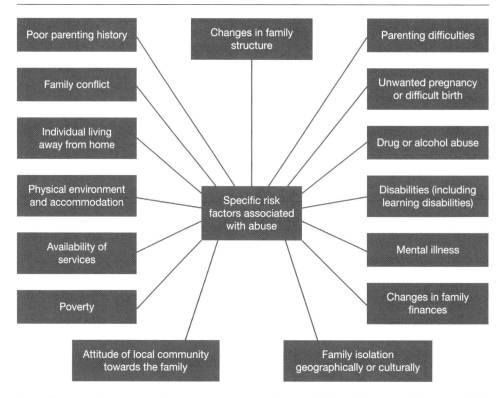

Figure 12.1   Specific risk factors for abuse, adapted from Rogers (2003) and Walker and Thurston (2006).

ACTIVITY

Reflect upon the different families that you work with/know.

Highlight the different styles of family structure.

Analyse each structure, exploring the strengths and weaknesses.

Are there any common themes for the families?

You may have considered some of the following themes:

- Families are social groups sharing accommodation, economic cooperation and reproduction (they share a household, resources and responsibilities).
- Families include adults of both sexes at least two of who maintain a socially approved sexual relationship (in Western society this is mainly through marriage).
- Families include children either born to the family or adopted (the couple reproduce).
- All families are essentially based around and are variations of the nuclear family:

    - Monogamy – when one individual is married to one individual (at a time).
    - Polygamy – when an individual is married to more than one individual (at the same time).

- The nuclear family – is seen to primarily consist of an adult man and woman, in a socially accepted sexual relationship with children (either their own or adopted).
- Extended family – like the nuclear family, consists of an adult man and woman, in a socially accepted sexual relationship with children (either their own or adopted), but also may include grandparents and grandchildren or siblings and cousins, and other kin.
- Beanpole family – like the extended family, it can include grandchildren and grandparents, but the relationships tend to be linear, possibly without partners, making it similar to lone-parent families.
- Lone-parent family – as the name suggests, these are made of a single parent with their children (biological or adopted).
- Reconstituted family – when a couple with children from previous relationships marry, resulting in step-parents, stepchildren and stepbrothers/sisters. There may also be children produced from that relationship.
- Gay/same-sex family – this type of family has only formally been allowed in the Western world in modern times – slowly Western countries are allowing same-sex marriages and as a result have to consider the same-sex family.
- Cohabitation – when two people decide to live together on a long-term basis in a relationship. The term is generally applied to a couple who are unmarried, but can be broadened to mean any number of people living together.
- Singles – someone who is unmarried and lives on their own.

Protective factors can also come from within the family, including the skills of a caregiver to support and protect the vulnerable individual; this can include close family members who can also offer appropriate care. Within the home the encouragement to develop independence, also having a strong faith or belief, can give individuals a sense of stability even during personal, family or community crises. Finally, the community itself can offer protective factors which can include having a supportive person in the neighbourhood, who may be a relative, family friend or peer – someone they can go to for support. This support enables the individual to create a secure and safe environment for them.

RESEARCH NOTE

Abuse and Neglect of Older People: Prevalence Survey Report

(O'Keeffe *et al.* 2007)

O'Keeffe *et al.*, with support from Comic Relief, undertook a study into the prevalence of abuse in the elderly. This was explored using interviews with individuals over the age of 66 years living in private households as '*evidence suggests that mistreatment is likely to be higher among such individuals*'. The study found that abuse and neglect of the older individual in the UK is similar to other Western countries. While the figure highlighted of 2.6 per cent seems low, and because it was a sample study, the team commented that this should be seen as conservative. Once the broader society, such as friends and neighbours are considered, the figure rises to 4.0 per cent and highlights the social environment as an element link to abuse.

An encouraging finding from the research is the extent to which older people who are living in the community, regardless of mistreatment, have regular social contact with friends and family outside the household. That is, the survey findings question the view that those who are mistreated are necessarily socially isolated.

(O'Keeffe et al. 2007: 85)

Another finding is the extent to which people sought help, whether this request for support was aimed at family friends or healthcare professionals. The main issue seems to be the inability of the older person's carer to care and the reasons highlighted were often complex, either socially or interpersonally, but infrequently wilful. Therefore early prevention and intervention including respite care is recommended by the research team, along with further research into the prevalence.

This research on elder abuse highlights the need for agencies to put greater effort into communication and understanding the relationships between family members and other professionals (Reder and Duncan 2004). As healthcare professionals there is a need to prioritise work in safeguarding individuals as highly as learning new procedures, computer data systems and legislative guidance (Walker 2013).

Process of protecting vulnerable individuals

It is possible to highlight the stages through which a potential abuse case may proceed. Often this does not pass beyond the assessment stage. Not many reach the stage of legal proceedings. At each stage the system asks whether the person is likely to suffer significant harm. If there is a positive answer the investigation will proceed further. Often the individual drops out of the system. The series of stages within any safeguarding system is as follows:

A COORDINATED INVESTIGATION NEEDS TO BE UNDERTAKEN

1   Reporting, to a single referral point.
2   Recording, with sensitivity to the abused person, the precise factual details of the alleged abuse.
3   Initial coordination, involving representatives of all agencies which might have a role in a subsequent investigation and could constitute a strategy meeting.
4   Investigation, within a jointly agreed framework to determine the facts of the case.
5   Decision-making, which may take place at a shared forum such as a case conference (Department of Health 2000).

Investigation

The process begins with accessing records about the person and their family. All relevant databases and records should always be checked. Any specialist service involvement including mental health, drug addiction rehabilitation and social services should be contacted to place the challenges in context. In Britain, police checks reveal if any member of the household has been convicted of serious crimes against children (Schedule 1 offences) (Walker 2013).

Recording and reporting

It is better to use professional judgement and report a concern rather than dismiss something that may have been seen. Lord Laming (Department of Health 2003) found that there were a number of occasions when Victoria Climbié could have been involved in the safeguarding process, if professionals had not excluded her because they did not see her experiences as abuse. Frequently this is caused by professionals being too optimistic, feeling that abuse to any individual could not happen in their class, patient list or caseload. A second factor that might hold a practitioner back from acting on a suspicion of significant harm is called cultural relativism. This is where the practitioner suspects that something is wrong, but this is excused as normal in that culture, family or community (Walker 2013). In the Jones family case study, the abusive relationship between Daisy and her son Frank could be seen as normal in families where members are unemployed. The most appropriate approach is to ensure that there is coordination of assessment and intervention to one referral point (or person). This will ensure that all the information is accessible in one place and a more complete picture can be seen. Often this is a social worker who is the 'Key Worker' and will draw the professionals together.

Investigation and initial assessment

A properly co-ordinated joint investigation will achieve more than a series of separate investigations. It will ensure that evidence is shared, repeated interviewing is avoided and will cause less distress for the person who may have suffered abuse. Once the facts have been established, an assessment of the needs of the adult (sic) abused will need to be made. This will entail joint discussion, decision and planning for the person's future protection.

(Department of Health 2000: 29)

While issues of confidentiality are important and only appropriate professionals should have the information, there is a need to protect the individual, which transcends the need to secure information. While this is often difficult for healthcare professionals, especially if a health intervention may be at risk, it is important to share knowledge to ensure that vulnerable individuals are protected. The referral stage is often the first stage of interagency cooperation and communication and can set the scene for the interactions that subsequently occur. Referrals can be made to social services, the NSPCC or to the police. When the referral is made, a conflict of expectations sometimes arises. The referrer often comes from a non-social work agency, or is sometimes a member of the family or the public talking with a health and social care professional. Making such a referral is an unusual, often stressful event, during which they require reassurance and time to discuss their concerns. The worker needs to elicit the maximum amount of hard information about the case in order to judge whether it is an appropriate referral or not (Walker 2013).

Types of abuse

There are a number of types of abuse:

- Physical
- Emotional
- Sexual
- Neglect and acts of omission
- Discriminatory
- Financial or material abuse.

Abuse can occur alone, but often there may be more than one type of abuse happening at the same time. Emotional abuse will usually occur in conjunction with other forms of abuse. It is difficult to physically abuse an individual without also inflicting emotional abuse. Also, when a child, young person or vulnerable adult is being sexually abused, there is often an element of emotional abuse as the perpetrator may well coach or groom the individual into performing the abuse. All types of abuse can be seen on a continuum from slight to severe and in a number of cases especially when physical this can be fatal.

COMMON FORMS OF PHYSICAL ABUSE

- Shaking the individual violently
- Hitting, punching or beating the individual
- Throwing the individual
- Kicking
- Throwing objects at the person
- Scalding and/or burning
- Grabbing, squeezing or crushing parts of the individual body
- Fabricated or Induced Illness (FII) by proxy
- Scratching, pinching or twisting parts of the individual body
- Poisoning (this could include prescribed drugs)
- Drowning
- Smothering or suffocating the individual
- Breaking bones
- Beating the individual with an object
- Biting
- Stabbing or cutting the individual (adapted from Walker and Thurston 2006).

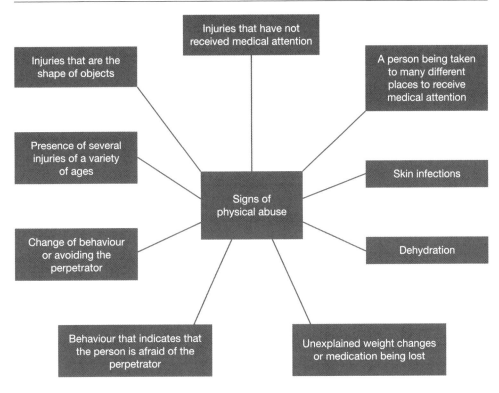

Figure 12.2 Signs of physical abuse.

CHARACTERISTICS SHOWN BY ABUSER WHO EMOTIONALLY ABUSES

- Deprives the individual of emotional comfort
- Humiliation of the individual
- Shows the individual a persistent negative attitude
- Verbal abuse of the vulnerable individual
- Inappropriate development expectations of children or vulnerable individuals
- Inability to recognise child's individuality
- Emotional rejection of the individual
- Telling the person they are unloved
- Frightening the individual
- Threatening the individual
- Inability to recognise the individual psychological boundaries
- Forcing cognitive distortions and inconsistencies on children or vulnerable individuals
- Corrupting and exploiting children or vulnerable individuals
- Ridiculing the individual
- Denying the individual's achievements (adapted from Walker and Thurston 2006).

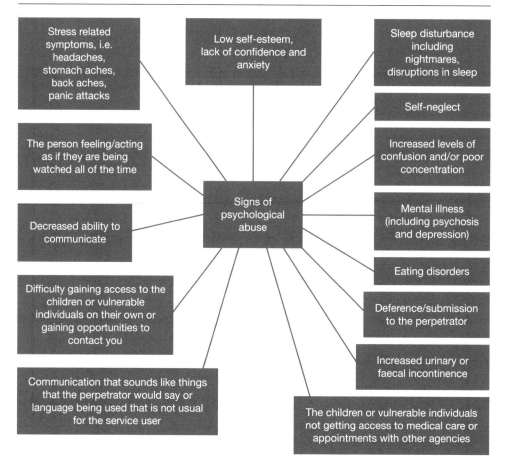

Figure 12.3   Signs that psychological abuse is taking place, adapted from Walker and Thurston (2006) and Local Government Association (LGA) (2015).

SEXUAL ABUSE

- Sexual assault
- Child or vulnerable individuals pornography, where sexual abuse is recorded
- Forced sexual intercourse, vaginal or anal
- Showing children or vulnerable individuals pornographic material
- Rape
- Involving children in sexual activities
- Masturbation of children or vulnerable individuals or of the perpetrator by the children or vulnerable individuals
- Touching, fondling, or kissing the children or vulnerable individuals in a sexual manner
- Oral sex with children or vulnerable individuals or of the perpetrator by the children or vulnerable individuals

- Indecent exposure
- Forced prostitution of children or vulnerable individuals
- Sexual activity with other children or vulnerable individuals
- Coerced sexual activity with animals or objects
- Images of the abused child on the Internet (adapted from Walker and Thurston 2006).

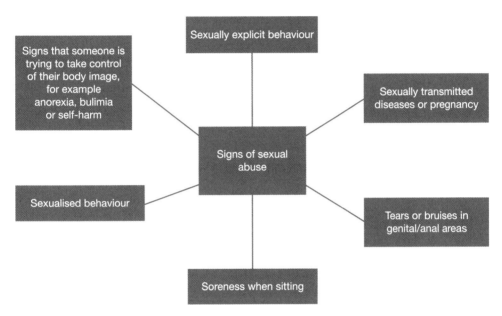

Figure 12.4   Signs that sexual abuse may be taking place, adapted from Walker and Thurston (2006) and LGA (2015).

NEGLECT AND ACTS OF OMISSION

- Inadequate or inappropriate food
- Inadequate or inappropriate clothes or bedding
- Denying or failing to provide the children or vulnerable individuals with adequate warmth and shelter
- Not responding to the requirements of a child's or young person's developmental stage, e.g. not toilet training the child
- Failing to wash or bath the children or vulnerable individuals
- Failing to provide children or vulnerable individuals with clean clothing and a hygienic environment
- Failing to supervise children or vulnerable individuals in potentially dangerous situations

- Failing to seek medical attention when children or vulnerable individuals are ill or injured
- Faltering growth of babies or young children (was Failure To Thrive [FTT])
- Failing to ensure attendance at school or employment for children or vulnerable individuals (adapted from Walker and Thurston 2006).

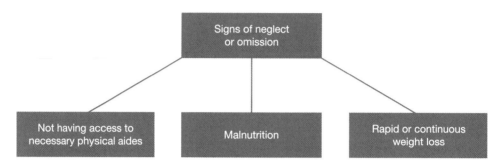

Figure 12.5 Signs that neglect and acts of omission may be occurring.

DISCRIMINATORY ABUSE

- Racist slurs
- Slurs or harassment on the basis of a disability
- Sexist slurs
- Slurs or harassment on the basis of sexual preference
- Age discrimination is also a form of abuse.

FINANCIAL OR MATERIAL ABUSE

- Theft
- Pressure concerning wills, property, inheritance or financial transactions
- Fraud
- The misuse of property, possessions or benefits by someone who has been trusted to handle their finances or who has assumed control of their finances by default
- Exploitation.

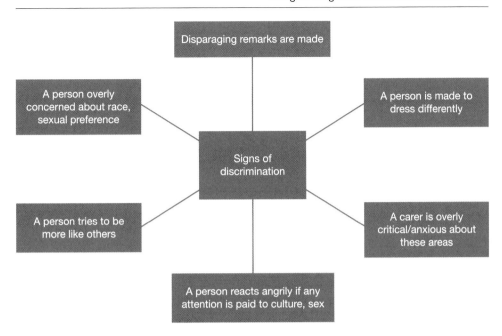

Figure 12.6 Signs that discrimination may be taking place, adapted from LGA (2015).

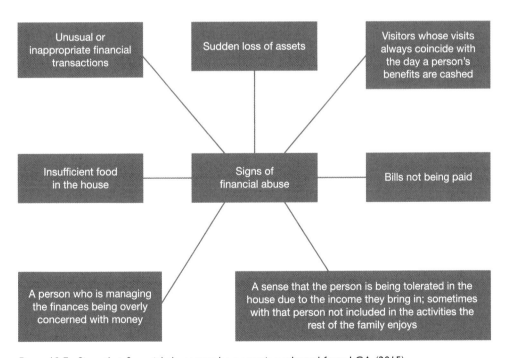

Figure 12.7 Signs that financial abuse may be occurring, adapted from LGA (2015).

Additional information for investigation into financial abuse:

- You will need to establish the vulnerable person's financial situation, for example, his/her pension, benefits, savings.
- Find out who has been responsible for handling/cashing pension, bank account and the like.
- Has anyone been appointed as an agent, appointee or with power of attorney?
- Is anyone refusing to give the person his or her pension book, bank book or similar?
- If there is any doubt about the situation, contact the appropriate Department of Work and Pensions office immediately.
- If it is suspected that financial abuse is occurring and the vulnerable person is asking for help to regain possession of a benefits book, the professional should ask the Department of Work and Pensions to put a hold on the benefit and issue a new book to the vulnerable person.
- If the vulnerable person is asking for someone in authority to take on his or her financial affairs, establish whether this should be someone in the local authority, for example Home Care, or another professional.
- Acquire the appropriate forms, either appointee forms from the Department of Work and Pensions or Court of Protection forms from the Office of the Public Guardian.
- Liaise with anyone who has been involved in the vulnerable person's financial affairs, such as his/her bank manager or solicitor (adapted from LGA 2015).

ACTIVITY

Using the meanings of the above behaviours, how do you think this is acted out in the family in the case study?

When exploring the behaviour of Frank who is emotionally and financially abusing Daisy, reflect on how this may make her feel.

When thinking about Daisy's situation it is worth bearing in mind that the fear which often accompanies emotional abuse can be just as traumatic as physical violence and not only affects an individual psychologically but can also affect them physically. Remember that some of the effects on the individual may not initially be linked to abuse; rather to the individual's other problems, especially when linked to behavioural or physical difficulties.

Inter-professional working

The use of the inter-professional team for Daisy and her family's situation is a necessary requirement, as collaboration and cooperation will ensure that her health needs are explored. This will include investigations and health assessments that the team require for support to continue seamlessly. While social work colleagues will follow up with social support and financial advice, housing colleagues may also be involved to explore issues related to the accommodation available. When challenges occur which are difficult to resolve then Local Safeguarding Boards, either for children or adults, need to be contacted for guidance or support.

Guidance on when to flag concerns:

- A practitioner feels that others need to know the important information that cannot appear on the database
- That this information may affect the types of services made available to the person
- The practitioner who has completed an initial assessment wants to discuss their findings.

Responsibilities of Local Safeguarding Boards:

- Developing local procedures
- Auditing and evaluating how well local services work together
- Putting in place objectives and performance indicators for protection
- Developing effective working relationships
- Ensuring agreement on thresholds for intervention
- Encouraging evidence-based practice
- Undertaking Part 8 reviews when a child/vulnerable adult has died or been seriously harmed
- Overseeing interagency training
- Raising awareness within the community (Walker 2013 in Thurston 2013).

ACTIVITY

Obtain a copy of your workplace's safeguarding procedures and practice guidelines.

Make a note of the contents.

- Examine it carefully and make sure you know how and to whom you should refer in cases involving protection.

Barriers to inter-professional collaboration

- Poor communication between agencies
- Power struggles between key professionals involved in the individual's care
- Traditional thinking with regard to services offered by specific agencies
- Lack of motivation by individuals to invest time in working together
- Different values and beliefs surrounding professional practice
- Different and competing priorities with regard to outcomes for the family
- Geographical location of offices or services
- Differences in terminology used across agencies
- Different philosophical frameworks used across agencies
- Lack of priority given to joint service planning
- Agencies' differing interpretation of their safeguarding responsibilities
- Concerns about client confidentially across agencies
- Lack of knowledge and stereotyping of practitioners from other agencies

- Inaccessibility of staff across agencies due to different work practices
- Budget restraints on local services
- Individual practitioners not able to incorporate interagency policies into their practice
- Different threshold criteria across agencies for making decisions
- Inconsistent levels of commitment of various professionals, especially following case conference
- Diverse pre-qualifying educational curriculum input on safeguarding (adapted from Walker and Thurston 2006).

Individual strategies for case conference or inter-professional meetings:

- Collect evidence from all colleagues who work with the family
- Follow up your intuition with a non-judgemental investigation of the facts
- Prepare the report in plenty of time and be familiar with the contents
- Be honest with the family before the conference
- Ensure information is kept in chronological order and is as complete as possible
- Actively listen to other members of the group and keep an open mind
- Be assertive and clear when presenting your information
- Be prepared to constructively challenge other members
- Be prepared to receive constructive criticism
- Remember to use professional judgement rather than emotive statements
- Give a sensitive but honest opinion of the situation
- Do not let the potential for intimidation hold back your professional opinion.

Table 12.1 Advantages and disadvantages of inter-professional working, adapted from Walker and Thurston (2006).

Advantages	Disadvantages
Collective sharing of responsibility	Time-consuming consultation
More efficient use of staff (enabling development of specialists)	Increase in administration and communication costs
Effective service provision (overall service planning)	Conflicting and different leadership styles, values and language
Satisfying working environment (more relevant and supportive services)	Reduced independence and autonomy of practitioners
Better risk management, auditing of services and research	Difficult for professionals to make individual decisions
Ease of access for families	Inequalities in status
Development of new ideas, roles and ways of working	Minimises the importance of professional differences
Opportunity for shared supervision	Risk of professional collusion
Enhancement of professional skills	Separate educational backgrounds
Avoidance of isolation for practitioners	Blurring roles
Efficient sharing of education and resources	Promotes professional openness

- Show respect and value everyone's view regardless of whether they match your own
- Do not be afraid to bring conflict to the group
- Remember the vulnerable person should be the main focus
- Maintain an anti-discriminatory focus
- Professional judgement should override any personal dislike
- Ensure you receive regular supervision to discuss issues raised at a conference (adapted from Walker and Thurston 2006; Wilson and James 2007; Munro 2008).

Strategic ways of working together:

- Joint education: both during pre-qualifying education and for continuous professional development
- Joint policy: for undertaking assessments, reviews or interviews
- Joint research: both locally on issues for local population and nationally for general trends
- Joint commissioning: both of universal service for families and specific services for individuals in need or at risk
- Joint agreements: for agendas, with consensus of opinion for aims and objectives
- Joint protocols: across agencies for sharing of information
- Joint sharing: of early concerns to encourage preventive or early intervention (adapted from Riley 1997; British Association of Social Work 2003; Children Act 2004; Walker and Thurston 2006).

To work closely and satisfactorily with families requires good communication skills. To work as an advocate requires an ability to negotiate with other members of a team and across agencies, which again requires effective communication skills. Finally, to empower a family means having the awareness to give information freely to ensure informed consent. In short, good communication is the oil which enables the inter-professional team to function smoothly and successfully for both the individual and the family. For an individual to voice their fear of abuse takes great courage and while most professionals appear to take into account the person's problems, welfare decisions are often made *for* the person (especially if they are older or seen as vulnerable), rather than *with* them. Professionals need as a team to put the individual's rights first when making decisions and only when this occurs can all healthcare professionals believe that protection policies truly protect the person and their rights. Great strides have been made, but with the knowledge about gaps in services leaving individuals at risk, professionals need to continuously monitor procedures and policies of interagency working to ensure that decisions are made in the person's best interest. Guidance suggests that staff should receive more comprehensive safeguarding training that equips them to recognise and respond to a person's welfare concerns. Thus the policy aspiration to foster closer collaborative working between agencies involved in safeguarding people faces serious obstacles (Walker 2013 in Thurston 2013).

There is a myth, subscribed to by most agencies and professional groups involved in safeguarding, which suggests that while at work one can leave the self or the personal part of the practitioner at home. However, those personal histories and feelings travel to work with the professional every day. The split between the professional and the personal is largely false, and the myth of the personal–professional split is likely to reduce rather than increase our individual and collective effectiveness. It is assumed that there is no need to care for staff who are engaged in safeguarding, as that comforting process should take place solely in the private life of the individual concerned, or somehow dissipate within the office (Walker 2013).

PRACTICAL GUIDELINES – HEALTHCARE INTERVENTION IN SAFEGUARDING

- Optimally non-intrusive
- Compatible with the promotion of individual potential and personal responsibility
- Balances both rights and risks, and care and control
- Recognises risks to health and social carers.

ACTIVITY

With a colleague, discuss ways in which health and social care workers pose a risk to patients/service users and how those risks could be minimised.

For example, be open and trust each other in a discussion about which patients make you feel angry or despairing and how you manage and process those feelings. You will find most other health and social carers have similar feelings. Sharing and reflecting on these feelings will make them much easier to handle and serve as important material for supervision from line managers.

PRACTICAL GUIDELINES – SKILLS AND KNOWLEDGE FOR SAFEGUARDING

Enhance integrated practice in safeguarding families through development of knowledge and skills.

Effective communication and engagement – includes establishing rapport and respectful, trusting relationships; understand non-verbal communication and cultural variations in communication; active listening in a calm, open and non-threatening manner; summarising situations to check understanding and consent; outline possible courses of action and consequences; ensuring people feel valued; understand limits of confidentiality and relevant legislation; report and record information.

Safeguarding and promoting the welfare of the family – includes ability to recognise overt and subtle signs of harm by considering all explanations for sudden changes in mood or behaviour; involve the family in promoting welfare and recognising risk factors; develop self-awareness about the impact of abuse; build confidence in challenging oneself and others; understand legislation, guidance and other agency roles; share information in the context of confidentiality; appreciate boundaries of your knowledge and responsibility; respond appropriately to conflict, anger and violence and understand that assumptions, values and prejudice prevent equal opportunity.

Multi-agency working – includes effective communication by listening and ensuring that you are being listened to; work in a team and forge sustaining relationships; share experience through formal and informal exchanges; develop skills to ensure continuity for the person; know when and to whom to report incidents or unexpected behaviour changes; understand how to ensure another agency responds while maintaining a focus on the persons best interests.

Sharing information – includes making good use of available information; assess the relevance and status of different information and where gaps exist; use clear unambiguous language; respect the skills and expertise of others while creating a trusting environment and seeking consent; engage with people and their families to communicate and gain information; share confidential information without consent where a vulnerable individual is at risk; avoid repetitive questions and assessment interviews; appreciate the effect of cultural and religious beliefs without stereotyping; understand the principles governing consent; distinguish between permissive information sharing and statutory information sharing and their implications (adapted from Walker 2013 in Thurston 2013).

ACTIVITY

Working with families across different professional groups has advantages and disadvantages.

What information is required to enable a better understanding of how the overall picture of support services fits together?

If better communication is to happen it is essential that the practitioner or agency concerned behaves in an assertive way by explaining the reasons behind a judgement or opinion to the rest of the interagency group. You must never attempt to take over another agency's role or sphere of activity. It is helpful to use the technique of predicting positive or negative outcomes for the proposed courses of action. Where possible aim for compromise if not consensus. Where there is a sense that one side has forced a decision through, the probability of positive interagency cooperation being achieved around that decision is extremely low.

CASE STUDY REVIEW – THE JONES FAMILY

There is a requirement to engage the whole family by addressing needs for safety and protection. While the main focus of intervention must be on the care and safety of Daisy, practitioners also need to engage Frank by addressing his own needs for finance and accommodation.

Domestic abuse interventions

Daisy is aware that her family will be under scrutiny and financial pressure if she leaves so she is stuck in an impossible dilemma. If Daisy stays, the practitioner will allege that Daisy is unable to protect herself. If she decides to leave she will potentially isolate herself from her family.

If staff acknowledge this dilemma in an uncritical way without blaming Daisy or by pretending that there is a simple solution, then they are more likely to begin the process of gaining her confidence and working collaboratively rather than coercively. Encouraging Daisy to attend an older person group would be a positive strategy. Daisy's health and social care needs should be openly discussed in a safe way without giving the false impression of knowing how she feels or by signalling discomfort or embarrassment at such sensitive matters.

Being part of a family

Engaging Daisy in conversation about her experiences as a wife and mother and comparing her life with how it is now will open up a rich seam of information which simultaneously can serve a therapeutic purpose.

Getting Daisy to list her worries and concerns about the family will help the professional to appreciate the emotional aspects of her experiences.

Attempts to engage her son need to be made but not at the risk of inflaming the situation or putting her at risk.

You can then help her consider ways of tackling these worries in small, practical ways before addressing the major issue of her complex relationship with her family.

Holistic overview of the review

The review needs to examine every element of the plan, check whether it is happening, which agency is responsible for what element, what impact the intervention is having on each person in the family and whether additional needs have emerged or alternative interventions need to be considered.

The review should check whether the plan is addressing and meeting each individual's needs, and mental health and emotional well-being, as well as their collective needs as a family.

The wider family context should be explored to see what pattern of relationships exist with a view to encouraging increased supportive contact.

If no immediate family exists then a wider definition of 'family' could identify religious, spiritual or social support networks. Daisy may not be able to manage every aspect because it feels overwhelming. For example, the older person's group may be too noisy or controlled by people who cannot meet her particular needs.

Thought needs to be given to finding the right group for her particular needs rather than just the first available resource. By establishing a solid platform for her to feel supported, empowered and capable of defining her needs she will be more likely to feel strong enough to deal with her son.

Evaluating the family's progress

If the situation became more risky then the practitioner would need to confront Daisy with the likely consequences of inaction on her part. However, this needs to be done alongside offering maximum support by all agencies involved in a coordinated package. Effective review and closure will more likely happen if a collaborative relationship with Daisy has developed which will enable her to seek further help in future if required.

By being proactive about potential problems and difficulties much goodwill can be generated and misconceptions dealt with before they occur during stressful situations. For practitioners involved in safeguarding situations it is important to acknowledge the powerful feelings aroused during this stressful work. Providing a safe environment with a neutral facilitator can be very helpful for the professionals involved, by providing support and reducing barriers to communication.

The journey towards good practice begins with the acknowledgement that all agencies and practitioner groups have something to offer the safeguarding process, and is followed by striving to let others participate in the fullest possible way in the process, combating the urge to think and work in unilateral ways (Murphy 2003; Walker 2013).

Table 12.2 The potential safeguarding plan summary for the Jones family

For Daisy	For son	For daughter-in-law
Physical	Physical/emotional	Physical
• Continue the physical support from daughter-in-law • To have assessment from district nursing team to assess Daisy's personal and medical needs	• Frank to attend anger management course	• Continue physical support for Daisy
	Neglects and acts of omissions	Neglects and acts of omissions
	• Support from housing to review accommodation	• Support from housing to review accommodation
Neglects and acts of omissions	Financial or material abuse	Financial or material abuse
• Daisy to attend day centre a few times a week	• Frank to attend job seekers club	• Liaise with anyone who has been involved in Daisy's financial affairs such as her bank manager or solicitor
Financial or material abuse		
• Liaise with anyone who has been involved in Daisy's financial affairs such as her bank manager or solicitor		

Chapter summary

- Safeguarding vulnerable adults is integral to working in healthcare.
- Having an understanding of the complexity of safeguarding issues and why they may occur will aid in escalating concerns in a supportive manner.
- Health and social care staff working with vulnerable individuals need to learn about, understand and engage critically but positively with other agency staff responsible for safeguarding.
- Different values, knowledge bases and skills in perceptions of the needs of families, who are or may be at risk of significant harm, need to be acknowledged.

Further resources

Victim Support. Available at: www.victimsupport.org.uk/.
Action on Elder Abuse. Available at: www.elderabuse.org.uk/.
Care Quality Commission. Available at: www.cqc.org.uk/.
Dignity in Care Network. Available at: www.dignityincare.org.uk/.

Further reading

Department of Health. 2004. *Every Child Matters: Change for Children*. London: HMSO.
Department of Health. 2008. *Laming Inquiry into the Death of Baby P.* London: HMSO.

References

Action on Elder Abuse. n.d. *Action on Elder Abuse* [online]. Available at: www.elderabuse.org.uk/ [Accessed 6 October 2013].
British Association of Social Work. 2003. *BASW Response to the DfES Green Paper: Every Child Matters*. Birmingham: BASW.
Children Act. 2004. London: HMSO.
Corby, B. 2006. *Child Abuse: Towards a Knowledge Base*, 3rd edn. Buckingham: Open University Press.
Department of Health. 2000. *No Secrets: Guidance on Developing and Implementing Multi-agency Policies and Procedures to Protect Vulnerable Adults from Abuse*. London: HMSO.
Department of Health. 2003. *Laming Inquiry into the Death of Victoria Climbie*. London: HMSO.
Department of Health. 2005. *Responding to Domestic Abuse: A Handbook for Health Professionals*. London: HMSO.
Devon County Council. n.d. 'Safeguarding Vulnerable Adults' [online]. Available at: www.devon.gov.uk/index/socialcare/adult-protection [Accessed 6 October 2013].
House of Commons Health Select Committee. 2004. *Elder Abuse. First Report of Session 2003–04. Volume 1, Report Together with Formal Minutes*. HC 111-I. London: HMSO.
Kay, J. 1999. *A Practical Guide: Protecting Children*. London: Cassell.
Local Government Association (LGA). 2015. *Adult Safeguarding and Domestic Abuse, A Guide to Support Practitioners and Managers*, 2nd edn. London: LGA.
Munro, E. 2008. *Effective Child Protection*, 2nd edn. London: Sage Publications.
Murphy, M. 2003. 'Keeping Going', in Harrison, R., Mann, G. and Murphy, M., eds, *Partnership Made Painless*. Lyme Regis: Russell House.
O'Keeffe, M., Hills, A., Doyle, M., McCreadie, C., Scholes, S., Constantine, R., Tinker, A., Manthrope, J., Biggs, S. and Erens, B. 2007. *UK Study of Abuse and Neglect of Older People Prevalence Survey Report*. London: National Centre for Social Research, King's College London, prepared for Comic Relief and the Department of Health.

Reder, P. and Duncan, S. 2004. 'Making the Most of the Victoria Climbie Inquiry Report.' *Child Abuse Review* 13: 95–114.

Rogers, C. 2003. *Children at Risk 2002–2003: Government Initiatives and Commentaries on Government Policy*. London: National Family and Parenting Institute.

Riley, R. 1997. 'Working Together: Inter-Professional Collaboration.' *Journal of Child Health Care* 1 December: 191–4.

Thurston, C., ed. 2013. *Essential Nursing Care for Children and Young People*. London: Routledge.

Walby, S. and Allen, J. 2004. *Home Office Research Study 276 – Domestic Violence, Sexual Assault and Stalking: Findings from the British Crime Survey*. London: Home Office.

Walker, S. and Thurston, C. 2006. *Safeguarding Children and Young People: A Guide to Integrated Practice*. Lyme Regis: Russell House Publishers.

Walker, S. 2013. 'Safeguarding Children and Young People', in Thurston. C., ed., *Essential Nursing Care for Children and Young People*. London: Routledge. Ch. 5.

Women's Aid. n.d. *Statistics: Domestic Violence Women's Aid* [online]. Available at: www.womensaid.org.uk [Accessed 31 August 2013].

Wilson, K. and James, A. 2007. *The Child Protection Handbook*. London: Bailliere Tindall.

Chapter 13

Teaching and assessing

Dr Anne-Marie Reid

LEARNING OUTCOMES

By the end of this chapter you will be able to:

1 Demonstrate a basic understanding of principles of learning.
2 Apply this to learning and teaching in different settings.
3 Explore methods of providing and receiving one-to-one support for learning.
4 Identify the key principles of assessment.
5 Review good practice in providing feedback.

Introduction

In every professional area of health and social care, staff are involved in their own continuous learning and development as well as in supporting others. Most healthcare staff provide both mentoring support for new or more junior colleagues and also contribute to the teaching of learners from a variety of disciplines in placement activities. Much of this support involves informal teaching in practical skills but it may also include more formal teaching to support the development of others who are studying for work-based qualifications such as NVQs and foundation degrees. Effective teaching is underpinned by assessing others, both formally and informally, and in giving feedback which is helpful in promoting further learning and development. Moreover, health and social care staff are frequently involved in teaching patients/ clients to improve their self-care skills in areas such as in wound care, self-medication and giving dietary advice, as well as teaching the correct use of aids to promote independence. For these reasons, teaching, assessing and giving constructive feedback are key elements in sharing knowledge and understanding within the practice environment to support the development of the whole team.

This chapter aims to provide an overview of current understanding of how we learn, key skills in teaching individuals and groups in different settings, planning teaching and developing appropriate resources, assessing others and giving feedback effectively. The chapter initially outlines key principles of good teaching and then uses case studies from practice situations to demonstrate how the principles are applied. In this way the chapter aims to improve your understanding so that you become a more effective learner and to act as a practical guide to equip you as a more effective teacher in the workplace.

Approaches to teaching and learning

Before considering the ways in which learning occurs, it will be helpful for you to reflect on your own experiences as a learner. We can then relate these to some examples of theoretical perspectives on how we learn.

ACTIVITY

Consider your own recent learning experiences:

- What was your best/worst experience of learning?
- What contributed to making it like that?
- What did you learn from it?
- How could it have been improved?

Feedback

You will of course have your own individual experience of positive and negative learning experiences. From my experience of more than 20 years of teaching a variety of learners on vocational and professional programmes, a number of words and phrases have consistently been used by learners to describe positive and negative learning experiences. These are summarised in Table 13.1.

I expect that you can identify with many of these points, and you may have others which are not included. Considering both positive and negative descriptions of learning experience allows us to establish some principles of good teaching which will run as a thread through this chapter. These apply to a variety of situations including teaching in small groups, teaching

Table 13.1 Positive and negative descriptions of learning

Positive descriptions of learning	Negative descriptions of learning
Aims of lesson made really clear	Not clear what we were supposed to be covering until half-way through
Stimulating and fun	Boring
Informative	Too complicated
Teacher was enthusiastic	Teacher was uninspiring
Teacher was very knowledgeable	Teacher seemed unsure and lacked confidence
Enjoyed discussion with other learners	Not enough time to interact with other learners
Enjoyed trying out practical activities as well as watching demonstration	Shown how to do activities but didn't get the chance to practise
Had good feedback on how to improve my performance	It wasn't made clear to me what I needed to change
Information paced with time to do my own reading and research	Too much was covered in a short time
Very relevant to what we needed to learn	Did not see relevance to my course or job role

practical skills, teaching and mentoring in one-to-one situations, teaching patients, assessing learning and giving feedback effectively.

PRINCIPLES OF EFFECTIVE TEACHING

1   Learners should be active contributors to the educational process.
2   Learning should be closely related to understanding and solving real-life problems.
3   Learners' current knowledge and experience need to be taken into account.
4   Learners should be encouraged and supported to use self-direction in their learning.
5   Learners should be given opportunities for practice with reflection on their own learning and feedback from teachers and peers.
6   Learners should be encouraged to analyse and assess their own performance to help them to develop new perspectives.
7   Teachers should model good practice in their teaching as this will help the next generation of practitioners to become more effective teachers and lead to better patient and client care (adapted from Cantillon *et al.* 2003).

How do we learn?

Historically, learning has been understood as individual acquisition of knowledge, and teaching has centred on the assumption that the teacher is the 'expert' and learners are 'empty vessels waiting to be filled' with knowledge. This is the **transmission** view of knowledge which assumes that learning is transferred unchanged from teacher to learner. Teaching methods built on this view have centred on the teacher transferring knowledge through written notes and through speech to the learner who is a relatively passive participant in the process. More recent understandings have emphasised **learner-centred learning** as being more effective, where learners are active participants in the process, are required to engage with the materials and discover how to apply learning to different situations (Petty 2009).

The process of actively participating in learning activity through engaging thoughts and feelings is linked to the idea of **experiential learning**. This is based on Kolb's (1984) learning cycle illustrated in Figure 13.1.

Kolb's cycle indicates how actively learning helps us to construct new ideas which inform how we approach situations in the future. Kolb's model has value but has been critiqued on the basis of being too simplistic because it suggests learning just at the individual level and learning as a straightforward, cyclical process (Jarvis 2006). In reality, learning is more messy than this with a variety of factors affecting what is learnt at different stages in the cycle, including the impact of other people and the situation around us. However, Kolb's model is helpful in suggesting how we develop skills in analysis, evaluation and abstract thinking which are key to becoming an effective reflective practitioner. This is described in more detail in other chapters in this book (see Chapter 2: Work-based learning). In order to help you to understand Kolb's cycle more fully, a case study example is provided below.

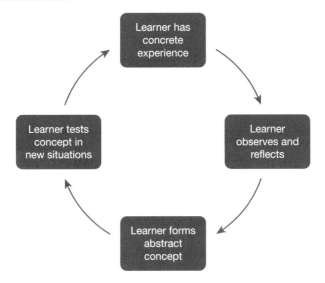

Figure 13.1 The Kolb cycle, adapted from Kolb (1984).

CASE STUDY EXAMPLE – SAJIT

Sajit is a second-year trainee nurse who is working on a hospital medical ward on placement. He has been asked to write an essay on 'informed consent' using a case study example from his recent placement experience. Prior to the placement Sajit was taught about the topic of informed consent through a lecture and small group tutorial on the topic (stage 1).

During the placement Sajit observed a consultant and senior nurse gaining consent from a patient. The consultant was concerned that the patient was not showing any improvement with her current treatment and wanted to try out a different drug regime. During the consultation the patient seemed upset and angry, saying that she had been told the drugs she was already taking would make her better. Sajit observed the sympathetic manner adopted by the staff and the way in which they listened very carefully to the patient's concerns. The consultant explained the problem in lay terms to the patient and carefully discussed the treatment options available. Sajit later reflected on the way in which the consultant described how she expected the new treatment to help but did not make any promises to the patient or put any pressure on the patient to make a decision. He also noted that the senior nurse took time after the consultant had gone to reiterate the information and provide emotional support (stage 2).

When writing about this in his essay, Sajit realised how tempting it might be to persuade a patient to try a new treatment when you are very keen to help them and to see their condition improve. He thought about how important it is for the patient to be given full information, and to be involved in the decision as much as possible. Sajit realised that informed consent is a more complex issue than he had first thought, and that there may be different challenges according to the individual patient and the situation. Sajit's understanding of the concept of 'informed consent' develops into one which involves deal-ing with emotions as well as making logical decisions (stage 3).

The next day on placement Sajit is asked to change a dressing for a patient who has been in an accident. The patient is upset at being kept in hospital because he 'hates' doc-tors and hospitals and is afraid of the sight of blood. Sajit introduces himself and explains why the dressing needs to be changed. He listens carefully to the patient's story and starts to understand the reasons behind his fear of medical treatment. Sajit reflects on what he learned from observing how the consultant and senior nurse dealt with the emotional aspects of gaining informed consent the previous day. He stays very calm in speaking to the patient, explaining in simple terms the procedure involved in changing the dressing. Sajit notices that the patient gradually starts to relax, and eventually the patient agrees to let him proceed. Sajit is now able to gain informed consent and successfully complete the procedure (stage 4).

Taking the example of Sajit, the steps in Kolb's cycle can be summarised as follows:

1   Sajit is introduced to the concept of informed consent – concrete experience.
2   He reflects on the meaning of informed consent when observing senior staff with a patient in practice – observe and reflect.
3   He develops his ideas about applying informed consent in real situations and the complex emotional issues involved – form abstract concepts.
4   He applies this learning to a new situation of gaining informed consent from an upset patient – test in new situations.

Using Sajit as an example, this process describes how learners construct their own individ-ual meanings within the learning situation which prepares them for meeting similar situations in the future. This idea is referred to as **constructivism** (Jarvis 2006) which involves learners in passing through stages of development, in which they 'construct' personal theories. As a concept is 'constructed', new ideas are assimilated within existing mental models. How each learner constructs new ideas obviously depends on what they already know, their motivation to learn, the effectiveness of their approach to learning and the support they have from others. Teaching effectively involves finding ways which encourage learners to construct knowledge by actively engaging with new ideas and developing understanding, not just memorising facts. This allows learners to apply knowledge in a meaningful way in the context of practice and deal with new situations by drawing on previous learning and experience.

Self-directed learning

Self-directed learning is key to developing independent learners who become equipped as **lifelong learners**, able to adapt to changing roles and changing demands in the workplace. Initially learners may need quite extensive guidance and monitoring in order to be clear about the intended learning outcomes and how these might be achieved. In general terms, learners can be encouraged to become more self-directed as they become more confident and more experienced as constructivist learners. This is enhanced by providing opportunities for **peer learning**, working with others on self-directed tasks. In general terms, there needs to be a balance between the type of self-directed learning and the readiness of the learner. Where too little guidance is given, a learner may give up the task quickly because they feel that they don't know how to get started. Careful monitoring by the teacher can help by assessing the progress of the learner and providing more guidance and constructive feedback as needed. Setting achievable goals helps to develop the learner's confidence and enables them to take on increasingly more complex tasks.

Planning teaching, developing resources and teaching practical skills

The most effective teaching in any situation relies on careful planning and preparation to ensure that the purpose of the teaching is clear, and that the methods and resources used are appropriate to the task. The principles of planning involve a number of steps which are briefly outlined below:

1   Identifying the needs of the learner.
    *   This will depend on the course or training programme involved as well as the stage of development and individual characteristics of the learner, any specific learning difficulties or needs and previous experience.
2   Setting aims and objectives which include the purpose and goals to be achieved. The aim is generally what is intended by the teacher, the objectives are the specific goals that will be achieved by the learner.
3   Planning appropriate resources and methods/activities which will enable the objectives to be met.
4   Designing the assessment to check learning and provide evidence that the objectives have been met.
5   Evaluating the session, which involves assessing how effective the teaching has been and identifying any future learning needs.

These steps are applied to a case study example of a one-to-one teaching situation where Elaine, a senior healthcare assistant, is supporting a more junior colleague, Louise, in the workplace. We will work through each of the steps and use the example of Elaine and Louise to explain these in more detail (Table 13.2). Later in the chapter we will apply the same steps to two other teaching situations in different settings.

CASE STUDY – ELAINE AND LOUISE

Elaine is a senior healthcare assistant who is working alongside Louise, a trainee healthcare assistant. In the course of work Louise tells Elaine that she would like to learn to monitor blood pressure as she needs to develop competence in this skill. Elaine suggests to her that she can observe Elaine the next time she takes a blood pressure reading for a patient. Elaine will then supervise Louise while she learns to do the procedure by herself.

1   **Identifying learner needs** – the learner is a trainee healthcare assistant, Louise. In order to identify her learning needs Elaine asks Louise what she knows about blood pressure and why it is important to monitor it. Louise explains that she has been taught about why blood pressure is monitored and she knows the range of normal readings. She has observed the procedure but has not had the chance to learn how to do it. Elaine concludes that Louise has theoretical knowledge about blood pressure but needs the practical skills of taking readings.

2   **Devising aims and objectives** – Elaine aims to teach Louise how to monitor blood pressure on a range of patients. The specific objectives are for Louise to be able to apply a blood pressure cuff correctly, take accurate readings and to be able to perform this consistently in practice.

3   **Planning resources and methods/teaching activities** – the appropriate resources required are a blood pressure cuff and stethoscope as well as a range of the patients whose blood pressure is to be recorded. The teaching methods, in the case of Elaine and Louise, involve observing a practical demonstration of the technique to be used with an explanation of what is happening. As the demonstration involves patients, it is essential that informed consent is gained before carrying out the procedure. After observing the technique, Louise will practice by herself with supervision and feedback from Elaine the first few times that she performs the skill. Elaine adopts this model to teach Louise how to take blood pressure accurately on a range of patients.

4   **Designing the assessment** – Elaine needs to check that Louise has a good understanding of the procedure and that she can perform this consistently well. Elaine is able to assess this through observing how well Louise is able to perform the skill and asking her questions as she is doing it. When this is being done informally on the ward while Louise is practising, this is known as formative assessment. Elaine gives Louise feedback on how well she is doing and any ideas for improving her technique. Louise also needs to demonstrate competence in this skill for the qualification she is working towards. Later she is formally assessed on her ability to take accurate blood pressure readings consistently on the ward. This is known as summative assessment. Different forms of assessment for different purposes are described in the Assessing Others section of this chapter.

5   **Evaluating learning** – Elaine checks that Louise now feels confident about taking blood pressures and asks her if there is any further support she might need.

Teaching practical skills

The case study illustrates an example of teaching practical skills, an important component of much of the teaching in the workplace. A model which is valuable in teaching practical skills, and one which was used by Elaine as she taught Louise, is **Peyton's four-stage approach** (Walker and Peyton 1998).

This approach builds on the principle of experiential learning described previously and provides guidance to supervisors on how to teach practical skills effectively.

One-to-one teaching

Opportunities for learning in professional and vocational education often involve one-to-one relationships of the type involving Elaine and Louise above. These types of work relationships may be described in different ways depending on the purpose and nature of the relationship:

- Coaching
- Mentoring
- Supervision.

Table 13.2 Steps in planning teaching: Elaine and Louise's case study

Steps in planning teaching	Case study example (Elaine and Louise)
Identifying the needs of the learner • Learner needs are dependent on the course or training programme involved as well as the stage of development and individual characteristics. • The identification of needs should take into account any specific learning difficulties or needs and previous learning experience.	Louise has an understanding of blood pressure and has observed it being taken. She needs to learn how to perform the skill herself.
Aims and objectives should be stated to outline what the learner can expect to be covering. • The 'aim' is what is intended by the teacher. • The 'objectives' are the specific targets to be achieved by the learner.	The **aim** of the coaching is to teach Louise how to monitor blood pressure. The **objectives** are that by the end of the coaching Louise will be able to: 1 Apply a blood pressure cuff correctly. 2 Take an accurate reading. 3 Perform consistently on a range of patients.
Resources should be planned beforehand to provide as effective a learning experience as possible. • Resources are planned to meet specific objectives as appropriate to task and situation The method is the teaching strategy and activities which are appropriate to meet learning objectives.	Elaine identifies a suitable patient and gets the blood pressure cuff and stethoscope ready. She explains the purpose of each to Louise. • Elaine gains informed consent from the patient for the procedure and for the demonstration. • Elaine carries out the demonstration according to Peyton's four-stage approach described below (Figure 13.2).
The assessment checks learning and may be designed by the teacher or set by another party (assessment is covered in more detail in the Assessing others section of this chapter).	Elaine informally (formatively) assesses Louise performing the task on a patient. Over the next few days Elaine supervises Louise carrying out blood pressure readings on a range of patients, giving feedback on how well she is doing. Once Louise is able to carry out the task consistently she is formally assessed (summatively) for her NVQ portfolio and has this competence signed off.
Evaluation of the learning event concerns an assessment of the extent to which the learner's needs are met.	Elaine checks that Louise needs no further help with taking blood pressures and asks her what support in other areas she might need.

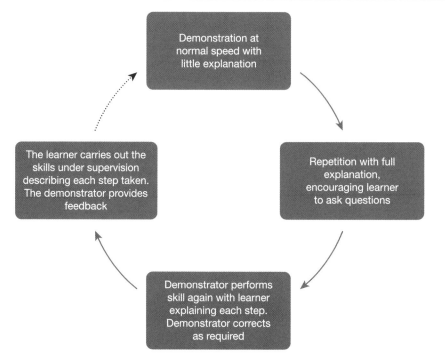

Figure 13.2 Peyton's four-stage model for teaching practical skills, adapted from Walker and Peyton (1998).

Work-based coaching

The purpose of coaching is to bring out the best in the individual in order to maximise their performance. This may be an aspect of the training involved in performance management, but often this happens within a much less formal structure, for example supporting more junior colleagues who are still in training. Coaching is often 'on the job' where the coach allows the trainee to identify particular needs or goals they would like to meet. The case of Elaine and Louise above is a good example of coaching in the workplace, teaching particular skills and providing guidance as the need arises in the course of day-to-day work. Coaching is similar to mentoring in the workplace but often differs in the type of relationship between the people involved.

Work-based mentoring and preceptorship

A mentor is someone who supports and guides another. The relationship can be formal, for example, learner nurses have a **mentor** assigned to them when they are undertaking work placements. The role of the mentor is to provide education, role modelling and feedback with the aim of supporting the mentee's performance and confidence. Once qualified, during the first year of their practice experience, junior nurses have a more senior colleague assigned to them to carry out this role who is known as a **preceptor**.

Formal mentoring – the mentor or preceptor provides guidance according to the requirements of a specific training or study programme in order to support the learner in meeting these requirements. It is very helpful to set ground rules to establish what each party expects of the relationship and to keep a record of meetings. Although mentoring is largely a supportive role, the mentor may also be required to assess the mentee's competence as part of the workplace assessment. An example of this is given in the case study below.

CASE STUDY – ISMAIL AND EVE

Ismail works with adults with learning disabilities and is currently undertaking a healthcare course. His mentor Eve is required to teach Ismail how to promote independence in clients in a way which is appropriate to each individual's needs and abilities. In order for Ismail to achieve his competence, Eve is also required to assess Ismail's ability to do this against the appropriate competency standard. Eve will sign the assessment as completed when she has been able to observe Ismail over a period of time and has seen him demonstrate this competence in his work consistently.

Informal mentoring – this type of relationship arises where a trainee or junior employee naturally develops a positive relationship with a more senior colleague who provides them with advice and guidance. The mentoring may be directly related to work tasks, understanding of organisational policies and procedures or in relation to managing relationships at work.

Peer-mentoring – this is a mutually agreed relationship between two people at a similar level of training or stage of study who support each other. The mentee will identify a challenge or problem and the mentor will ask helpful questions to prompt the mentee to reflect on the situation, identify different courses of action and decide how to take things forward. The peer mentoring relationship is an equal relationship where both parties learn from one another but it is still important to respect confidentiality to maintain mutual trust.

STUDENT TIP – PEER MENTORING

Try and identify a peer with whom you can develop a peer mentoring relationship. This can help you to learn quicker and also increase your motivation as it can be more enjoyable to set targets and work together.

Work-based supervision – supervision may have different connotations depending on the purpose and the nature of the relationship involved. In a formal educational situation, supervision most commonly refers to an ongoing relationship where the teacher is supervising learners who are engaged on fairly lengthy projects such as degree dissertations. The supervision normally centres around providing academic support and guidance to provide regular feedback on progress. In the workplace, supervision generally refers to a more formal process of providing one-to-one support for professional development and/or performance management. In some health and social care professions such as social work, psychiatry and psychotherapy, all practitioners have regular extended supervision meetings to help them to deal with challenging work with complex client cases. This is referred to as **professional supervision** (Scott and Spouse 2013). A case study example of Allan, a social worker who is supervised by Tracy, is described below.

CASE STUDY – ALLAN AND TRACY

Allan is a social worker who works in the area of safeguarding children and he has been qualified for three years. He has a case load which is demanding and he often has very difficult decisions to make. Every six months (or more often if required) Allan meets with his social work supervisor, Tracy, to reflect on his work. He has the opportunity to talk through difficult cases and his decision-making in dealing with these. Discussing the challenges with Tracy provides support for him and the opportunity to reflect on any areas for improving his practice and on his career development.

In other situations, **managerial supervision** is associated with closely monitoring the progress of an individual for whom you have management responsibility. This may be when they are undergoing a period of training, at which point they may need more one-to-one support with taking on new tasks and responsibilities. In other cases, **performance management** (Armstrong 2012) may need to be carried out where performance is falling below expected standards. It is important in the latter case to set out exactly what is expected of the individual according to their role in the organisation and their job description. Performance may not be as expected because the individual is unclear about their role or needs training in a particular area. It is helpful to set out expectations of both parties with regard to the purpose of the supervision and role of the supervisor. Training needs should be identified and a clear plan of action should be drawn up together with a written record of the meeting. These provide the basis on which the employment continues, where the individual responds well to additional support and training or, in the worst case scenario, where evidence is recorded which gives grounds to terminate the employment. In either case, the Human Resources (HR) department of the organisation should be fully involved to ensure that the employee is given the opportunity to improve, and to ensure that any remedial action taken is in accordance with employment law and the policies of the organisation.

Irrespective of the type of supervision, coaching or mentoring involved, there are key principles of one-to-one support which develop effective relationships and lead to positive outcomes. These are summarised as follows:

KEY PRINCIPLES OF EFFECTIVE ONE-TO-ONE SUPPORT

1   Set out 'ground rules' at the start which outline expectations of the relationship agreed by both parties.
2   Keep the discussions confidential except where this is not appropriate, e.g. if it transpires that one of the parties is at risk or if a law has been broken.
3   In a formal supervision or mentoring relationship it is recommended to keep notes of regular meetings.
4   Asking helpful, open-ended questions supports the learner or trainee in reflecting and finding their own answers.
5   Give positive and constructive feedback on performance and on ideas.
6   Avoid giving too much advice – offering small snippets frequently works much better than overloading.
7   Refer to more senior colleagues or other forms of support as appropriate.
8   Set clear action points and pick these up in future meetings to check progress.

Teaching patients and clients

Patient education is perhaps the most important form of teaching in which healthcare professionals are involved. Underpinning this is the principle that good patient care involves working in partnership with patients to empower them and to encourage self-care where possible, as described in other chapters of this book. Key principles involved in teaching patients and clients are:

- Teaching should aim to empower patients/clients with knowledge which allows them to make informed decisions about their own care.
- Effective teaching is underpinned by effective communication.
- Effective teaching is likely to lead to better understanding and conformance to treatment plans.
- Effective teaching motivates patients/clients by encouraging self-care and improving quality of life.
- Working in partnership with patients and clients is congruent with policy on the 'Expert Patient' (Department of Health 2001).

Much of the teaching of patients and clients involves ongoing one-to-one support where bite-sized chunks of information may be given or reinforced as part of normal day-to-day care. In other instances the teaching may be deliberately planned in advance where the patient/client is being given in-depth information about their particular disorder, being given health promotion advice or they are being taught an element of self-care. Many of the principles outlined above regarding effective one-to-one support apply equally to teaching patients and clients. A case study example of John who is supporting Edith in the community is described below.

CASE STUDY – JOHN AND EDITH

John works as a healthcare assistant in the community in supporting patients and clients with long-term conditions. He is currently undertaking a foundation degree in healthcare and has been learning about type 2 diabetes. He works with a number of patients with the disorder. One of John's clients is Edith who has arthritis and who has also recently been diagnosed with type 2 diabetes. Edith tells John that the doctor has explained the condition to her, but at the time she was feeling upset and confused and didn't fully understand what the doctor was saying. She asks if John could tell her more about the condition.

John listens carefully to Edith and agrees that it can be very confusing when we are given a lot of new information and it is normal to require information to be repeated to fully understand what is being said. John suggests to Edith that she speaks to her doctor during the next visit to express her concerns and to ask him to explain the disease and treatment again. In the meantime, John promises to find some helpful patient information material for Edith which explains type 2 diabetes and to go through this with her during his next visit. John plans out how he will teach Edith more about her condition and how to deal with it in line with the steps in planning teaching we covered earlier in the chapter. John discusses his plan with his supervisor before he next visits Edith. A copy of John's plan is shown in Table 13.3.

Table 13.3 Steps in planning teaching: John and Edith's case study

Steps in planning teaching	Case study example (John and Edith)
Identifying the needs of the learner • Learner needs are dependent on the course or training programme involved as well as the stage of development and individual characteristics. • The identification of needs should take into account any specific learning difficulties or needs and previous learning experience.	Edith is the learner in this case. She has an expressed need for clear information on type 2 diabetes at a level appropriate for a lay person.
Aims and objectives should be stated to outline what the learner can expect to be covering. • The 'aim' is what is intended by the teacher. • The 'objectives' are the specific targets to be achieved by the learner.	John's **aim** is to teach Edith more about her condition and how to deal with it. The **objectives** are that by the end of the visit Edith will have: 1 Developed an understanding of diabetes, appropriate to a lay person. 2 Appreciated the need for treatment. 3 Explored how she might best deal with living with diabetes.
Resources should be planned beforehand to provide as effective a learning experience as possible. • Resources are planned to meet specific objectives as appropriate to task and situation. The method is the teaching strategy and activities which are appropriate to meet learning objectives.	John identifies patient education material on diabetes which will be helpful for Edith. • They read through this together. • John explains some key terms. • John explains the lifestyle advice which is given to patients with the condition. • They explore how this advice might apply to Edith's situation.
The assessment checks understanding. It may be designed by the teacher or set by another party (assessment is covered in more detail in the Assessing others section of this chapter).	At the end of the visit John checks Edith's understanding of what they have discussed. He leaves her with the patient education leaflets to read again.
Evaluation of the learning event concerns an assessment of the extent to which the learner's needs are met.	On the next visit John checks to see if Edith has any further questions about her condition. He asks how she is managing to follow the advice on coping with diabetes and asks her about any further support she requires.

Afterwards, Edith tells John that she now has a much better understanding of her condition and feels more able to cope with the diabetes and with the lifestyle changes that she is making.

Teaching small groups

Many of the key principles involved in providing one-to-one support apply equally well when dealing with small groups of learners. However, teaching small groups differs in as much as there may be a variety of learning needs within the group and so different teaching methods may be required to meet these needs. Creating an effective learning environment which ensures that everyone is contributing and is able to meet the objectives of the teaching is important. The aim of this section is to explain techniques in teaching small groups effectively in formal or informal situations including classrooms, training facilities, practice settings and other sites of learning.

ACTIVITY – LEARNING IN SMALL GROUP SITUATIONS

Think back to your recent experiences of learning in a small group situation.

- What made this an effective learning experience or otherwise?
- Who did you learn more from – the teacher or other learners?
- Did you feel that everyone had an opportunity to contribute?
- Did you feel comfortable asking questions?

Feedback

Hopefully, your recent experiences of group learning have been positive and you have benefitted from both the expertise of the teacher and also from sharing experience and working on tasks with other learners. In any teaching situation it is important to create a positive relaxed atmosphere where learners feel motivated to learn, feel that the topic is relevant and of interest to them and are encouraged to recognise that they have something valuable to contribute. In order to illustrate this, we will apply the steps in planning teaching effectively to a case study example of teaching a small group in a healthcare setting. Rahima is the teacher as stated and her plan is illustrated in the case study below.

CASE STUDY – RAHIMA

Rahima is a qualified staff nurse based on an acute medical ward. She has been asked to be involved in induction for three Trainee Assistant Practitioners who are based on the ward. Rahima has been asked to teach them about Hospital Acquired Infection (HAI) in line with the hospital's policy. It makes sense to go through the information and procedures with all of them together and so she sets aside one hour to do this. She takes time to plan the session in advance to ensure that that the teaching is effective (Table 13.4).

1 **Identifying learning needs** – Rahima knows that the learners are undertaking the first year of a Foundation Degree in Health and Social Care. They need to know about HAI and minimising risks in line with hospital policy.
2 **Devising aims and objectives** – Rahima aims to explore HAI and ways of reducing this in a hospital setting. The specific objectives are that by the end of the session the learners will be able to identify common bacterial agents involved in HAI and the relative risk associated with these, identify the main sources of infection, outline measures to reduce risk and appreciate the hospital policy on infection control and their role in reducing this.

3   **Planning resources and methods/teaching activities** – Rahima considers carefully how she can put across the information in a learner-centred way which engages learners and allows them to contribute and share experience. She starts by exploring what the learners already know by brainstorming ideas and she notes these down on a flipchart. She then shows the learners a video on HAIs which is part of the induction package. She allows time for discussion and answering questions. She gives the group a practical demonstration of effective handwashing to reduce HAIs. She asks the learners to repeat her technique and supervises while they practise, giving feedback to individuals as appropriate. She finishes the session by summarising the main points and gives the learners a handout to reinforce these. Rahima considers how long each part of the session is likely to take and builds this into her planning.

4   **Designing the assessment** – Rahima assesses the learning by checking that each learner is able to perform the correct technique following her demonstration. She also asks questions during the session and at the end to check understanding. She asks the learners to repeat her technique and supervises while they practice, giving feedback to individuals as appropriate.

5   **Evaluating the learning** – Rahima asks the learners if they have found the session useful and understood everything. She asks if they have any suggestions as to how she could improve her teaching next time. She checks to see if the learners need any further information or guidance on HAIs.

The role of the teacher in small group sessions is to facilitate the learning process and to do this effectively Rahima needs specific skills including the ability to ask good questions; questioning effectively is a skill often underestimated. Asking open questions is generally more fruitful than asking closed questions which require a single answer. Encouraging the learner to give some detail in their response is helpful in understanding their thinking processes and allows the teacher to probe further. Helpful questions often start with 'why' 'what' and 'how'.

STUDENT TIP – ASKING GOOD QUESTIONS

Asking open questions helps to promote learning:

- Why do you think that might be the case?
- What do you think are the implications of this?
- How do you think that might apply in other situations?

These questions encourage learners to think more deeply, to develop higher-level thinking skills and form abstract concepts which helps them to relate this understanding to new situations as described in Kolb's cycle. These types of questions should elicit evidence of learning and allow constructive feedback to be given to move learners further forward.

Questions can also be directed towards different learners according to their individual needs. For example, it is helpful to ask an under-confident learner relatively easy questions which allow them to demonstrate knowledge, this gives a sense of accomplishment and helps them to build their confidence. A very able learner will benefit from more challenging, probing questions which encourage them to think more deeply. When answers are provided it is

Table 13.4 Steps in planning teaching: Rahima's case study

Steps in planning teaching	Case study example (Rahima)
Identifying the needs of the learner • Learner needs are dependent on the course or training programme involved. • Learner needs depend on the stage of development, individual characteristics and previous learning experience. • Identification of needs should take into account any specific learning difficulties.	The learners are undertaking the first year of a Foundation Degree in Health and Social Care. They need to know about Hospital Acquired Infection (HAI) and minimising risks in line with hospital policy.
Aims and objectives should be stated to outline what the learner can expect to be covering. • The 'aim' is what is intended by the teacher. • The 'objectives' are the specific targets to be achieved by the learner.	**Aim**: to explore HAI and ways of reducing this in a hospital setting. **Objectives**: by the end of the session the learners will be able to: 1 Identify common bacterial agents involved in HAI and the relative risk associated with each of these. 2 Identify the main sources of infection. 3 Appreciate measures to reduce risk including effective handwashing. 4 Identify hospital policy with regard to infection control and their role in reducing this.
Resources should be planned beforehand to provide as good a learning experience as possible. • Resources are planned to meet specific objectives as appropriate to task and situation. The method is the teaching strategy and activities which are appropriate to meet learning objectives.	Resources and methods: • Initial discussion to identify what the learners already know (10 min). • A short video which outlines common bacterial agents and the relative risks (15 min). • A discussion on main sources of infection (10 min). • A practical session on effective handwashing (15 min). • A handout summarising the hospital infection control policy. • A question and answer session to summarise key points (10 min).
The assessment checks understanding and may be designed by the teacher or set by another party (assessment is covered in more detail in the Assessing others section of this chapter).	Understanding is assessed informally (formative assessment) in discussion throughout the session. The learners must complete an online quiz on infection control as part of mandatory training requirements after the session (summative assessment).
Evaluation of the learning event concerns an assessment of the extent to which the learners' needs are met and any areas for improving on teaching.	Rahima checks to see if the learners need any further information or guidance on HAIs. She also asks if they have any suggestions as to how she could improve her teaching next time.

important to give an element of positive feedback even if the answer is not the one expected. If possible, simplify the question or give a hint to allow the learner to move closer to where you would like them to be. Asking questions in this way is an important means of assessing understanding during teaching, mentoring or coaching sessions.

FACILITATOR SKILLS

- Appropriate attitude during group teaching
- Good preparation
- Organised and well-structured
- Ability to control the group
- Good questioning
- Effective listening
- Probing further
- Explaining
- Summarising

In this section we have considered lesson planning in detail including how to write aims and objectives, choose methods and resources and to think about assessment to check learning. We are now going to consider how to plan assessment, and different types of assessment, in more detail depending on the type of learning which is being 'measured'.

Assessing others

Principles of assessment

Before considering in detail the principles of assessment, it is helpful to consider the various purposes the assessment might serve:

- To support learning.
- To determine whether learning objectives are met.
- To improve teaching.
- To award a certificate or judgement of competence.
- To satisfy regulatory bodies and the general public that standards are being met.

The reasons for assessing learners in vocational and professional education, as in other areas of education, are multiple. These relate not just to the theoretical purpose of the assessment, but also to meeting the needs of the various stakeholders involved. Some examples of potential stakeholders and what they might need from the assessment are listed below:

Learners – assessment provides feedback on progress which supports further learning needs. Success in assessment increases confidence and motivation and gives reward in the form of a certificate/qualification.

Teachers – assessment provides evidence of understanding and competence of individual learners. Across a group it provides evidence on whether the learning objectives of the module/course as a whole are being met. In this way it demonstrates evidence of effective teaching and indicates any areas where teaching may be improved.

Institutions – learner performance in assessment acts as a benchmark for the institution as to how well it is doing in comparison to previous performance and to other institutions.

Regulators – regulators such as the Nursing and Midwifery Council (NMC) or Health and Care Professions Council (HCPC) use evidence of assessment standards and levels of qualification to ensure a properly trained workforce. For example, they set a target for the numbers of care workers who should have achieved NVQ 2/3 level in a care setting.

Patients/public – reassurance of standards of competence of healthcare staff. The public want assurance that the staff treating them will provide a good standard of care.

Consequently, setting and maintaining high standards of formal assessment is important in meeting the needs of learners and ensuring that all stakeholders involved are satisfied that the assessment processes are 'fit for purpose'. Of course, much assessment in the workplace is much more informal as part of a process of mentoring, coaching and supervising more junior colleagues, as indicated earlier, in the section on one-to-one teaching.

Before discussing how to design assessment and provide effective feedback in more detail we will consider the role of **formative** and **summative** assessment. Formative assessment is also known as 'assessment for learning' as the emphasis is on learning from the feedback rather than on the testing itself. Summative assessment is also known as 'assessment for progression' (Black *et al*. 2003) as the emphasis is on making a judgement which affects a learner's progression to the next stage, although of course constructive feedback should also be given to support future learning. Key differences between formative and summative assessment are shown in Table 13.5.

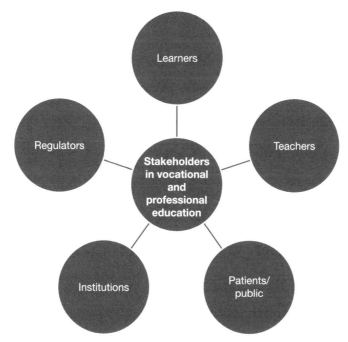

Figure 13.3 Stakeholders in professional and vocational education.

Table 13.5 Formative and summative assessment

Formative assessment	Summative assessment
Assessment to monitor ongoing learning.	Assessment for progression to next stage.
May take the form of 'in-course' tests, interactive quizzes, 'mock' examination, portfolio exercises.	'High stakes' assessment such as end of module written exams, multiple-choice examinations, OSCEs.
Intended to shape future learning.	Provides a summary of performance.
Emphasis is on providing the learner with good detailed feedback to reflect on their performance and identify strengths and limitations.	Emphasis is on using the result to make progression decisions.

In the case study examples given previously we have seen some examples of both formative and summative assessment:

- In Elaine and Louise's case study – Louise was assessed **formatively** when practising taking blood pressure from patients while Elaine was supervising her. Once Louise was ready to carry out the task consistently by herself she was assessed **summatively** in order to have this competence signed off for her portfolio.
- In Rahima's cases study, Rahima's learners were assessed **formatively** through questioning during the session to check their understanding. They were also assessed formatively on using the correct handwashing technique. They were assessed **summatively** after the session by completion of an online quiz on infection control as part of mandatory training requirements.

Types of assessment

As indicated previously, assessment is an integral part of planning and should be considered in advance in order to judge the extent to which the learning objectives are being met. It is helpful to consider assessment types in relation to the **domains** of learning involved. The domains of learning may be categorised with reference to knowledge/cognition, behaviour and skill/attitudes. The categorisation is not perfect as it suggests that thinking, attitudes and skills are all separate from one another, and yet we use these in combination when acting as a 'whole' person. However, it is helpful in analysing some of the complexities of the learning process and considering what is being assessed. This is illustrated by Miller's Pyramid (1990) in Figure 13.4.

The base of the pyramid is concerned with what the learner *knows*, with a progression to the judging if the learner *knows how* – for example, knows how to perform a task; then the next level *shows how* refers to the ability to demonstrate this to others, with, finally, a synthesis of all of these whereby the learner *does* the task competently on a routine basis.

In order to illustrate this we will return to our case study examples:

- In Elaine and Louise's case study, Louise is being assessed formatively at level 3 – '*shows how*' when she first demonstrates her ability to measure blood pressure in a patient. When she is being assessed summatively for her NVQ portfolio she is assessed at level 4 '*does*' to show how she has developed competence in performing this skill as part of everyday practice.

Assessment Theory

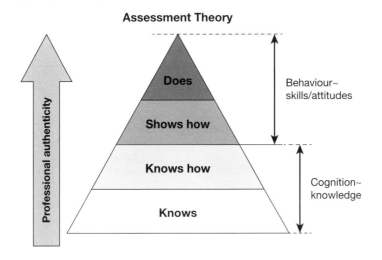

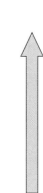

Level 4.	Learner integrates knowledge and skills through an authentic independent performance, within day-to-day work practice
Level 3.	Learner demonstrates their knowledge through action (involving cognition and behaviour) such as demonstrating taking blood from a mannequin
Level 2.	Learner explains how to perform a skill
Level 1.	Learner acquires the knowledge required for their future practice

Figure 13.4 Miller's Pyramid, adapted from Miller (1990).

- In Rahima's case study, Rahima's learners were assessed formatively at level 3 *'shows how'* when they were asked to demonstrate correct handwashing technique during the session. They were assessed summatively at level 1 *'knows'* when they had to answer questions online after the session as part of their mandatory training.

The types of assessment which might be included in a vocational or professional course in healthcare are as follows:

- Written essay/report
- Multiple-choice examination
- Workplace assessment
- Portfolio assessment
- Objective Structured Clinical Examination (OSCE).

These different types of assessment may be considered at different levels on Miller's Pyramid in Figure 13.5 to indicate the domains being tested in each case.

When planning assessment it is important to consider the domain of knowledge being tested and to plan the assessment across the whole course of a vocational or professional programme to test knowledge across all domains where possible.

What we assess

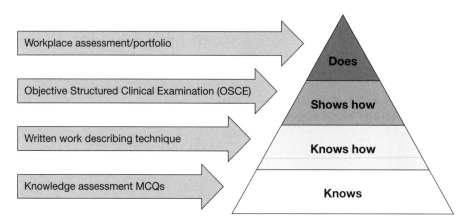

Figure 13.5 What we assess, adapted from Miller (1990).

ACTIVITY – PLANNING A TEACHING SESSION

Imagine that you are planning a lesson for a small group of your fellow learners.

- Choose a topic which is of relevance to your area of work and plan a short lesson (30–45 minutes).
- Decide on the aim and learning objectives.
- Choose appropriate methods and resources to meet these, given the nature of the session and time available.
- Design an appropriate assessment which will enable you to check learning – try to incorporate more than one domain from Miller's Pyramid.
- Decide on a suitable way of evaluating the lesson.

How we assess

Marking criteria

When it comes to judging the value of an assessed piece of work and awarding a grade, this should be driven by the **marking criteria** for that particular assessment and the course involved. In academic work much of the assessment is graded as a percentage mark or it may be judged at a 'Pass, 'Merit' or 'Distinction' level. In order to establish what this standard means, the marking criteria should be explicit about what components are being judged with indicators on how a mark at various levels will be awarded. Some examples of criteria used to judge written work are as follows:

- Good structure and logical flow.
- Well-written and well-referenced.

- Effective use of theory.
- High level of critical analysis.

Criteria used to judge an oral presentation will be somewhat different, with the following likely to be included:

- Clear articulation.
- Good pace/flow.
- Good eye contact and audience engagement.
- Good use of visual aids and resources.

The extent to which the learner meets the criteria will determine the mark given for the individual component with all of these contributing to the overall mark. Learners should be given clear guidelines on the assessment beforehand and have access to a copy of the marking criteria (usually in a handbook or available online) so that they are well-informed about what is expected of them.

STUDENT TIP – LEARNING FROM ASSESSMENT

Next time you have an assessment to complete, read the marking criteria carefully before you hand in the work.

Try to assess your own work against the criteria and identify areas for improvements.

Hopefully, reading the marking criteria carefully and considering how your work is marked against this will help you improve your own work and assess the work of others. Having considered this, we will now move on to explore how to give feedback effectively after the assessment in order to support the learner in their further development.

Giving feedback

The learner needs to know the answers to the following questions:

- What did I do well?
- What did I do less well?
- Why did I get this particular mark (or pass/fail) this assessment?
- How can I improve next time?

In providing feedback the role of the teacher is to be clear in supporting the learner to find the answers to these questions. Good practice in giving feedback generally follows the rules of the 'feedback sandwich':

1   A positive assessment of the strengths of the work (even with poor work there are some strengths that can be identified and it is important to look for and emphasise these).
2   A realistic assessment of the work including an indication of where specifically marks have been lost with a discussion of how improvements can be made.
3   Finish on a positive note with reference back to strengths.

This approach is based on an understanding that a very negative account leaves the learner feeling very downhearted; they may lose so much confidence that it is difficult for them to have the motivation to continue. Emphasising some positives gives the learner a foundation to build on. However, being too positive (unless the work is virtually perfect) leaves the learner confused about why they have lost any marks and may not provide them with a target to aim for in future.

Often written feedback is given, in which case the written feedback should address the questions by clarity in the writing and sufficient detail to address the points in the 'feedback sandwich'. It is important to give specific points from the work to illustrate this and to refer to the marking criteria. For example, if you have said that some of the writing is muddled, indicate examples by giving the page number and paragraph. It is good practice to annotate the work at the appropriate point to make this clear as the learner reads back through the marked work.

Ideally, there will also be an opportunity for verbal feedback and this will certainly be the case in work-based assessment.

STUDENT TIP – THE FEEDBACK SANDWICH

When giving feedback remember to:

* Emphasise positive aspects.
* Give specific feedback on where to improve.
* End on a positive note with reference back to strengths.

Work-based assessment

The same principles of giving feedback effectively apply in the workplace and here you may also find Pendleton's Rules helpful:

Pendleton's Rules

* Ask the learner to describe their positive achievements.
* Respond positively and if possible describe further examples of good practice you have observed.
* Ask the learner to describe how they are dealing/coping with their problem areas.
* Add your own suggestions for dealing with problems and for improving practice (adapted from Scott and Spouse 2013).

When providing feedback on a work-based assessment or task, you will inevitably be discussing performance on a more personal level. For example, Elaine will be commenting on Louise's ability to communicate effectively with patients and her professional approach, as well as her practical skills in taking blood (Elaine and Louise's case study). Similarly, Eve will be commenting on Ismail's attitude towards clients and his communication skills

Table 13.6 Giving feedback, adapted from Norcini and Burch (2013)

Methods of feedback to be avoided	Helpful methods of feedback
Being overly critical which creates a difficult atmosphere.	Creating a calm, respectful atmosphere.
Not giving the learner time to give their views first.	Asking the learner how they think that they performed before commenting yourself.
Being judgemental or making personal remarks.	Being non-judgemental.
Making very general comments such as on an individual's general behaviour.	Giving feedback on specific points such as an instance of behaviour.
Giving too much feedback at once.	Breaking feedback down into manageable chunks.
Basing feedback on personal opinions.	Making clear reference to marking criteria, performance criteria or specific goals.
Not indicating where the learner should go next.	Suggesting ideas for improvement.

(Ismail and Eve's case study). This means that the supervisor giving the feedback has to be sensitive in how areas for improvement are communicated. It is important in these cases to comment on specific behaviour rather than making remarks which sound critical of the person. For example, Elaine might say 'you explained the procedure really well to Mr Smith but you handled his arm a little roughly when you were applying the blood pressure cuff'. This would give Louise a clear idea of how to improve her technique but reassures her that she is communicating well with the patient.

Another aspect which is important in giving feedback is timing. It may not be appropriate for Elaine to give Louise detailed feedback on the ward in the presence of the patient. It is more appropriate to make a brief comment at the time, and then to arrange an appropriate time and place to give fuller feedback. Another tip is to avoid giving too much information at once. This is not effective as the message gets muddled and may be overwhelming; little and often is much more effective.

The points covered in this section are summarised in Table 13.6.

Chapter summary

This chapter set out with the intention that through studying it you would have met the following objectives:

- Developed a basic understanding of principles of learning.
- Applied this to learning and teaching in different settings including patient education.
- Explored methods of providing and receiving one-to-one support for learning.
- Identified the key principles of assessment.
- Reviewed good practice in providing feedback.

Further resources

Higher Education Academy. Available at: www.heacademy.ac.uk/.
JSTOR. Available at: www.jstor.org/.
InfEd. Available at: www.infed.org/.

Further reading

Day, K., Grant, R. and Hounsell, D. 1998. *Reviewing Your Teaching*. Edinburgh: Centre for Teaching, Learning and Assessment.

Elen, J., Clarebout, G., Leonard, R. and Lowyck, J. 2007. 'Student-centred and Teacher-centred Learning Environments: What Students Think', *Teaching in Higher Education* 12(1): 105–17.

Hocking, C., Brett, P. and Terentjevs, M. 2012. 'Making a Difference – Inclusive Learning and Teaching in Higher Education through Open Educational Resources', *Distance Education* 33(2): 237–52.

Leach, L. and Zepke, N. 2011. 'Engaging Students in Learning: A Review of a Conceptual Organiser', *Higher Education Research & Development* 30(2): 193–204.

Light, G. and Cox, R. 2001. *Learning and Teaching in Higher Education: The Reflective Professional*. London: Paul Chapman.

Nicklin, P. J., Kenworthy, N. 2002. *Teaching and Assessing in Nursing Practice: An Experiential Approach*. Toronto: Balliere Tindall.

Springhouse. 1998. *Patient Teaching Made Incredibly Easy*. New York: Springhouse Corporation.

References

Armstrong M. 2012. *Armstrong's Handbook of Human Resource Management Practice*, 12th edn. London: Kogan Page.

Black, P., Harrison, C., Lee. C., Marshall, B. and William, D. 2003. *Assessment for Learning: Putting it into Practice.* Maidenhead: Open University Press.

Cantillon, P., Hutchinson L. and Wood, D. 2003. *ABC of Learning and Teaching in Medicine*. London: BMJ Medicine.

Department of Health. 2001. *The Expert Patient: A New Approach to Chronic Disease Management for the 21st Century*. London: Department of Health.

Jarvis, P. 2006. *Towards a Comprehensive Theory of Human Learning*. Oxford: Routledge.

Kolb, D. A. 1984. *Experiential Learning*. Englewood Cliffs, NJ: Prentice Hall.

Miller, G. E. 1990. 'The Assessment of Clinical Skills/Competence/Performance', *Academic Medicine* 65: 63–7.

Norcini, J. and Burch, V. 2013. *Work-based Assessment as an Educational Tool*, AMEE Guide 31. Dundee: Medical Education in Europe.

Petty, G. 2009. *Evidenced-based Teaching: A Practical Approach*, 2nd edn. London: Nelson-Thornes.

Scott, I. and Spouse, J. 2013. *Practice Based Learning in Health and Social Care: Mentorship, Facilitation and Supervision*. Chichester: Wiley & Sons.

Walker, M. and Peyton, J. W. R. 1998. 'Teaching in the Theatre', in Peyton, J. W. R., ed., *Teaching and Learning in Medical Practice*. Rickmansworth: Manticore Publishers, 171–80.

Index

abuse 257; child abuse 258; discriminatory 264, 268–9; domestic abuse 258; elder abuse 258; emotional 264, 265; financial or material 264, 268–70; neglect and acts of omission 264, 267–8; physical 264, 265; psychological 259, 266; reasons for 259; risk factors 259–62; sexual 264, 266–7; social psychological 259; sociological 259; statistics 258; types 264–70
active immunity 230
active listening 79
Acts of Parliament, stages for passing 132
ageism 120
agenda-mapping 250
alcohol 254
anonymised direct quotes 212
antenatal and newborn screening programme 227
Ashley, Jack 165
assessment 7–9; feedback 301–3; formative 297, 298; guidelines 8; institutions 297; learners 296; marking criteria 300–1; method 300–3; patients/public 297; principles of 296; regulators 297; summative 297, 298; teachers 296–7; types 298–9; work-based assessment 302
assessment for learning 297
assignments 8
Assisted Dying Bill 172
associations/correlations 194, 195
attitude 246; formation 111–12
audit cycle 151–2
authors 44–5
autonomy 168, 175; respect for 119–20
avoiding blame culture 100

bar charts 209, 210
beanpole family 261
Beauchamp, Tom 168
beneficence 119, 168–9
Bentham, Jeremy 118, 164–5
bias 200, 207
bibliography 38, 39

bivariate graph 223, 224–5
blinding 193
Bolam v Friern Hospital Management Committee (1957) 174
bonding capital 222
books: library 10–11; literature searching 20, 22–3
Boolean operators 27–8; AND 27, 29; NOT 28; OR 28
Borton's educational framework 64–5
Bournewood Case, HL v UK [2004] 177
bridging capital 222
Bristol Royal Infirmary 152
bullying 96
burnout 106–7

Caldicott, Dame Fiona 181
campaign work 253
cancer: prevention 221; screening programme 227
candour, duty of 100
Care in the Community 137
Care Quality Commission (CQC) 136
case conferences 272
case study 35
cervical cancer 230; screening 228, 254
Chadwick, Edwin 217
challenging 100
child abuse 258
childhood immunisations 155
Children Act 1989 180
Childress, James 168
chlamydia screening programme 227–8
Choose and Book 136
Choosing Health 129, 139
citation 26
CiteUlike 46
citing 38
clarifying questions 73
Climbié, Victoria 263
clinical audit: definition 151–3; stages 153; undertaking 153–4

Clinical Commissioning Groups (CCGs) 136
clinical governance 150–4
closed-ended questions 202, 203
closed questions 73
cluster sampling 199
coaching 287, 288
Cochrane Database 213
codes of conduct 117
cohabitation 261
collaboration 103
Comic Relief 261
Commission for Patient and Public Involvement
    In Health 139
Commission for Quality In Healthcare (CQC)
    150
Commission on Human Medicines (CHM) 158
communication 69–92; active listening 79;
    applying skills 88–9; barriers to 80, 81–2,
    89; with clients 83–8; culture and 82–3;
    definitions 70–1; electronic 76–8; email
    77–8; face-to-face 72, 74; interactional
    approach 89; methods 71–2; models 89–90;
    non-defensive 98–9; non-verbal 75–6, 79;
    para-verbal 74; phatic 73–4; planning 88;
    principles 79–83; reflections 89–90; settings
    82; teamwork and 97–8; telephone 77;
    transactional approach 89; types of questions
    73–4; verbal 72–3
community development 253
confidentiality 180–1, 263
confirmability 207
confounding variable 191, 192
consent 174–5
consent form 175
consequentialism 118
constructive criticism 99–100
constructivism 284
containment 229
contents page 61, 62
control group 192
convenience sampling 200
correlations 194, 195
course guide 8
crash calls 155
credibility 207
critical analysis 36
critical thinking 36–7
cross-sectional survey 195
cultural relativism 263
culture 111; communication and 74, 82–3
curriculum vitae (CV) 62

data 191
data collection tools 191, 202–3; validity and
    reliability of 207–8
Data Protection Act (1998) 59

database 25–6; health and social care 25, 26;
    searching 25–6
decision-making 120
Declaration of Helsinki (1964) 167
Declaration on the Promotion of Patient Rights
    In Europe 116
dementia, communication and 84
demographics 126–7
dentists 138
deontology 118
Department of Health Public Health Outcomes
    Framework 219
dependability 207
dependent variable 191, 192
depersonalisation 99
deprivation of liberty 178
descriptive qualitative research 195
descriptive research design 194
descriptive statistics 209, 211
'deteriorating patient' intervention 159
diary, reflective 53, 58
digital libraries 9
Dignitas clinic 172
dignity 110, 115–17; definition 115; importance
    of 116–17
disclosure 99
discrimination 120, 122–3
discriminatory abuse 264, 268–9
diversity 120
domains of learning 298
domestic abuse 258
double blinded RCT 193
Driscoll developmental framework 64–5
drug use 224–5
duty-based ethical thought 166–8
duty of candour 100

e-books 9, 24
e-journals 9
Ebola virus 169
editions 45
elder abuse 258, 262
electronic books (e-books) 9, 24
electronic communication 76–8
electronic journals (e-journals) 9
email 9, 77–8
emotional abuse 264, 265
empathy 82, 96, 99
empirical research 187
Endnote 46
environmental health 219–21
epidemiology 127–8, 223–4
equality 120, 122
essays 8; types of 35
ethics 110, 117–18; principles 119–20; research
    208; theories 118–19

ethnography 195, 201
European Convention of Human Rights
    169–70
European Court of Human Rights 170, 171,
    177
Ewles and Simnett's five categories for health
    promotion approaches 239–40
examinations 8
exclusion criteria 192
exercise 237–8
experiential learning 282
experimental design 191–2, 193–4
experimental group 192
extended family 261
extraneous (confounding) variable 191, 192

face-to-face communication 72, 74
face-to-face interview 204
Facebook 31
Falconer, Lord 172
Family Law Reform Act 1969 180
family: beanpole 261; cohabitation 261;
    extended 261; gay/same-sex 261; lone-parent
    261; nuclear 260, 261; reconstituted 261;
    singles 261
feedback 38, 293–6, 301–3
feedback sandwich 302
financial abuse 264, 268–70
fines, library 10
First Class Service, A 151
fiscal welfare 129
fixed response questions 202
Flying Start NHS 93
focus group 204
formal mentoring 288–9
formative assessment 297, 298
Foundation Trusts 136, 137
four principles approach 168–9; autonomy
    168; beneficience 168–9; justice 169;
    non-maleficence 169
Francis, Robert, QC, report 69–70, 101, 104,
    150, 154
frequency 194
frequency distribution table 210
future tense 36

general practitioners 138
generalisability 200
Gibb's reflective cycle 65
Gillick v West Norfolk & Wisbech Area Health
    Authority 1985 180
Glass v UK 2004 180
glossary 47, 48
Goody, Jade 228
Google 12, 15, 17, 24
grammar checker 38

graph 209; bivariate 223, 224–5
Green Book 230
grounded theory 195

Harvard system of referencing 39, 41
health and safety 160–1
Health and Safety at Work etc. Act 1974 160
Health and Social Care Act: 2001 139; 2008
    130; 2012 216
health belief model (Hochbaum) 242–3
health education 247
health improvement 225
health information 253
health promotion 235–54; approaches to
    239–40; barriers to healthy living 237–9;
    behavior choice and 236; communities 253;
    controversies 249; definition 239; groups
    252–3; healthy living 235–6; individuals 250;
    patients and 249–53; priority areas 253–4;
    theories for 240–9
health protection 225, 247
health screening 226–7; condition 226;
    programme 226–7; test 226; treatment 226
healthcare delivery 135–40; day-to-day
    running of 137–8; demographics 126–7;
    epidemiology 127–8; factors influencing 126;
    public and patient involvement in 139–40;
    roles within 138–9; social policy 128–33
healthcare policy 133–5
healthy living 235–6; barriers to 237–9
Hippocratic Oath 180
HIV 232
homelessness 218
homophones 37–8
HPV vaccination 230
Human Fertilisation and Embryology Authority
    180
human rights 169–72, 257
Human Rights Act 1998 169–72, 181;
    deprivation of liberty 171; key articles 170–2;
    private and family life 171; protection against
    torture 171; right to life 170–1
hypothesis 190, 191

immunisation (vaccination) 229–30
in-text referencing 41
incident reporting 155
inclusion criteria 192
independent variable 191, 192
individuality 121
inferential (descriptive) statistics 209, 211
informal mentoring 289
informal welfare 129
information, evaluation of 30–1; age 31;
    authorship 30; content and coverage 31;
    reason for information 31; source 30

information sources 11
information technology 31
informed consent 284
Inter-Library Loan service 41
inter-professional meetings 272
inter-rater reliability 207
Internet resources, quality of 12–13
interventional (experimental/quasi-experimental)
    design 191–2, 193–4
interventional design 192
interviews 202, 204–5; advantages and
    disadvantages of 204–5; face-to-face
    204; semi-structured 204; structured 204;
    unstructured 204
intimate space 75
intra-rater reliability 207

Jade Goody effect 228
Jenner, Edward 229
journal articles 24, 25, 26–7
justice 20, 169

Kant, Immanuel 118, 166–7
Keogh, Bruce 152
key workers 263
Kolb's learning cycle 282–4, 294

labelling 123
Laming, Lord 263
Lasting Power of Attorney (2014) 176
leadership and management 104–6
leadership in teams 104
leadership skills 104–5
leading questions 73
learner-centred learning 282
learning: experiential 282; learner-centred 282;
    lifelong 51–2, 58, 284; peer 284; positive and
    negative descriptions of 281; process 282–4;
    self-directed 284–5
learning agreements 54–5
learning contract 54
learning disabilities, communication and 84
learning goals 54, 57, 58
learning logs 9
legislation 230–2
library, effective use of 9; borrowing books
    10–11; fines 10; information sources
    11, 12–16; library website 9; logins and
    passwords 9; quality of Internet resources
    12–15
life course analysis 221–2
lifelong learning (LLL) 51–2, 58, 284
Lifting Operations and Lifting Equipment
    Regulations 1998 (LOLER) 133
Likert scale 203
listening 79, 95, 100

literature searching 16–29; advanced 29; books
    20, 22–3; combining words 27–9; database
    25–6; e-books 24; journal articles 24, 25,
    26–7; key concepts, words/phrases for 17–19;
    key elements 17; locations 20; mind map
    17, 18, 19; planning 17; reading list 16, 20,
    22–3, 24; recording 30; refining 29; results,
    relevance of 29–30; scope 21–2; strategies
    27–30, 32
Liverpool Care Pathway 133
Local Involvement Networks (LINks) 139
Local Safeguarding Boards 270–1
lone-parent family 261
longitudinal study 194

Makaton 84
managerial supervision 290
Manual Handling Operations Regulations 1992
    133
marking grid/criteria 8
Marmot report 219
material abuse 264, 268–70
Maxwell-Fyfe, Sir David 170
mean 209
median 209
medication errors 157–8
Medicines and Healthcare Products Regulatory
    Agency (MHRA) 158
MENCAP 84
Mendeley 46
Mental Capacity Act 2005 173–8, 179
Mental Health Acts 129; 1959 129; 1983 129,
    171, 177, 178–9
mentor/supervisor, role of 60–1
mentoring 287, 288–9
Microsoft Office Referencing Application
    46
Mid Staffordshire Hospital inquiry 69–70, 101,
    104, 150
Mill, John Stuart 118, 166
Miller's Pyramid 298–300
mind mapping 17, 18, 19, 76, 83
mode 209
Model of Health Promotion (Tannahill) 247,
    249
MONITOR 136
monogamy 260
morals 117
motivational interviewing 250–1
multiple-choice examination 299
myocardial infarction 231

narrative data 195
National Health Service 137–8
National Institute for Clinical Excellence
    (NICE 1999) 165

National Institute for Health and Care
    Excellence (NICE 2013) 133, 137, 141, 151,
    165, 185
National Institute for Health and Clinical
    Excellence (NICE 2005) 151, 165
National Patient Safety Agency (NPSA) 155
National Reporting and Learning System
    (NRLS) 155
National VTE Prevention Programme 160
neglect and acts of omission 264, 267–8
NHS Act 1946 129
NHS Commissioning Board Special Health
    Authority 155
NHS Constitution 100, 167, 172–3
NHS e-Referral Service 136
NHS Trust Development Authority 136
NHS Trusts 136, 138, 139
Nicklinson, Tony 172
non-defensive communication 98–9
non-formal learning 52
non-interventional design 191, 194–5
non-maleficence 119, 169
non-probability sampling 201
non-verbal behaviour 95
non-verbal communication 75–6, 79
note taking 32–3, 36
notional character 123
nuclear family 260, 261
numerical data 191

obesity 130, 133–5, 222, 254
objective structured clinical examination
    (OSCE) 9, 299
observation 202, 205; advantages and
    disadvantages of 206; non-participant 205;
    participant 205
observational design 191, 194–5
observatory interactive maps 225
occupational welfare 129
one-to-one teaching 286–7, 290
open-ended questions 73, 202, 203
open-mindedness 82
organisational resilience 154
outreach work 253
Overview and Scrutiny Committees 139

paraphrasing 36, 37, 79
para-verbal communication 74
parental responsibility 179–80
passive immunity 230
password, library 9
Pasteur, Louis 229
Patient Advice and Liaison Services (PALS)
    139
Patient and Public Involvement in Health Forums
    (PPIFs) 139

patient centredness 147
patient safety 154–60; medication errors 157;
    Seven Steps to 156–7
Patient Safety First 159, 160
patient safety incident (PSI) 154
patient safety solution 154
peer learning 284
peer-mentoring 289
perceived barriers 243
perceived benefits 243
perceived control 246
perceived severity 243
perceived susceptibility 242
performance management 290
personal development plan (PDP) 51, 56–9, 63
personal space 75
Peyton's four-stage model for teaching practical
    skills 286, 288
pharmacists 138
phatic communication 73–4
phenomenology 195, 201
physical abuse 264, 265
pie charts 209
place of publication 45
placebo 193
plagiarism 40
polygamy 260
Poor Law Acts 129
population 198
portfolio 8, 58–9, 61–7; additional evidence
    63; assessment 299; body 62; competences
    63; contents page 61, 62; curriculum vitae
    (CV) 62; final section 62, 63; front sheet
    61, 62; job description 63; module learning
    outcomes 61; written assignments 63
post-test design 193
poverty 223
power analysis 200
praising 100
pre-test design 193
preceptorship 288–9
prejudice 82, 122
present tense 35–6
presentations 8
Pretty, Dianne 172
prevalence 194
prevention 247
primacy effect 81
primary referencing 41–2
private welfare 129
probability (P) 199, 211
probing questions 73
professional supervision 289
prospective events 194
proxemics 74
psychological abuse 259, 266

public health, improving 216–32; assessing
    determinants of health 223–8; definition
    217–19; history 217; theoretical approaches
    219–23
public space 75
Pubmed 26
Puente, Omar 172
Purdy, Debbie 172
purposive sample 201
Putnam, Robert 222

qualitative data 204
qualitative research 191, 195–8
qualitative sampling 201
Quality and Outcomes Framework (QOF) 151,
    152
quality assurance 145; programmes 145–8
Quality Assurance Agencies 150
quality in healthcare 144–61; cost of 149;
    dimensions 145–6; objectives 148
quality measurement domains 146
quality of life 190
quantitative research 191–5, 197; sample size in
    200–1
quantitative sampling 199–200, 201
quasi-experimental design 191–2, 193–4
questionnaires 202, 203–4, 223; advantages and
    disadvantages of 203–4
quick response (QR) codes 10
quotes, direct 36

racism 120
Rainbow Model of Health (Dahlgren and
    Whitehead 1991) 220, 240–1
randomised controlled trials (RCT) 193
range 209
rating scale 202, 203
reading: effective 3–4; skills 1–3; skim 3, 4–6
reading list 16, 20, 22–3, 24
recency effect 81
reciprocal determinism 241
reconstituted family 261
reference list 38, 39
referencing 26, 38–47; authors 44–5;
    bibliography 38, 39; definition 38; editions
    45; information for 43–4; key tips 47;
    management 46; need for 40; place of
    publication 45; primary and secondary
    (second-hand) 41–2; recording 42–6;
    reference list 38, 39; in research articles
    213; style 39–40; in-text 41; Web resources
    45
reflection 63–7, 89–90, 96
reflection-in-action 63, 64, 67
reflection-on-action 64, 65, 67
reflective account 35

reflective listening 250
reflexive practice 67
reflexivity 100
RefWorks 46
reliability 207–8
Reporting of Injuries, Diseases and Dangerous
    Occurrences Regulations 2013 (RIDDOR)
    133
representative sample 199, 200
research: definition 187; developing knowledge
    using 186
research articles 188–214; abstract 189; data
    collection tools, validity and reliability of
    207–8; discussion and conclusion 212–13;
    inferential statistics 211; introduction 189;
    methodology 191–8; qualitative results
    211–12; quantitative results 209–11;
    references 213; research ethics 208; research
    questions 190; results 208–12; sampling
    198–206; systematic review 213; title 189
research cycle 188
research design 191
research ethics 208; understanding the process
    187–8
respect 110
retrospective events 194
risk compensation hypothesis 232
risk displacement 232
role modelling 101
rotavirus vaccination 230
Royal Society for the Prevention of Accidents
    (ROSPA) 231

Sackett, David 184
'Safe Surgery Saves Lives' global challenge
    155
safeguarding; barriers to 271–2;
    inter-professional working 270–4;
    skills and knowledge for 274–7
Safety in Doses Reports 157
sample 198–9
sample size: in qualitative research 201–2;
    in quantitative research 200–1
sampling 191, 198–206; cluster 199;
    convenience 200; data collection tools
    202–3; non-probability 201; probability 199;
    quantitative 199–200, 201; single random
    199; stratified random 199
sampling error/bias 200
saturation, data 201
Savage v South Essex Partnership NHS
    Foundation Trust (2010) 170–1
scanning 3, 4–6
Scarman, Lord 180
screening 254
search engine 12, 15

seat belt legislation 231–2
secondary (second-hand) referencing 41–2
self-awareness 61, 89, 96, 106, 110
self-determination theory 246–7, 248
self-directed learning 284–5
self-efficacy 241
self-fulfilling prophecy 103
semi-structured interview 204
Seven Steps to Patient Safety 156–7
sexism 120
sexual abuse 264, 266–7
Sidaway v Board of Governors of the Bethlem
    Royal Hospital 1985 174
Signalong 84
single person 261
single random sampling 199
skills book 8
skim reading 3, 4–6
small talk 74
SMART principles 57, 58
SOCAT 223
social actors 75
social capital 222–3
social cognitive theory (Bandura) 241–2
Social Enterprises 137
social learning theory 241
social marketing 228
social media 31
social policy 128–30; development of 130–3;
    legislation 129
social space 75
social welfare 129
soler mnemonic 79
sources 40
spatial distance 74, 75
spellchecker 37
spider diagram 17, 97
spidergram 61, 62
Stages of Change Model (Prochaska and
    Diclemente) 244–5
standard deviation 209
standards 145
statistical significance 211
statistics 191, 223–5
stereotyping 122–3
stratified random sampling 199
structured interview 204
student handbook 8
suicide 129
Suicide Act 1961 129, 172
summarising 79
summative assessment 297, 298
supervision 287
supporting 100
Surgical Safety Checklist 155, 156
survey 194; workplace 58

SWOT analysis 56–7, 58, 62, 63
systematic review 213

tables 209
Talking Mats 84
target population 198
teaching 280–96; approaches to 281–2; effective
    282; feedback 281–2, 293–6; one-to-one
    286–7, 290; patients and clients 291–2;
    planning 285–90; practical skills 285–6,
    288; resources 285; small groups 292–3;
    work-based mentoring and preceptorship
    288–9
team work 93–108; avoiding blame culture
    100; collaboration 103; communication
    within 97–8; constructive criticism 99–100;
    influence behaviour in 100; leadership and
    management 104–6; leadership in teams
    104; leadership skills 104–5; non-defensive
    communication 98–9; recognition of
    burnout 106–7; reflection and empathy 96;
    relationships within 94–6; role modelling
    101; tribalism 101–3; whistleblowing 101
telephone 77
tense 35–6
theoretical sample 201
theoretical writing 35
theory of planned behaviour 246
theory of reasoned action 246
transferability 207, 212
transmission view of knowledge 282
Transtheoretical Model (TTM) 244–5
tribalism 101–3
trustworthiness 207
tuberculosis 254
Twitter 31

UK Study of Abuse and Neglect of Older People
    Prevalence Survey Report 261–2
unemployment 223
Universal Declaration of Human Rights (1948)
    169
unstructured interview 204
username 9
utilitarianism 118–19, 164–6

validation 85–6
validity 207–8
value-based judgements 113
value system 111, 114
values: in decision-making 113; definition
    111; formation 111–14; importance of
    114–15
Vancouver system of referencing 39
variables 190
venus thromboembolism (VTE) 160

VERA acronym 84–8; activity 87–8; emotion 86–7; reassurance 87
verbal communication 72–3
virtual learning environment (VLE) 9, 16
vocabulary 6–7
voluntary welfare 129
vulnerable individuals, protection of 262–3; investigation 262–3; investigation and initial assessment 263; recording and reporting 263

W v Egdell [1990] 2 wlr 471 181
Web 2.0 31
Web resources 45
welfare services 128–9
whistleblowing 101
Widgit 84
willingness to learn 82
work-based coaching 288
work-based learning (WBL) 51–61; definition 52–3; learning agreements 54–5; learning goals 54, 57, 58; mentor/supervisor, role of 60–1; personal development plans 51, 56–9; portfolio evidence 58–9, 61–3
work-based mentoring 288–9
work-based supervision 289
Working For Patients 145
workplace assessment 299
World Bank 223
World Health Organization (WHO) 135, 145, 155, 231, 235, 239
writing skills 34–9; audience 35; direct quotes 36; fact vs opinion 32; feedback 38–9; note taking 36; objectives 35; paraphrasing 36, 37; structure 34, 35; tense 35–6; types of 35
written assignments 63
written essay/report 299

yellow card system 158–9

Zotero 46